You and Your Health
Volume 2
The Human Body
Diseases
Symptoms

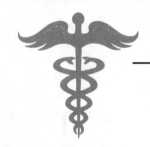

VOLUME 2
New Edition

You and Your Health

The Human Body
Diseases
Symptoms

In three volumes, illustrated

Harold Shryock, M.A., M.D., and
Mervyn G. Hardinge, M.D.,
Dr.P.H., Ph.D.

In Collaboration With 28 Leading Medical Specialists

Published jointly by

PACIFIC PRESS PUBLISHING ASSOCIATION
Boise, ID 83707
Oshawa, Ontario, Canada
Montemorelos, N. L., Mexico

REVIEW AND HERALD PUBLISHING ASSOCIATION
Washington, DC 20039-0555
Hagerstown, MD 21740

ISBN 0-8163-0534-X

CONTENTS

Volume 1—More Abundant Living

Volume 2—The Human Body; Diseases; Symptoms

Volume 3—More Diseases; First Aid; Emergencies

SECTION I—The Glands and the Nervous System

The Glands — Endocrine Gland Disorders — The Nervous System — Diseases of the Nervous System — Mental Illness: Neuroses and Psychoses

SECTION II—The Sensory System

The Organs of Sensation — Pain — Diseases of the Eye — Diseases of the Ear, Nose, and Throat

SECTION III—Cancer

Characteristics of Cancer — Manifestations of Cancer

SECTION IV—Dietary Problems

Deficiency Diseases — Disorders of Regulation

SECTION V—Allergies and Infections

Allergic Manifestations — Infections — Viral Diseases —

INTRODUCTION

The three volumes of You and Your Health are a continuum. As for content, all three could well have been bound into a single book. But such a book would have been too large to handle.

Volume 2 picks up where volume 1 leaves off, but it has unique characteristics. Section I, consisting of the first four chapters of volume 2, enables the reader to stand off and take a broad look at the advantages modern medical science provides in combating disease. Section II brings the reader a little closer to the actual problems of illness by explaining the body's automatic defenses against disease (chapter 5) and then by listing the ways in which the body signals with symptoms to indicate that it is sick (chapter 6).

Beginning with section III and continuing through the remainder of volume 2, several organ systems are described. Then following each description, the diseases that may affect that particular system are listed and the appropriate treatments summarized.

At the back of volume 2 the reader will find detailed four-color plates illustrating the anatomy of a number of organs and systems. He will also find a complete index covering all three volumes of You and Your Health. Thus, in looking for a certain topic, for the description of a certain organ, or for the manifestations and treatment of a certain illness, the index will indicate the location either in volume 2 or in either of the other two volumes.

SECTION I

Combating Disease

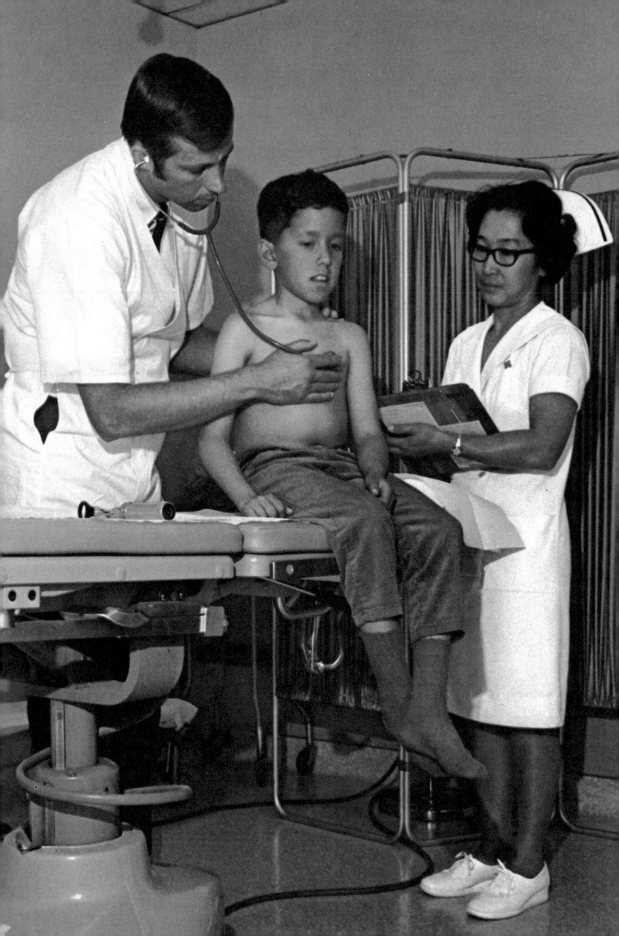

Progress in Medicine

Medical science during the last century has kept abreast of civilization's progress and continues in today's jet age to make spectacular advances. Average life expectancy in the United States has increased from 49 years (in 1900) to more than 70 years. This addition has come about largely because control of epidemics and infections has virtually wiped out onetime major killers and because treatment of disease is now based on a knowledge of fundamental causes.

A Backward Look

Roll back the calendar to 1875. Imagine yourself living back then. What do you see?

Homes are lighted by candles and kerosene lamps. Streetlights burn gas and have to be lighted each evening by the town's lamplighter. There are no telephones. Telegraph is the accepted way to send urgent messages. Typewriters are not yet in general use.

Tuberculosis was the major killer then, causing approximately one out of every five deaths. It affected people of all ages—babies, teenagers, young adults, and oldsters.

At mention of "tuberculosis," we can almost hear some modern schoolboy ask, "What's that?" But in 1875 the word struck terror to many families. Physicians were baffled, for as yet they did not know the cause of the "white plague."

René Laënnec, the inventor of the stethoscope, the instrument that so greatly aided in the diagnosis of tuberculosis of the lungs, had died of this disease at the age of 45. Physicians were more than ordinarily susceptible, it seemed, probably because of their close contact with patients.

Another major health problem in 1875 was infection. A high percentage of the deaths among soldiers in the then-recent Civil War had resulted from germ-infected wounds.

Germs?—Yes, physicians were beginning to read about the work of Pasteur and Koch. Pasteur was beginning to see germs in the microscope, and Koch was learning to cultivate colonies of them in the laboratory. But as yet scientists did not recognize the various kinds of germs, except the rod-shaped organism that causes anthrax and the organisms involved in fermentation as demonstrated by Pasteur. How germs could invade open wounds and then spread throughout a person's body to threaten his life they did not yet understand. (See pictorial supplement at the back of this volume for painting and write-up of Pasteur and six other persons famous in the early and ongoing development of medical science and practice.)

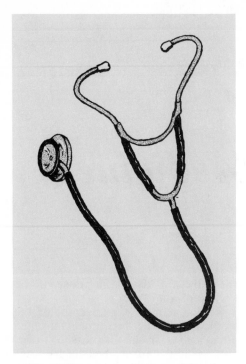

The stethoscope, invented in the nineteenth century helped immeasurably in the diagnosis of disease.

In 1875 surgeons wore their street clothes when they performed operations. They carried their instruments in a bag as they went from one patient to the next. The instruments were usually wiped "clean" before being used again, but in doing this, nobody thought of germs.

About 20 percent of the surgical operations performed were amputations, and about half of the patients died of infections that followed. Surgeons shrank from performing operations that required opening of the body cavities. The reason was simple—practically all such cases died of infection even though the surgical procedure may have been done skillfully.

See What Happened

In 1880, Dr. Edward Trudeau became the promoter in the United States of a revolutionary method of treating tuberculosis. A few years earlier he had cared for a brother who died from tuberculosis. Then Dr. Trudeau developed the disease. The treatment in those days consisted of bleeding, of the application of leeches to draw blood, of blistering of the skin, and of the administration of such drugs as compounds of antimony. Patients were kept in seclusion in dark rooms with no ventilation.

But once Dr. Trudeau became ill he reasoned that if he were going to die, he might as well die happy. Earlier in his life he had spent a few weeks on a hunting trip in the woods of the Adirondacks in upstate New York. Now he determined to return to Paul Smith's hunting camp and enjoy the outdoor life while he lasted. But instead of dying within a few months, Trudeau lived on and even improved. So, as he became able, he resumed his practice of medicine, specializing now in the treatment of tuberculosis by encouraging a way of life which promoted the patient's resistance to the illness.

In 1882 the germ that causes tuberculosis was identified. In 1896 the X ray came into use and since then has been a great help in the diagnosis of tuberculosis and in following either the progress of the disease or the progress of the cure, as the case might be.

By the 1940s and 1950s surgical methods were in use by which one lung, when affected by tuberculosis, could be collapsed so that it could rest while healing took place. But the big breakthrough came with the availability of isoniazid, often used in combination with other drugs. It stifles the growth of the germs that cause tuberculosis.

Notice what has happened. From being a major killer in 1875, by 1900 tuberculosis had dropped into second place as a cause of death in the United States. By 1937 it was in sixth place. By 1950, in seventh place. And now it is not even listed among the major causes of death. But tuberculosis still occurs, with about 30,000 new cases registered each year and about 5000 deaths.

A similar, remarkable improvement

has occurred in the control of wound infections. Joseph Lister, professor of surgery at the University of Glasgow in the 1860s, introduced primitive methods of killing the germs that contaminated open wounds. He began by dipping surgical dressings into carbolic acid (phenol). This practice helped to kill the germs in the wounds, but the carbolic acid also damaged the tissues with which it came in contact. By 1880 it was demonstrated that the germs which cause wound infections are readily and more easily killed by heat than by contact with antiseptic solutions. It was then that the present method of sterilizing surgical dressings and instruments was introduced. But the greatest

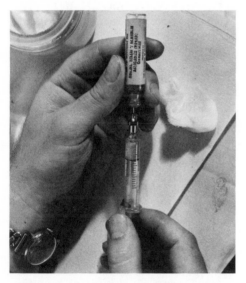

The development of sulfonamides and antibiotics during the 1940s proved to be a great advance in the control of infections.

advance in the control of wound infections came with the development of the sulfonamides in the 1930s and the antibiotics, beginning in the 1940s.

Infectious Diseases

Of the various infectious diseases, most of which have virtually been conquered within recent years, smallpox stands as the classic example. It is hard for the present generation to understand the terrors of smallpox epidemics that used to ravish whole countries at a time. During the eighteenth century smallpox was responsible for the death of an estimated 60,000,000 people in Europe, one out of every three deaths among children under ten years of age being caused by it. It ravaged America too. One epidemic after another overtook Boston. In the epidemic of 1721, more than half the inhabitants of the city contracted smallpox, and one out of every seven patients died.

But vaccination and the cooperation of health agencies throughout the world has changed the picture so completely that smallpox is now the first of the various contagious diseases to be listed as conquered. Supposedly, the last case of naturally occurring smallpox was reported in Somalia in 1978. It is therefore no longer recommended that children in the United States be vaccinated for smallpox. Would that there might be better cooperation than now exists in the use of the available vaccines so that many of the other contagious diseases could be similarly stamped out!

Great progress has been made, however, with certain other infectious and contagious diseases. For example, only a few cases of the dread disease of diphtheria show up each year in the United States, and these always among those not immunized or whose immunity through immunization has waned by virtue of passing years. A still more recent success story is that of polio, with only eight cases being reported in the United States in 1976.

But the flip side of this success story gives cause for alarm. Of the more than 50 million children younger than fifteen years of age in the United States, about 20 million have not been immunized adequately for protection against the following seven diseases: polio, measles, rubella (German measles), pertussis (whooping cough), tetanus, diphtheria, and mumps. It is among these that the illnesses will occur, if and when they do. And these unprotected people are the ones who will be responsible for a future epidemic, should there be one.

While speaking of infectious diseases, we must mention one group of serious illnesses with a blemished record. The blemish, however, is not due to lack of progress in medical science, but rather to the inclination of human nature to indulge in sensual ventures regardless of consequences. We are speaking of the sexually transmitted (venereal) diseases, which are increasing rapidly and running virtually out of control.

Other Triumphs

Diabetes has not been conquered or eradicated, but modern medicine has developed an understanding of the disease. This knowledge, along with the identification and production of insulin, has enabled diabetics to improve their life expectancy and to live almost normal lives.

Arteriosclerosis, high blood pressure, and stroke are still with us, but progress has been made in the care of persons with tendencies to these illnesses so that lives are prolonged and the occurrence of serious complications reduced.

Progress in the early detection and treatment of cancer is saving thousands of lives each year, as discussed more adequately in volume 3, chapters 10 and 11.

Spectacular progress has been made in developing ways of caring for patients acutely ill or suffering from chronic, life-threatening illnesses. These new methods, many of them in the field of surgery, are discussed later in this chapter.

New Emphasis: Preventive Medicine

For centuries it was assumed that the job of the physicians was to *treat* disease. They were cast in the role of repairmen trained to patch up the human organism once it had been injured by disease or accident. It was considered foolish to consult a doctor unless a person was actually sick.

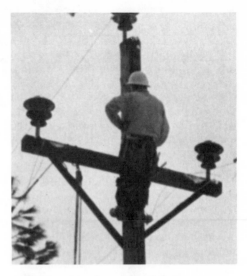

For centuries physicians were looked upon as repairmen rather than as educators in preventive medicine.

But with the advance of medical science has come an increasing understanding of the causes of disease. Knowing the cause, the next logical step is to remove it and thus prevent the disease. Preventing a disease always excels treating it after it has developed. Suffering is avoided. Complications and resulting handicaps are bypassed. The life-shortening influence of illness is prevented.

With the knowledge of how to prevent disease has come a relatively new branch of medical science called "preventive medicine."

People laughed at physicians and medical research workers when they began placing emphasis on preventing disease. They said, "You doctors are about to run yourselves out of business." But physicians are happy for the change.

Even though the average person lives longer today than a few decades ago, people still suffer from accidents, from the wear-out diseases, and even from those illnesses which could have been prevented. But physicians now can give more attention to the relief of suffering, to making their patients' lives more enjoyable, and to preventing many of the ordinary illnesses.

Disease Prevention Requires Cooperation

In order to help his patients stay well, a physician must have their cooperation. Unless they use the methods of disease prevention he teaches them, they will not be able to rise above the dangers of illness.

Imagine a person who has just inherited a large fortune. This newly rich person is not trained in business methods. He realizes the danger, however, of losing his fortune unless he invests it properly. If wise, he will seek out an investment counselor. Even though not trained in business himself, he then can expect to receive satisfactory returns.

Similarly, every normal human being is "wealthy" by having inherited a healthy body. If he uses this "wealth" wisely, he will be rewarded by years of good health and resulting happiness. To "cash in" on this advantage he should consult his family physician on how best to "invest" and preserve his valuable health asset.

Examples of Preventing Illness

1. *Coronary Heart Disease*. Coronary heart disease is a major killer, especially among men. If present trends continue, one man out of five in the United States will suffer a heart attack before he reaches 60. The actual heart attack which carries a high risk of either sudden death or a persisting health handicap is the culmination of the arteriosclerosis developed in the person's body over many years, ever since he was a youth.

Several "risk factors" underlie the possibility of heart attack. The presence of any one of these makes a person more susceptible to coronary heart disease. With two or more present, the probability is multiplied accordingly.

So elimination of these risk factors should be a major consideration in preventing coronary heart disease. Here's what to concentrate on: (1) abstain from or discontinue the use of ciga-

rettes (see chapter 54, volume 1); (2) maintain normal blood pressure, even when this requires a physician's supervision (see chapter 9, volume 2); (3) use a diet designed to maintain normal weight (avoiding obesity) and at the same time retard the development of arteriosclerosis (see chapter 53, volume 1); and (4) follow a program of active physical exercise (see chapter 52, volume 1).

2. *Cancer*. People used to have a fatalistic attitude toward cancer, assuming that it strikes those unfortunate enough to have inherited such a predilection. True, cancer sometimes seems to run in families, this hereditary factor still generally recognized by modern medical scientists as a cause for susceptibility.

However, in most cases another factor must be added—an environmental insult of some kind, such as smoking. About one out of ten individuals has an inherited susceptibility by which the continuous use of cigarettes causes

Lung cancer could be largely prevented if cigarette smoking could be eradicated.

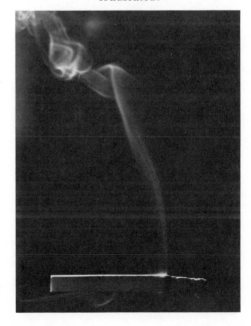

lung cancer. Logical conclusion: Many forms of cancer are preventable—preventable by avoiding the environmental factors which trigger the susceptibility to cancer. More is explained about the causes and susceptibilities to cancer in volume 3, chapters 10 and 11.

3. *Chronic Lung Disease.* The term "chronic lung disease" refers to the conditions of emphysema and/or chronic bronchitis, either one of which may or may not be complicated by asthma. Chronic lung disease is considered in greater detail in chapter 13, volume 2. Suffice it to say here that the destruction of lung tissue which occurs in chronic lung disease results from prolonged irritation of the delicate tissues of the respiratory organs. The offending irritants are introduced as contaminants in the air regularly breathed.

The normal tissues of the lungs and air passages possess a considerable and effective resistance to irritating particles carried by the air. Such common contaminants include asbestos, beryllium, silica, coal dust, and the irritating substances contained in smog as an element of air pollution.

The use of cigarettes makes the lung tissues much more susceptible to the destructive effects of these air contaminants. A nonsmoker may tolerate them for a lifetime, often experiencing little effect on his lung tissues except as he may suffer from repeated infections of the respiratory organs. But the smoker tolerates these air contaminants poorly.

It is important that workmen in industries in which the air is contaminated with irritants such as mentioned above should take definite precautions against lung damage, like wearing appropriate masks. By far the greatest protection, however, consists of abstaining from the use of cigarettes.

4. *Complications of the Use of Alcohol and Drugs.* It used to be thought that the use of alcoholic drinks did comparatively little harm to the tissues of the body. The harm supposedly consisted merely of making the drinker careless in his conduct and more susceptible to accidents. But now, as pointed out in chapter 54, volume 1, the hazard of alcohol is recognized to be much greater. Taken into the body, it compounds the effects of certain drugs so that the combination produces a greater and more tragic effect than the simple action of the drug plus the alcohol. An estimated five hundred unintentional deaths a year occur in the United States on this account. The use of alcohol by an expectant mother may cause certain physical deformities and various degrees of mental retardation in the child.

Alcohol is now recognized to be a "multisystem toxin" which affects not only the liver to produce cirrhosis but also other organs, such as the brain and the heart. The damage to the heart is progressive with the continued use of alcohol, producing in its final stages a condition of congestive heart failure which ends fatally. Obviously, the means of preventing these tragic consequences is to abstain from alcoholic drinks.

The human tragedies resulting from the use of drugs are also discussed in chapter 55, volume 1. Just here, however, we are concerned with the growing problem of hepatitis, so common among users of the "needle" for self-administering their "fix." The virus causing hepatitis is easily passed from one person to another through the careless use of the hypodermic needle, only one of the many health hazards related to the use of drugs. Again, to prevent these health- and life-destroying complications makes much better sense than to try to treat them after life has been blemished.

Perpetuating One's Health

Life is progressive. It moves on year after year, regardless of whether the individual wants it to or not. And there is no turning back.

With the passing of time come advantages and disadvantages. Physically, the human body tends to wear out. This deterioration takes place at a faster rate if a person pursues a careless way of life and at a slower rate if he follows simple rules of conservative living.

Here are three principles which, as you follow them, will promote your health and help you to avoid illness.

1. *Exercise Consistently*. Muscles in action require more oxygen and more food material than muscles at rest. It is the blood that brings both oxygen and food to the muscles. So, during exercise the heart beats faster and more forcefully to propel greater volumes of blood. Breathing is also faster and deeper to provide the extra amounts of oxygen.

The arteries carry the blood from the heart to all parts of the body. Once the blood has served its purpose in the various tissues, it is returned to the heart through the veins. Blood flowing through the veins is under very little

Exercise as a consistent practice goes far in perpetuating health.

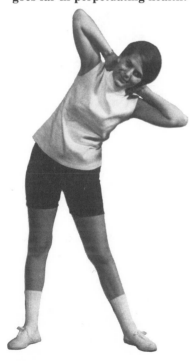

pressure. But the veins contain tiny valves which keep the blood from flowing backward. When large muscles contract, they squeeze the veins and so move the blood on its way toward the heart. This is how physical exercise actually aids in the circulation of blood.

Consider the way the muscles increase in size and in strength when used actively over a period of weeks. Likewise, the various vital organs of the body increase their capacities under the stimulus of exercise. The heart pumps more blood. The lungs can handle greater volumes of air. The digestive organs become able to satisfy the increased demands for food materials. Exercise is a wholesome stimulant to all tissues and organs of the body.

Make exercise a part of your way of life. Take the stairs instead of the elevator. When you need to go two or three blocks, walk instead of using your car. Go to bed a little earlier in the evening so you can rise the next morning in time for some active, physical exercise before breakfast.

2. *Cultivate Self-discipline*. Some of the things people do are detrimental to their health. Consider the excessive use of sugar. The average American craves sweetened soft drinks, prefers sugar-coated breakfast cereals, eats candy bars between meals, and indulges generously in pastries and desserts. Why? Because of cultivated habit.

From the standpoint of the body's cravings, it is just as easy to train the taste buds to enjoy the natural flavors of foods as it is to coach them in a compelling demand for sweets.

Alcohol takes its toll in the form of more than 25,000 traffic deaths a year in the United States. In addition, it damages the heart, the brain, the liver, and other organs in countless thousands of other people.

Cigarettes are responsible for the death of more than 100,000 persons a year in the United States by way of lung cancer. They also hasten the time of death of three or four times this many by increasing their susceptibility to such illnesses as coronary heart disease and emphysema.

Year by year physicians are becoming more aware of the hidden hazards of ordinary medicines. Better to discover and remove the actual cause of a headache than to stifle the discomfort by taking a tablet.

Promoting health requires that a person govern his pattern of living by what he knows to be best rather than yield to habits and customs.

3. *Radiate Optimism and Appreciation.* One day a long line of customers stood waiting to be checked out at the supermarket. It was a busy time and people were in a hurry. The atmosphere grew tense.

Suddenly an elderly customer, a man of foreign background, began singing in a lusty tone what could well have been his national anthem. He smiled as he sang and, presto, the whole atmosphere changed as everyone began to smile.

The human body consists of a group of organs which relate themselves very much as people in a group. And of all the organs, the brain carries the greatest influence over other organs. This causal relationship is logical, for the brain not only provides for a person's conscious experiences but it dominates the so-called "autonomic nervous system" which controls the functions of the body's tissues and organs.

When a person is unhappy, discontented, or downcast, the body's vital processes slow down and may even become disorganized. But when one's attitude is cheerful, when he feels courageous and optimistic, and when he manifests appreciation for other people, a vitalizing influence emanates from the brain so that all of the body's organs function efficiently.

Simple Rules to Live By

It is easy to agree to the three pinciples just listed. Putting them into practice can be a little more difficult. Here is a list of suggestions that will help you to cooperate with your doctor in promoting health and preventing illness:

1. Rise a few minutes earlier in the morning so as to have time for a brisk walk, a short jog, or some sitting-up exercises. Follow this workout with a hot shower topped off with straight cold water. The stimulating effect will be beneficial to your general health.

2. Eat a good breakfast and abstain from the ten o'clock sweet snack.

3. Eat simple, wholesome food at every meal in preference to gourmet fare.

4. Promote your physical fitness rather than taking recourse to pain-relieving drugs.

5. Develop attitudes of optimism and appreciation so that you will have

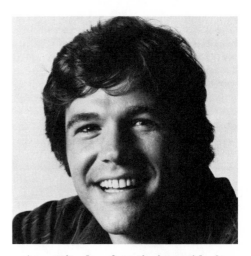

An attitude of optimism aids in maintenance of good health.

no need for chemical tranquilizers.

6. Take a neutral shower (at body temperature) before retiring, in preference to relying on sleeping pills.

7. Abstain from personal indulgences that would be harmful to your health.

Fads and Nostrums

We are dealing in this chapter with the progress that has been made by modern medical scientists in their efforts to combat disease. Much of this progress has originated in research laboratories and in teaching hospitals. But shifting the emphasis to prevention rather than cure depends on educating the public. Medical information must be shared in order for persons not medically trained to benefit.

But this commendable trend of sharing information has set the stage for many pseudoscientists to intrude. We could list various fads, cures, and nostrums being currently promoted. But within a few months the list would be out of date, some claims having been proved false and others replaced by new ones. So we will mention several general areas in which pseudoscientists promote their programs and wares; then we will conclude the section with a list of cautions that will help you to sort the true from the false.

"Cancer cures" have been and will continue to be numerous and appealing. It is understandable that a person with cancer will "grasp at a straw." Those who promote false methods of treatment are lavish with their claims and even with their promises. Reputable physicians, however, are careful not to raise the cancer patient's hopes beyond the limits of reality. So it is easy for the distressed cancer patient to turn to someone promoting a "cure." The tragedy is that valuable time is lost as the cancer patient relies on a supposed cure instead of cooperating with a trained specialist in his use of proven methods of treatment.

Diet fads have been with us for many years and, doubtless, will continue. Often a certain diet is promoted as the means of curing high blood pressure, arthritis, or obesity. Some diets, intended for weight reduction, are actually deficient and increase the risk of illness.

Supposed remedies for arthritis continue to attract a lot of attention. Mysterious beauty aids not only raise false hopes but may even damage the skin and cause permanent blemishes. And so it goes. Many persons are persuaded to part with their money in the hope of receiving some mysterious cure beyond what scientific medicine is honestly able to offer.

How can the nonmedical person recognize a harmful fad, an unproven cure, or a nostrum? Following is a list of precautions: Beware when (1) the product or service is promoted as a secret remedy; (2) the sponsor claims he is battling the medical profession which has, so far, refused to accept his discovery; (3) the remedy is being sold from door to door or promoted by newspaper and magazine advertisements; (4) the product or service is supposed to cure a wide variety of unrelated ailments; (5) the sponsor of the cure has an unusual degree supposed to qualify him as a specialist in his field; or (6) the claims of the sponsor seem too good to be true.

Modern Methods of Dealing With Disease

Remarkable advances have been made in recent years in the methods of treating disease. Limited space permits mention of only a few classic examples:

1. *Microsurgery.* Surgery involves the manipulation of the body's tissues. Originally, surgery consisted almost entirely of the removal of diseased or damaged tissues. Increasingly, however, surgeons have become concerned with restoring or transplanting tissues to a normal or more nearly normal relationship so as to improve their function.

The critical factor in any kind of tissue transfer is the continuing vitality of the tissue being transferred. In order for a transplanted tissue to continue to live, there must be provision for it to receive adequate blood at its new location.

Thus, surgeons have developed methods of joining blood vessels that have been severed so that the flow of blood can continue to a tissue even though it has been transferred to a new site. The joining of blood vessels requires meticulous work. Many vessels are so small as to be hardly seen by the naked eye. Microsurgery as it is now practiced requires that the surgeon observe his work through a microscope, that he use miniature instruments, and that he use needles and suture materials so delicate that they do not damage the small tissues being manipulated. For example, the suture material used in many microsurgical procedures is about half the diameter of a human hair.

It is the development of this branch of surgery (microsurgery) that now makes possible the reattachment of amputated fingers, hands, forearms, and other parts of the body. The surgical procedures are tedious, often requiring as much as ten to twenty hours of continuous effort.

Microsurgery has been expanded now to include the reunion of nerves when these have been severed. It is not possible for complete function to be restored after a nerve has been severed and then reunited. But the partial function usually realized is much better than no function at all.

The techniques of microsurgery are used by ear specialists to operate on the minute structures of the middle ear, and by this means the hearing of thousands of people has been restored or improved. Specialists in diseases of the eye have adapted the techniques of microsurgery to perform operations previously impossible.

2. *Organ Transplantation.* The next step in this advancement has been to take a tissue or an organ from one person and transplant it into another person. The news media has awakened the public's interest in this possibility even beyond what is possible on the operating table. A few years ago it was virtually assumed that a person with heart disease could "trade in" his damaged heart and have it replaced by a healthy heart salvaged from some young person who had died of an unrelated disease or accident.

Now we seldom hear of heart transplantation. What has happened? A conservative attitude toward the transplantation of organs has been

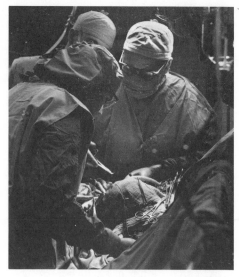

Organ transplantation is considered one of modern medicine's greatest triumphs.

forced upon the medical profession by the problem of tissue rejection, not by the technical problems of uniting the blood vessels, ducts, and nerves. The body's mechanisms for protecting itself against the invasion of germs works excellently in building up immunity against germs but works to the individual's disadvantage when it comes to the rejection of tissue from another person, even from a near relative.

Progress is being made in solving the problem of tissue rejection, but the progress is slow. Transplantation of the heart from one person to another is still being carried on in one or two medical centers, but the patients for this procedure are being very carefully selected. The relatively few patients now approved for this procedure are those who have such serious heart disease that they would not be able to survive on their own. Even in such cases, the patient's condition must be favorable with respect to other organs of his body.

Transplantation of the liver is being carried on in carefully selected cases. At the time of writing, between 25 percent and 40 percent of those receiving liver transplants have survived for at least one year, and many of these have excellent liver function.

Better success has attended the transplantation of a kidney from a donor to a recipient. The ultimate success of a kidney transplant depends upon many factors, a major one, of course, being the control of tissue rejection as mentioned above. The one-year survival rate for kidney transplants now stands at approximately 50 percent.

In dealing with persons who have serious kidney disease, the physician in charge now has a choice between kidney transplantation (the surgical procedure) and the use of dialysis (artificial kidney). The dialysis procedure requires that the patient must be present at a dialysis center at least two or three times a week and allow his blood to circulate through the artificial kidney equipment for approximately six hours at each visit.

3. *Open Heart Surgery*. For many years, even after abdominal surgery was practiced successfully throughout the world, surgeons hesitated to open the chest. When air was permitted to enter either side of the chest, the corresponding lung would collapse. Surgery on the heart was considered impossible because a person's life depends on continuous circulation of his blood.

But within recent years these difficulties have been overcome. Present methods of anesthesia keep the lung from collapsing even when the chest is open. As for the continuous circulation of the blood, the heart-lung machine not only maintains the circulation of blood throughout the body, independent of the heart, but provides for oxygenating the blood without its having to pass through the lungs.

These technical advances make it possible now for the heart surgeon to open the heart, repair its defects, close it again, and cause it to resume functioning. Congenital defects of the heart can now be repaired. Faulty heart valves can be repaired or even replaced by prosthetic devices. When the circu-

lation of blood to the heart muscle is curtailed by arteriosclerosis, a bypass procedure is arranged in which a vein taken from some other part of the body is inserted to carry blood around the diseased artery.

Heart surgery as now practiced has prolonged the lives of thousands of persons.

4. *Joint Replacement*. In some cases of fractured hip, the head of the thigh bone (femur) becomes separated from the source of its blood supply and thus the fracture will not heal. In such a case it is now possible to replace the head of the femur by a metallic prosthesis. Healing takes place normally, and the patient is able to walk again within a relatively short time.

Knee joints that have been damaged by accident or have become useless because of arthritis can be replaced with metallic joints which function quite normally. In some cases of deformity of a hand by arthritis, the orthopedic surgeon can reconstruct the hand, even transplanting certain joints of the fingers and relocating the tendons of muscles in such ways that function is restored.

5. *Feeding by Vein*. There are some conditions in which a sick person becomes unable to take food by mouth. The giving of fluid and even of glucose by vein has been a great help in tiding a patient over immediate problems. But glucose of itself does not supply nutritional needs for longer than a few hours.

Finally there has been developed a method which provides "total parenteral nutrition" over a prolonged period, and with which the patient may even gain weight and strength. The procedure must be a precise one so as to avoid infection. A catheter is introduced into the subclavian vein, and through this catheter the nutritional fluid joins the bloodstream just before it enters the heart. The nutritional solution consists of the simple amino acids (components of protein) together with glucose (a source of energy), plus vitamins and minerals. Emulsified fat is sometimes added by a supplementary route. The procedure must be monitored very carefully and must be conducted under precisely controlled conditions in the hospital. It is a life-saving procedure for patients who would otherwise starve because of their present inability to assimilate food through their digestive organs.

Conclusions

The authors of *You and Your Health* are thrilled that we live at a time in the world's history when medical science has made and is making such remarkable progress. Month by month new methods are perfected which not only add to the comfort of persons suffering illness but which serve to prolong their lives. Human life is priceless. Members of the health professions are dedicated to the continuing effort to preserve life and to relieve suffering.

Doctors and nurses receive satisfaction as they use their skills in caring for the sick and aiding the healing processes which make their patients well again. But it is even more important to deal with healthy people and encourage them to adopt the principles of rational living so that they can be spared from prevailing illnesses. Thus they can enjoy sustained vitality, both physical and mental.

What Your Doctor Can Do for You

It is natural and customary for every family and sometimes individual persons to have certain selected professional people that they go to for help as needed. A man has "my barber," and a woman has "my hairdresser." A family has "our pastor," and a husband and wife have "our banker." A businessman has "my lawyer." So it is logical that every family have "our doctor," and every single person have "my personal physician."

Now that medical science has developed in so many directions, doctors specialize in the various fields of medicine and surgery. Each specialist is trained and experienced in his own field, such as in the treatment of skin diseases, in problems relating to bones and joints, in the diagnosis and treatment of disorders of the endocrine glands, or in disorders of the nervous system.

But a family does not want a specialist as the family doctor. Rather, they need someone interested in the family's total well-being. It matters not what a person's ailment may be, the family doctor must be one who either treats the specific illness himself or helps to arrange an appointment with a physician who specializes in the treatment of the problem.

Time was when we spoke of personal physicians as "general practitioners of medicine." These were physicians who had completed the regular medical course and had become licensed as physicians, but had not chosen to take additional training in a specialty. People tended to regard these general practitioners as less qualified for diagnosis and treatment than those who had become specialists. But the picture has changed.

Medical educators and people in general have come to realize that the family doctor needs to be as fully qualified in the general field of medical science as does the specialist need to be well informed and experienced in his limited field. And so there has developed the profession of "family practice."

This "specialty" dates back to 1969 when the American Board of Family Practice was officially established. This professional organization supervises and certifies a period of training (usually three years) beyond the regular medical course for those physicians who select family medicine as their professional field of choice. The training of such a physician includes instruction and experience in handling emergencies, guidance in hospital procedures, supervision in common surgical procedures, and training in the behavioral sciences. The latter enables the family physician to evaluate the stresses under which persons in our modern society find themselves. He is qualified to give counsel on the problems of human relations. He evaluates illnesses, treats those that come within his range of experience, and refers others to the proper specialists.

This program of training for family practice has become popular among young physicians. Nine years after the establishment of the American Board of Family Practice, a total of 19,000 family practice physicians had been certified after training in this field. Furthermore, the American Board of Family Practice requires that its members keep up to date on the new developments in the science of medicine. They must take written examinations at occasional intervals in order to maintain their certification. They must allow an officer of the American Board of Family Practice to make a periodic review of their records to check on the quality of their practice of medicine. They must attend lecture courses totaling 300 hours during each six-year cycle.

Choosing a Personal or Family Physician

When new in a community, you may not know the physicians qualified as family physicians. In such a case, you can speak to the administrator or the chief of the medical staff of your local hospital. Ask for the names of qualified family physicians in your community. Make sure that the hospital where you inquire is an accredited institution. Another source of information is the office of the county medical society. If you live in an isolated area, you can contact the headquarters office of the American Academy of Family Physicians, 1740 West 92nd St., Kansas City, Missouri 64114, requesting a list of the certified family physicians in your area.

It is better, by far, to make your selection of a physician at a time when you and your family members are in good health, not waiting until some

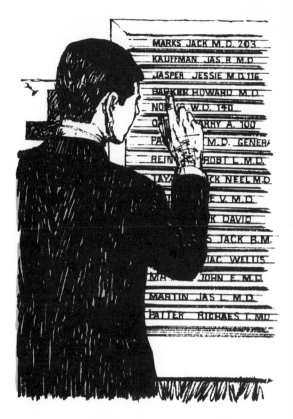

emergency requires you to seek a physician in haste. Your best interests are served by a physician who concerns himself with your total well-being at all times, not only when you are sick. He should be fully as interested in keeping you well as in treating you once you become ill. He should be the kind of person you can look to as a trusted friend rather than a mere technician.

With this in mind, you should talk to more than one physician, if available, before making your final selection. Speak to each one frankly about your desire to have a physician who will carry the responsibility for maintaining your health. Tell him that you are more interested in keeping well than in being treated after you are sick. Here are some questions that will guide you in your appraisals of the physicians among whom you must choose:

1. Is he certified by the American Board of Family Practice?

2. With what hospital is he affiliated,

and is he a member of the hospital's staff of physicians? Is this hospital accredited?

3. Is he a member of the local medical society? If so, this means that he is in good standing with his colleagues and that he adheres to the accepted standards of medical practice.

4. What are his arrangements for taking care of his patients' emergency illnesses at night, on holidays and weekends, or at times when he may not be personally available?

5. Does he see his office patients by appointment, or do they have to wait their turn in his waiting room?

Once you have selected your family physician, trust him, rely on him, and follow his recommendations.

Periodic Checkups

The emphasis on preventing disease and on detecting early evidences of illness, includes periodic checkups. In the past it has been recommended that a person have a thorough examination each year, including laboratory tests.

But such annual head-to-toe examinations plus laboratory tests carry a high price tag, both for the patient and for the time schedule of a busy physician. In many instances, the information gained one year will be the same as that obtained the previous year. And so the custom of the yearly health examination has come in for scrutiny by some leading medical authorities. Such organizations as the Canadian Medical Association and the American Cancer Society now recommend that the periodic checkup by the family physician be individualized to suit the needs of the particular person, especially when the individual sees the same physician year after year. In such cases, the physician becomes so well acquainted with the individual patient that he knows his particular weaknesses and tendencies to illness.

At his first contact with a patient, a physician makes a record of the patient's medical history and does a head-to-toe examination, in addition to arranging for a battery of laboratory

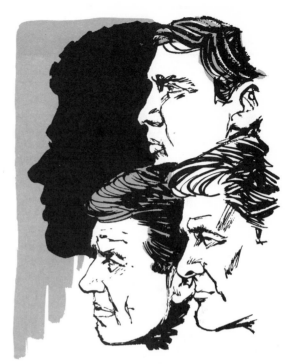

One in four of the nation's population will have cancer at some time.

tests, attempting to determine the most pressing problems. Later, the physician will make examinations and order tests as indicated by what he discovered previously. The patient may not yet have symptoms, but if he faces possible risk with a certain disease (as a smoker in respect to lung cancer) or if the record shows that his close relatives have been susceptible to a certain disease (as a family record of diabetes), then the physician will check on these possibilities at each of the patient's visits.

The following schedule is offered as a guide. It will be noted that certain procedures are more necessary at specific times of life. One's family physician will modify such a schedule to fit the needs of the individual. Whenever symptoms develop between regular appointments, these should be reported promptly to the family physician, who will then decide what examinations should be made at this time.

SUGGESTED SCHEDULE FOR PERIODIC CHECKUPS

Procedure	Value	Frequency
A. FOR INFANTS		
1. Search for congenital defects and endocrine disorders	To provide for early treatment as indicated	See chapter 6, volume 1
2. Establish a plan for immunizations	To protect the child against infectious diseases	See page 35 in this chapter
B. FOR CHILDREN		
1. Review schedule for immunizations	To maintain protection against infectious diseases	At age 5 and 15
2. General physical examination	To detect abnormalities or illness	At age 3 and 5 and every 3 years thereafter
3. Blood count and urinalysis	To detect anemia or kidney disease	At age 3 and 5 and every 3 years thereafter
4. Check hearing and vision	To correct and avoid handicap in school	At age 3, 5, and 8
5. Check teeth	For referral to dentist as needed	At age 3 and 5 and every 3 years thereafter
6. Check blood pressure	To detect beginnings of high blood pressure	At age 5 and 15
C. FOR ADULTS TO AGE 39		
1. General physical examination of heart, lungs, skin surface, and all body openings	To provide clues for beginning illness and to discover need for corrective procedures	Every 2 to 3 years
2. Check blood pressure	To detect beginnings of high blood pressure and to check on the heart's general function	Every 2 to 3 years; oftener if abnormal
3. Pap smear for women	To provide information on the general condition of the uterus, cervix, and vagina, and to signal the possible beginning of cancer	Every year for 2 to 3 years; if favorable, then at 3-year intervals
4. Electrocardiogram (EKG)	To detect changes in heart function and to provide a basis for comparison in later years	At age 35
5. Skin tests for tuberculosis	When there is a positive test after previous negative tests, further search should be made for the site of a tuberculous infection	Every 5 years
6. Tests for venereal disease	To provide opportunity for treatment even in the absence of symptoms	Every 2 to 3 years for sexually active persons

Procedure	Value	Frequency
D. AGE 40 AND THERE-AFTER		
1. General physical examination of heart, lungs, skin surface, and all body openings	To detect beginning disease and indicate the need for corrections	Every 2 to 3 years
2. Check blood pressure	To detect the beginnings of high blood pressure and to check on the general function of the heart	Every 2 to 3 years; oftener if abnormal
3. Sigmoidoscopy	This examination of the last portion of the large intestine provides a clue to the beginning of cancer in this area	Every 2 to 3 years
4. Blood count and urinalysis	To detect anemia or kidney disease	Every 2 to 3 years
5. Chemical blood tests	A check on the cholesterol level helps in determining the risk of arteriosclerosis; elevated blood sugar may indicate diabetes; level of urea nitrogen indicates kidney function; and level of calcium in the blood is a check on parathyroid function	Every 5 years
6. For women: physical examination of the breasts plus X ray (mammography) if lumps are present	These examinations by a physician supplement the woman's self-examination as a clue to cancer	Every 2 to 3 years; oftener if lumps are noted
7. For women: pap smear examination	To indicate the condition of the uterus, cervix, and vagina, and to signal the beginning of cancer of the cervix	Yearly for 2 years; then every 2 years, but oftener if abnormal
8. For men: prostate examination by palpation	For detection of beginning cancer	Every 2 to 3 years; oftener if abnormal
9. Stool examination for "hidden blood"	To check on the possibility of cancer or other bowel problems	Every 2 to 3 years
10. Check on hearing and vision	To indicate the need for referral to specialists in these fields	Every 5 years
11. Tonometry	This simple measurement of pressure within the eye can indicate beginning glaucoma and its threat to vision	Every 2 to 3 years; annually if family history of glaucoma
12. Electrocardiogram (EKG)	To indicate the quality of the heart's function	Every 10 years; oftener if abnormal
13. Immunizations for pneumonia and flu	To protect against illnesses which are serious for older persons	Every year for senior citizens

The Physician as a Health Counselor

Many of the diseases which cause suffering and premature death can be avoided if the factors in the environment or in the individual's life-style which cause these diseases are eliminated. And this observation brings us to a recognition of the importance of a physician's influence in helping his patients to avoid the factors that make them susceptible to disease.

Patients should feel free to ask about things that perplex them. Physicians realize, more and more, their responsibility to help their patients understand the principles of healthful living. It is at the occasion of the periodic examination, as described in the previous section, that the patient and his doctor have the best opportunity to consider these matters of healthful living.

Physicians as now trained for family practice have a knowledge of the various risk factors that make persons susceptible to illness. For example, the most frequent cause of death among men in their prime of life is coronary

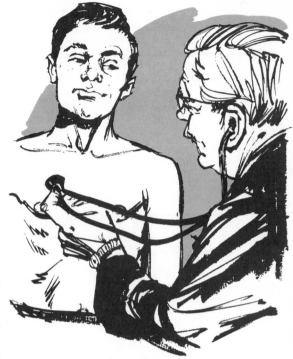

Do youth need periodic checkups? See accompanying schedule.

CAREFUL EXAMINATION CAN DETECT THESE AND OTHER DISEASES BEFORE THEY PRODUCE SYMPTOMS

*Heart disease—various kinds
*High blood pressure and hardening of the arteries
*Cancer: of the breast
          lung
          stomach
          colon
          rectum
          uterus
          skin
Lesions of the rectum and lower bowel
Anemia
Kidney disease
Diabetes
Tuberculosis
Glaucoma

*The first three on this list are today's "major killers." Valuable time can be gained and lives can be saved by discovering and treating them early.

heart disease. By reviewing the risk factors it can be predicted how susceptible a man is to this serious illness. For a list of these risk factors and a discussion of their significance, see chapter 8, this volume.

If a certain man presents only one or two of the risk factors and they in mild form, his physician can give him guidance regarding his life-style, thus helping him to prevent a heart attack. If, however, he is extremely overweight and smokes two packs of cigarettes a day and persists in eating too much food, he is an easy candidate for coronary heart disease, even though no history of this illness shows up in his family. His physician can help him develop a new life-style with controllable risk factors eliminated.

Motor-vehicle accidents are the second most common cause of death among men in their early forties. At first thought, it may seem that the physician has no responsibility in the matter of preventing vehicle accidents. But as we examine the risk factors, we observe that negligence in the use of seat belts is not the only risk factor that contributes to this problem. The use of alcoholic drinks or the use of narcotics and other medications make the individual more susceptible to accidents on the highway. The family physician, being acquainted with his patient and his pattern of living, is in a position to urge him to eliminate the risk factors that contribute to his prospect of an accident.

Why Do People Hesitate?

In the face of the obvious advantages resulting from periodic checkups and from receiving advice from their family physician, it seems strange that so many people ignore these opportunities to keep themselves in good health. Some, just naturally fatalistic, think that what is going to be will be. They read about persons who have had to give up important careers because of premature illness. But they still cling to the belief, "It can't happen to me."

Many persons have complained, after receiving a clear bill of health, "All I received in return for my money was the assurance that I am disgustingly healthy." But such a person will not hesitate to take his car to an automotive service center for its 5000-mile service and pay up to a hundred dollars. Probably the car runs very little better after the service than it did before. But its period of usefulness will be prolonged by the care which the periodic service provides. From a business standpoint, this is money well spent. Why should there be a difference, then, in spending money for a checkup of one's most valuable asset—his health?

Some people complain that they have to wait too long when an appointment is requested before they can get to see the doctor. He may be booked for several weeks in advance. But consider this: The time of waiting for a routine checkup does not put the person in jeopardy. But when a person waits for symptoms to develop before he requests an appointment with his doctor, every day of continued waiting allows his disease to progress that much farther and makes the treatment more difficult.

Immunization

Immunization provides protection within a person's body, rendering it less susceptible to contagion. But this protection is generally specific for each disease. That is, immunization against polio protects only against polio, not against diphtheria, whooping cough, or tetanus. Each disease requires a separate defense mechanism. So, in considering the advantages of immunization, we must consider the ways in which a person can be protected against each of the common communicable diseases. But first a word about immunization in general and the great advantage it offers.

Immunization is something like insurance—it removes the element of risk. But immunization is better than insurance. Insurance compensates for loss or tragedy, while immunization prevents the tragedy in the first place.

31

Thanks to medical science, many of the contagious diseases can be prevented now. But prevention is an individual matter, each person having to be immunized for each particular disease.

The Story of Smallpox

Smallpox was the first of the contagious diseases to be controlled. The story of how this came about provides good insight into the modern system of immunization for protection from the other contagious diseases.

Smallpox, in its day, caused millions of deaths. It sometimes caused blindness. In previous centuries, smallpox was a scourge to the entire world.

It was in the latter part of the eighteenth century that Dr. Edward Jenner, a young physician in England, became interested in verifying the rumor that milkmaids seldom contracted smallpox. In those days cows were milked by hand, and in England by milkmaids.

A disease called cowpox was prevalent among cows. Perhaps because of handling cows, milkmaids often contracted this disease, but only once. It was a mild disease, sometimes accompanied by a slight rash, from which the milkmaid soon recovered.

Dr. Jenner began to wonder whether cowpox and the more severe disease, smallpox, were related. He knew that a person who had had smallpox was also not susceptible to a second attack. He wondered, therefore, whether an attack of cowpox might not cause the same defensive reaction within the body as the more severe disease.

It took many years of convincing and persuading before Dr. Jenner's method of preventing smallpox was generally accepted and before his theory of the relationship between cowpox and smallpox was admitted to be correct.

His method of immunizing against smallpox was to transmit cowpox deliberately to a person who had never had smallpox. This would make the person slightly ill, but for a few years thereafter the person thus treated would remain immune to smallpox.

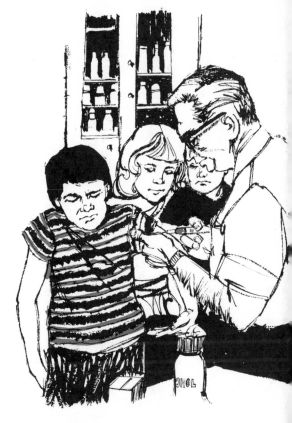

It is now understood that both smallpox and cowpox are caused by a virus—a disease-producing organism much smaller than ordinary bacteria.

Gradually vaccination for smallpox became standard throughout the world. The method of vaccination was simplified so that the doctor merely placed a small amount of purified vaccine on the skin of the person being immunized, usually on the left upper arm. Then with a needle he repeated pressure on the skin through the droplet of vaccine, thus introducing a small amount of vaccine into the skin. In a person not previously immunized against smallpox, a reddening of the skin at the vaccination site occurred a few days later, and a slight feeling of illness persisted for two or three days.

Thanks to the worldwide program of vaccination for smallpox, the World Health Organization declared on May 8, 1980, that smallpox has been eradi-

cated. It may now be considered to be a disease of the past.

Prevention of Certain Diseases

Many diseases feared in former decades as veritable scourges now can be prevented by the simple procedure of immunization. Thanks to the influence of our public-health agencies and other health-promoting organizations, programs of immunization have become quite widespread. We now list the common diseases for which immunizations have been developed:

1. *Pertussis (Whooping Cough).* For babies under three months of age pertussis (whooping cough) carries a 25 percent mortality rate; for children under four years of age, 5 percent. Also, serious complications frequently develop. For more information on pertussis, see volume 1, chapter 6.

Fortunately, an effective agent is available for immunizing against pertussis—a vaccine administered by injection. The immunity conferred is not as long-lasting as some others. Doctors therefore recommend repeated doses during the child's first six years, as recommended later in this chapter.

2. *Diphtheria.* Diphtheria is another communicable disease now under good control, thanks to widespread immunization. But this comforting knowledge carries with it the danger that persons may become complacent, willingly taking a chance rather than carrying through the proper procedure for immunization.

Immunization for diphtheria should be begun early in an infant's life and should be renewed at intervals thereafter, as specified in the recommended schedule appearing later in this chapter. For a discussion of this disease and its proper treatment, see chapter 18, volume 3.

3. *Polio (Poliomyelitis).* Many adult readers of this book will recall the days before the conquest of polio when this disease was a terror to every family and every community. Children were more susceptible, but many young adults were also affected. The principle manifestation of the disease was paralysis, and this accounts for the name by which it was often called —"infantile paralysis."

People everywhere rejoiced when polio was brought under control by immunization. In 1954 there were an estimated 38,000 cases in the United States. Vaccination for polio began in 1955, and that year there were about 29,000 cases. Then the number of cases dropped rapidly. By 1973 only 14 cases were reported, with three deaths.

In more recent years there have been a few minor epidemics of polio in localized areas. The persons involved in these epidemics were persons who had not been immunized!

The danger of polio still lurks. The polio virus is still around; but because people tend to forget the tragedies of the past, some seem less insistent now on vaccination for polio as compared with before. The first immunization for polio should be given to the infant at two months of age. Repeat immunizations should be carried out thereafter to age six as indicated in the recommended schedule in this chapter. For a further discussion of the disease, see chapter 16, volume 3.

4. *Tetanus.* Tetanus, commonly called lockjaw, is a dread disease. The toxin produced by the tetanus germs affects the nervous system, causing painful spasms of certain muscles, often those that close the jaw and that move the neck. Highly poisonous, even relatively small amounts of it can cause death.

Penetrating wounds, such as those caused by a nail or a splinter, may introduce the germs or spores of tetanus into the deeper tissues, where they multiply most readily in locations not exposed to air. The body's resistance to tetanus is not long-lasting; even an attack of the disease, if survived, does not confer permanent immunity. But with the present good methods of im-

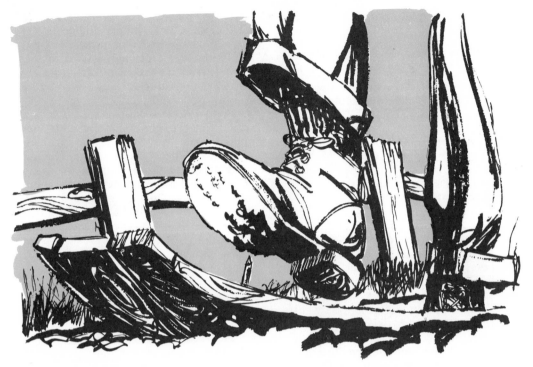

Tetanus germs, commonly present in barnyards, may be introduced into the body by a puncture wound such as caused by a nail.

munization, the body's resistance lasts more than five years. Because immunity to tetanus wanes as time passes, physicians recommend extra protection whenever they deal with a serious penetrating wound, even though the patient may have been previously immunized. With children, the possibility of penetrating injuries is so great that it is best to maintain an active immunity to tetanus throughout the years of childhood. Then later, have booster injections administered periodically as in the following schedule of immunization, or whenever a serious injury occurs.

The effectiveness of immunization against tetanus is attested by the experience of the United States armed forces during World War II. All service personnel were required to be immunized. As a result, only 15 cases of tetanus occurred among the two thirds of a million wounded men—a phenomenal improvement compared with previous wars, before availability of immunization.

For a further discussion of tetanus, see chapter 18, volume 3.

5. *Measles (Rubeola).* Measles, a common contagious disease in the United States before vaccination, still is more prevalent among children than among adults. Ordinarily the illness is mild. Some persons consider it best for a child to have the disease in routine fashion whenever he happens to be exposed. Thus the child builds his own immunity and will be protected from this illness for life. But measles carries the risk of serious complications, so to have a child immunized is better than to run the risk of such complications as pneumonia or encephalitis.

An effective vaccine to protect against measles was introduced in 1963. It is hoped that with the continued use of this vaccine, measles, as a disease, may be completely eradicated

from the United States within the next few years.

For a further discussion of measles, see chapter 16, volume 3.

6. *Rubella (German Measles).* Rubella is a mild contagious disease as far as the immediate illness is concerned. But when an expectant mother becomes ill with this disease during the first three months of her pregnancy, grave danger threatens that her unborn child will be so affected by the virus of this disease that it will not develop normally. Many congenital deformities of infants can be traced to such damage by rubella. A preventive vaccine for rubella became available in 1969. It is advised that all children should be immunized against rubella. It is also advised that susceptible women of child-bearing age should receive the vaccine. Inasmuch as the immediate effects of immunization are similar to those of the actual disease, women of child-bearing age who are immunized should avoid pregnancy for the next three months after receiving the vaccine.

For further information on this disastrous disease, consult chapter 16, volume 3.

7. *Mumps.* For children, mumps is a relatively harmless disease. In adulthood, however, serious complications may occur. These may involve the sex organs, either the ovaries or the testes, and may occasionally produce sterility. Other complications of mumps include pancreatitis and encephalitis.

A vaccine to protect against mumps is now available, and it is recommended that all children should receive this vaccine. The preferable time for this immunization, as mentioned in the schedule which follows, is one year of age.

The Official Schedule for Immunization

The program for immunizing a child against the diseases which have just been listed begins at two months of age and continues at stated intervals throughout the remainder of childhood.

The accompanying schedule for immunizations is proposed by The American Academy of Pediatrics and is sanctioned by the Center for Disease Control of the U.S. Public Health Service. Your family doctor probably has a copy of this schedule, for it is the pattern that most physicians follow in caring for their young patients. By consulting the schedule you will know when to take your child to the doctor's office for his next immunization.

A glance at the accompanying schedule reveals that immunization is an ongoing program that lasts throughout the years of childhood. It is important, therefore, that a careful record be kept for each child of the various immunizations he has received and the dates on which these have been administered. The family physician who administers the immunizations will doubtless keep such a record in his office. You are fortunate if you are able to stay with the same physician year after year. However, families tend to move from place

Recommended Schedule for Immunization of Infants and Children

2 months	DTP* and TOPV†
4 months	DTP and TOPV
6 months	DTP and TOPV
1 year	Measles, rubella, mumps‡
1¹/₂ years	DTP and TOPV
4-6 years	DTP and TOPV
14-16 years	TD§ and thereafter every ten years

*Diphtheria and tetanus toxoids with pertussis vaccine
†Trivalent oral polio vaccine
‡Combined vaccines
§Combined tetanus and diphtheria toxoids, adult type

to place as do also some physicians. Therefore, it is important that parents keep an accurate record for each child, giving the same information as is kept by the doctor in his office. For the reader's convenience, medical record forms have been included at the back of volume 1 of this set.

Immunizations for Other Diseases

Protection by immunization is also available for certain other contagious diseases. But these diseases occur under special circumstances, and so the related immunizations are not included in the official schedule already provided.

1. *Rabies*. This tragic disease, once it develops in a human being, is invariably fatal. It is caused by a virus transmitted to human beings by the bite of an infected animal, typically a "mad dog." Other animals besides dogs, such as bats and skunks, are susceptible to this disease and can transmit it to humans through their saliva when they bite.

Rabies does not occur commonly in human beings; therefore it is not recommended that immunization be carried out generally. There is a period of at least two weeks after a person has been bitten by a rabid animal before the disease becomes established. During this time it is important for the individual to be immunized and thus be saved from the development of the actual disease.

For additional information on rabies and for details on the modern method of immunization, consult chapter 16, volume 3.

2. *Influenza (Flu)*. Influenza is perhaps our most prevalent contagious disease. Several viruses may cause it, and the particular virus or combination of viruses that cause one epidemic may differ from that which causes another. Vaccines have been developed to protect against each of the viruses that can cause influenza; but, unfortunately, the vaccine which protects against one virus does not protect against the others.

It is customary in immunizing against influenza to use a "polyvalent" vaccine which consists of a mixture of vaccines for the various viruses that commonly cause this disease. Even so, unusual combinations of causative viruses are often present in a new epidemic of influenza. Manufacturers of vaccines are constantly on the alert to provide vaccines that will protect against the influenza viruses currently prevalent.

Another complication in the immunization for influenza is that the immunity is not of long duration. A person depending upon the immunity which influenza vaccine provides should have the immunization repeated each year. Those who need this protection most, either for their own safety or for the protection of those closely associated with them, are doctors, nurses, teachers of elementary schoolchildren, elderly people and those caring for them, and those who are caring for babies and preschool children. Also, patients with respiratory or cardiac conditions should have this protection. The preferred time of year for obtaining this immunization is early autumn.

The National Institutes of Health now recommends that amantadine (Symmetrel), an anti-viral drug, may be used effectively along with influenza vaccine as a means of preventing influenza.

For a further discussion of influenza, see chapter 16, volume 3.

3. *Rocky Mountain Spotted Fever.* This disease occurs in several countries. In the United States it is most prevalent in the Rocky Mountain area. The disease is transmitted by the bite of an infected tick. A suitable vaccine is available to protect against this disease, and its use is recommended for those who live or vacation in areas where the disease occurs, particularly those who have unusual opportunities for exposure to the infection.

For a further discussion of this disease, see chapter 17, volume 3.

4. *Q Fever*. This disease somewhat resembles pneumonia and occurs commonly among persons who have close contact with domestic animals or animal carcasses. It is relatively common in the southwestern part of the United States.

There is a vaccine available to protect against Q fever. However, the vaccine causes local reactions in some of those who receive it. It is therefore recommended that the vaccine be used only for persons at high risk of this disease, such as dairy workers, wool sorters, tanners, and slaughterhouse workers.

For a further discussion of this disease and the accepted treatment, see chapter 17, volume 3.

5. *Pneumococcal Pneumonia*. Various germs and viruses can cause pneumonia, one of the most common being the pneumococcus bacterium, of which there are 14 strains. In 1968, there was released for use a polyvalent vaccine which is effective in protecting against this type of pneumonia. Its use as a preventive measure is recommended for elderly people and those with serious chronic diseases. The protection offered by the use of this vaccine lasts for three to five years.

For a further discussion of the various kinds of pneumonia, see chapter 13, this volume.

When You Travel

Several serious contagious diseases prevail in certain parts of the world but not in others. These include cholera, epidemic typhus, yellow fever, typhoid fever, and plague. When a person travels to areas where these diseases occur, it is imperative, of course, that he be protected in advance. Travel agents and public-health officials can give advice on the particular immunization procedures to be followed and for what countries.

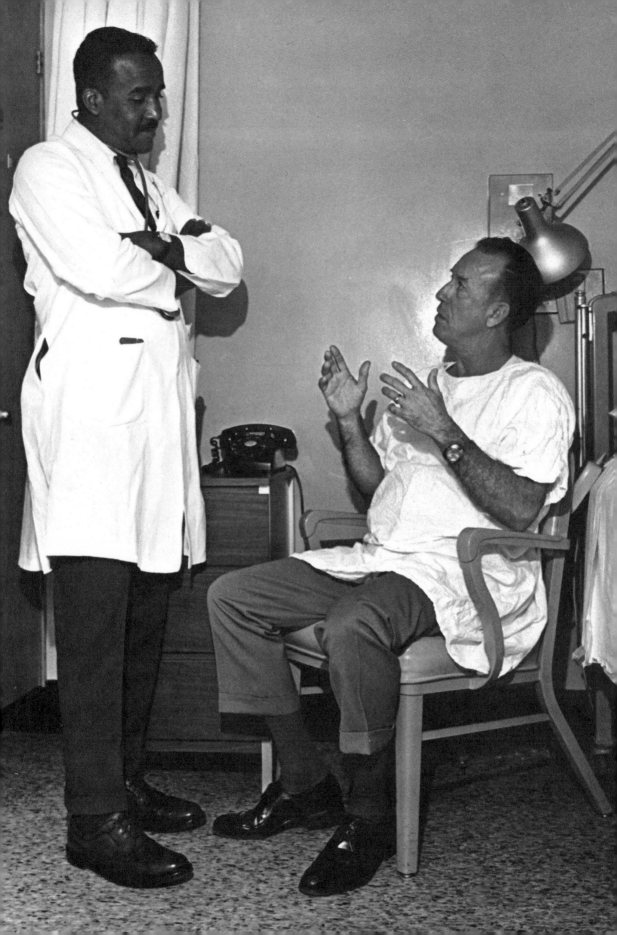

Helps for Diagnosis

The doctor's first consideration, when a person comes for help, is to find out why he came. If it is for a routine examination, then the doctor's task is to make a careful check into the person's health. If the results are good, the doctor reassures the patient. If evidences of something wrong show up, the doctor recommends remedial measures and a proper program for conserving health.

If a patient comes to the doctor because he is already sick, the doctor listens to his "complaints" (the symptoms the patient has noticed), asks questions that may help him to understand these complaints, examines the patient for other possible "signs" of illness, arranges for laboratory tests or diagnostic examinations, and then—once the diagnosis is made—outlines and supervises a program of treatment.

A doctor keeps a record for each of his patients. So when a person comes to the doctor for the first time, certain biographical items must be jotted down as a part of the record. Next comes the list of complaints and symptoms, with a story of how these developed. The doctor asks about previous illnesses, noting any possible relation to the present one. For instance, a child may have a rash resembling that of measles; but if he has already had measles, the doctor looks for some other reason for the rash. Or a patient may have had attacks similar to the present one. This would indicate that the disease is probably a recurrence of a previous ailment.

A doctor's office nurse often does much of the preliminary interviewing and recording. She takes the patient's "history," weighs and measures him, and checks his temperature, pulse rate, breathing rate, and blood pressure.

Temperature is usually taken by inserting the thermometer bulb under the tongue for a minute or two. Sometimes the thermometer is held in the armpit instead, but this method is less reliable. Rectal temperatures are the most reliable, but they are seldom taken except on young children and unconscious patients.

The pulse rate is usually counted by feeling its beat on the thumb side of the wrist. The doctor often counts the pulse rate by listening to the heart through a stethoscope, and the sound and rhythm give other important information at the same time.

Respiration is counted conveniently by observing the rise and fall of the chest wall while a patient lies on his back.

Blood pressure is measured by using a special instrument called a sphygmomanometer ("sphyg" for short). Its essential parts are an inflatable cuff that fits around the arm and a gauge or a

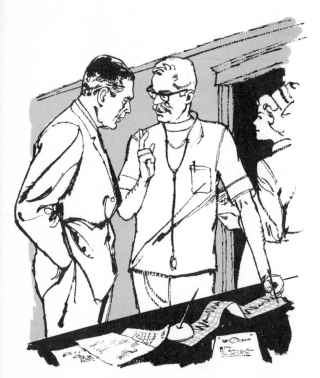

The doctor evaluates his observations and the special tests, makes a diagnosis, and advises the patient accordingly.

mercury-filled glass tube to measure the pressure. The figures used in recording blood pressure, like those used for recording barometric pressure, represent measurements in millimeters of mercury.

Classically, two figures, such as 120/80, are used to record a person's blood pressure. The higher figure (systolic) indicates the pressure within the arteries at the peak of the heart's action. The lower figure (diastolic) represents the lowest level to which the blood pressure drops between heartbeats.

The Physical Examination

In examining a patient, the doctor usually makes a general inspection first. He asks the patient to stand, walk a few steps, then turn around and walk back; that is, if he has not already observed the patient's posture and gait

sufficiently. Years of experience enable doctors to gather valuable information from a glance at patients as they walk into their examining rooms.

The doctor then observes the color and appearance of the patient's skin, especially that of the face. Any flushing or pallor is likely to show on the face more clearly than elsewhere, such as yellowing due to jaundice. Some diseases cause swelling or puffiness of the face, usually most marked below the eyes. Then, with the patient sitting up, the doctor examines his head, noting the hair and scalp.

The eyes are observed for their general appearance: possible cross-eye, "watering," yellowing or redness of the conjunctiva or the whites of the eyes, et cetera. Visible growths or inflammation involving the eyeballs or eyelids are noted. Then the lower lids are turned down and the upper lids turned inside out so that their lining membrane can be observed. The pupils are checked to see if they are round and of the same size. Both the "accommodation" and the light reflexes are checked. The first of these refers to the automatic control by which the eyeballs turn inward and the lenses change shape just enough to keep an object in focus when held close to the eyes. The second (the light reflex) permits the pupils to contract automatically and promptly when a bright light shines into the eyes.

The doctor may use an opthalmoscope to look into the patient's eyes. With this instrument the retina and its blood vessels can be seen. Conditions such as pressure within the eyes or pressure within the skull, as well as such systemic diseases as arteriosclerosis, diabetes, and nephritis are often suggested by what is observed through the opthalmoscope.

In the course of a physical examination a doctor may ask the patient about his eyesight; but when glasses are needed or when the eyes are diseased or have been injured, the patient is usually transferred to an opthalmologist— an eye specialist.

In examining the ears, the doctor first looks for any excess of wax in the external canals. If he finds any, he removes it so as to get a clear view of the eardrum through his otoscope. The appearance of the drum gives valuable information on whether the middle ear (beyond the eardrum) is normal or infected.

Two simple tests can be used to determine the extent of a patient's hearing loss, if any. One is to hold a watch at various distances from each ear to see how well the patient hears the ticking. The other is to hold a vibrating tuning fork near each ear and then to press its stem firmly against the scalp behind each ear and at various places on the head.

By these tests the doctor can discover any impairment in the hearing, in which ear the impairment is greatest, and whether the impairment is due to nerve degeneration or to obstruction along the pathway over which the sound waves must travel from the outer to the inner ear. With this knowledge, he can refer the patient to an otolaryngologist if advisable. This specialist has instruments that can give more complete information, and he can provide special treatment, including surgery.

A superficial examination of the nose will usually disclose any partial obstruction resulting possibly from an accident or fractured bone. Examination of the interior of the nasal cavities is usually aided by the use of a special type of forceps, or speculum, which stretches the nostrils so that light can shine in. A simple inspection will tell whether the septum (partition between the two nasal cavities) is crooked or set nearer one side than the other, whether the turbinates (three membrane-covered folds of bone on the sidewall of each nasal cavity) are normal, and what may be the condition of the lining membrane. The doctor will notice any discharge from the sinuses into the nasal cavities. He knows that any abnormality of the bones of the nose can seriously interfere with breathing. If he discovers such abnormalities, he can refer his patient to a nose and throat specialist for surgery.

The neck is examined externally for swellings or tender areas caused by possible diseased or inflamed lymph nodes. These are useful signs in helping to diagnose certain systemic diseases as well as ailments of the nodes themselves.

The interior of the mouth is easily seen, of course. The doctor usually needs only a flashlight and a "tongue blade" to examine it. The appearance of the lining membrane may give valuable information. The condition of the tongue is often helpful in diagnosis.

The tonsils, too, can be observed. Their size and appearance may indicate need for surgery. They cannot be seen clearly, however, while the back part of the tongue is in its usual position. For this reason the doctor asks the patient to say "ah." Making this sound automatically flattens the back of the tongue. If the flattening by this means is not sufficient, the doctor gently presses the tongue with the wooden blade.

If the larynx, including the vocal cords, is to be examined, the doctor will use a small mirror mounted at an angle at the end of a slender metal handle. When this instrument is held in the back part of the throat and lighted by the rays from a flashlight, the doctor can see into the larynx.

Examination of the shoulders consists of inspection plus observation while the patient moves his arms in various ways. A frequent cause of trouble in the shoulder is bursitis—inflammation of one of the bursae. A bursa is a tissue sac which contains a small amount of fluid and serves to cushion the moving parts of the area. In bursitis, movement of these parts cause intense pain. X-ray studies may help in differentiating bursitis from difficulties within the joints proper.

Methods of Examining the Chest

Examining the chest involves four classic procedures: (1) inspection (observing with the eyes), (2) palpation

41

(feeling with the fingers), (3) percussion (thumping), and (4) auscultation (listening through a stethoscope).

1. *Inspection.* The doctor first looks at the shape of the chest and observes whether it is symmetrical and whether its expansion and contraction during ordinary and forced breathing follow the normal pattern. With a woman patient he observes the breasts for the possibility of a retraction of either nipple or an abnormal dimpling of the skin—either of which is suggestive of an invading type of tumor.

2. *Palpation.* In using palpation the doctor relies on his sense of touch to determine what he can about the breasts (in both men and women) and the condition of the lungs and heart. The breasts are palpated to learn whether they contain a tumor or cyst, and if so, whether it is attached to the skin or to the chest wall (which is typical of cancerous growths).

Normally, when a person speaks in a firm, deep voice, vibrations are set up within the chest which carry through to the overlying skin. Accumulations of fluid in the chest or disease of the lungs change the vibrations in ways the doctor can detect as he places his fingers firmly against the skin.

3. In *percussion* the doctor lays a finger against various parts of the patient's chest and thumps sharply on the back of his finger with the tip of a finger on his other hand. He pays careful attention to the sound thus produced. The chest wall overlying healthy lung tissue gives a characteristic resonance when examined by percussion. Consolidation of the lung tissue or cavity formation or collections of fluid change this characteristic resonance.

The part of the chest wall which overlies the heart gives out a characteristic flat sound when percussion is used. By carefully marking the spots where the general resonance changes to this flat sound, the doctor can determine the borders of the heart. When a

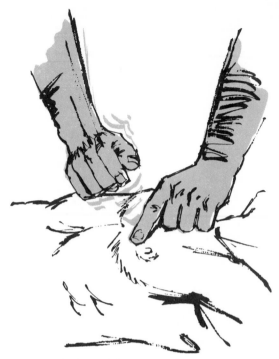

Sounds heard in percussion procedure give the doctor clues regarding the patient's health.

more precise measurement is needed, measurements by X ray are made.

4. The stethoscope used in *auscultation* is a simple instrument consisting of a chest piece or "bell" placed against the patient's skin, a double earpiece which the doctor fits to his own ears, and a pair of rubber tubes which convey the sounds picked up by the bell to the earpiece.

Normal breathing can be heard through the stethoscope as a soft, blowing sound. So when air is not entering some part of the lung, no "breath sounds" are heard over this area. With a stethoscope, the doctor can detect a "cavity" in the lung (except a small one). If a bronchial tube is partly filled with fluid or mucous discharge, it produces characteristic whistling, wheezing, or bubbling sounds. Examining the lung by auscultation is very important in diagnosing and following the progress of tuberculosis of the lungs.

A stethoscope gives information about the heart as well as about the lungs. It provides the easiest way to judge the rate and rhythm of the heart's action. It enables the doctor to hear the closing of its valves and the peculiar sounds ("murmurs") that may occur when a valve is not closing tightly.

The four methods of chest examination—inspection, palpation, percussion, and auscultation—are useful in examining other parts of the body also. Inspection is valuable in examining any visible part of the body and palpation can be used even when the part being examined is not visible. Percussion is of little use except for body parts that are hollow, such as the chest. Auscultation is useful in examining these parts, too, and can be used to check on the blood flow through large arteries, as can palpation if the arteries are near the body's surface.

Examination of the Abdomen

All four methods of physical examination are used in examining the abdomen. Inspection will tell whether it is normal or abnormal in shape, revealing any unusual distention. It will also detect abdominal movements associated with breathing. Palpation is of more use here than with the chest, because the chest is enclosed in a bony cage, which prevents feeling the organs and possible tumor masses by hand pressure.

The liver normally occupies a position high up on the right side of the abdomen, and the spleen a corresponding position on the left. Neither organ extends far enough down to be felt below the lower border of the ribs unless it is enlarged. But in specific diseases these organs may be enlarged, so an attempt to palpate them should be a part of every physical examination. Either or both may be enlarged without becoming abnormally hard, or they may become both larger and harder. The liver becomes nodular in some cases and this may be detected by palpation.

Obviously, if there are tender areas in the abdomen, possibly indicating inflamed, infected, or otherwise diseased organs, these can be located by palpation, especially if pressure is applied. Peptic ulcer, inflamed gallbladder, and appendicitis are often detected in this way. Firm and deep pressure in the central portion of the abdomen may detect the pulsations of the aorta. It is much easier to feel these pulsations in thin people than in the stout. The same is true of the ropelike colon deep in the left side of the abdomen of patients afflicted with chronic colitis or spastic constipation. Tumor growths of any considerable size usually produce masses that can be detected by careful palpation.

By inspection the doctor can detect any excessive fat deposit in the abdominal wall, but by palpation he gets a better idea of the thickness of the fatty layer and can know whether the patient should reduce. A person with a broad frame and heavy bones may not be overweight, even if the height-weight tables indicate that he is. But too thick a fat pad in front of the abdomen shows that the person weighs more than he should, no matter what his actual weight may be. If a fold of this pad, pinched up between the thumb and fingers, is as much as an inch (2.5 cm.) thick, weight reduction is in order. The tendency for this pad to increase in thickness increases with age, and so does the risk of damage to health from overweight.

Some diseases make the muscles of the abdominal wall rigid, a fact particularly true in acute appendicitis and following bites by black widow spiders. Such rigidity can be detected easily by palpation.

A small amount of gas is normally present in the intestine. This accounts for a slight drumlike sound when the abdomen is tested by percussion. The sound is likely to be stronger in some areas than in others, because the gas is not evenly distributed. If more than the usual amount of gas is present, the sound will be louder; but a thick abdominal fat pad will tend to deaden it.

Special Examinations for the Heart

We have mentioned earlier in this chapter how the physical examination and X ray help the doctor to know the size and shape of a patient's heart. By using the stethoscope he can even tell, reasonably well, how the heart's valves are functioning.

The heart is such an important organ and difficulties with it often so threatening to the patient's well-being that physicians and other scientists have with great ingenuity devised precise methods of determining the heart's condition. We will mention several of these: electrocardiography, angiography, cardiac catheterization, and echocardiography.

Electrocardiography. In electrocardiography a sensitive instrument records the minute electric currents associated with the contraction of the heart's muscle tissue. Variations in these tiny currents are recorded by the machine in the form of continuous ink tracings—an electrocardiogram (EKG).

For the patient the making of an elec-trocardiogram is simple. To begin with, several "leads" (small electrodes) are placed in certain key positions on his skin. He lies quietly while the tracing is being made. The currents being measured are so small that he feels nothing unusual while the electrocardiography is in progress.

The electrocardiogram provides important information on the sequence of events that take place in the heart with each heartbeat. Damage to the heart causes alterations in the "normal" electrocardiographic tracing. The electrocardiogram is useful, therefore, in estimating the damage done by a heart attack, and the extent and possible rate of recovery thereafter.

Angiography. The procedure of angiography makes the flowing blood visible by X ray. To accomplish visibility, a harmless chemical substance which casts an X-ray shadow is injected into a blood vessel. Its course, as it moves along with the flowing blood, is recorded by X-ray pictures taken in moving picture fashion. This procedure can be used to study the

A patient undergoing heart catheterization as an aid to the doctor in diagnosing defects.

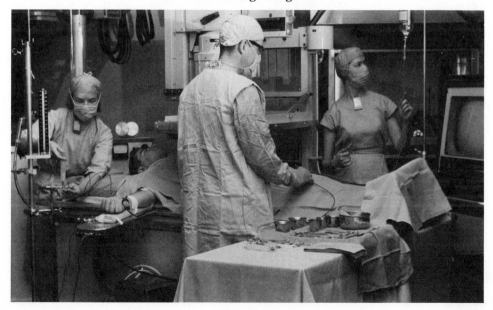

blood vessels in various parts of the body. When used as part of a study of the heart, the course of blood through the heart, whether normal or abnormal, can be followed. Angiography can be used in connection with cardiac catheterization (see the following paragraphs), with the chemical substance being inserted through the catheter when it is within the heart.

Cardiac Catheterization. Cardiac catheterization was mentioned in chapter 17, volume 1, because of its usefulness in connection with the treatment of congenital defects of a child's heart. The procedure is useful in examining the hearts of adults as well. Cardiac catheterization was developed as an adjunct to heart surgery. It is valuable in determining, prior to heart surgery, the exact condition of a deformed heart.

The doctor introduces a very small, metal-tipped tube (catheter) into one of the patient's blood vessels and, using the blood vessel as a guide, he passes it directly into the chambers of the heart. The position of the catheter can be double-checked at all times by observing its metal tip as revealed by X ray.

Abnormal openings in the heart's internal walls are indicated when the catheter wanders beyond normal boundaries. Such openings, when present, permit the blood within the heart to travel by abnormal routes. In so doing, freshly oxygenated blood just returned from the lungs may be mixed with that having a high content of carbon dixoide.

To find out how much of such mixing of the two streams of blood has taken place, small samples of blood are drawn through the catheter from various locations within the heart. Analyses of these samples for their carbon dioxide and oxygen content provide the heart surgeon with information which helps him to plan his surgical procedure.

Echocardiography. Echocardiography is a procedure in which ultra-high-frequency sound waves are directed into the region of a person's heart. As these waves encounter tissues of contrasting densities, they send back echoes which are converted to visual images on an oscilloscope screen in a manner similar to the images on a radar screen. Echocardiography is harmless to the patient and provides information to the examiner comparable to what he would obtain if the heart were being explored at surgery.

Methods of Examining the Brain

From a practical standpoint, the brain is even more inaccessible for examination than the heart. Its action cannot be heard through the stethoscope, and an ordinary X-ray film of the head shows the skull but gives very little information on the condition of the brain. Of course, it is quite easy to know when a person's brain is not functioning correctly: he may not think clearly, the things he talks about may not make sense, or he may even be unconscious. But even these evidences do not give the physician enough data on what is the matter with the brain as an organ. So certain special methods of examining the brain have been developed.

Electroencephalography (EEG). This procedure involves making tracings of the minute electric currents that pass through the brain, just as electrocardiography does with the heart. A specialist in electroencephalography is acquainted with the normal "brain waves" and also understands the meaning of abnormal tracings. The method helps in determining how much the brain has been damaged in case of head injury. When repeated it gives information on what progress the patient is making.

Another use of electroencephalography is in evaluating a patient who has convulsions. It is useful also in determining whether a person's brain contains a tumor or an abscess.

Air Encephalography. In this procedure, air is introduced by needle either into the space (within the meninges) that surrounds the brain or into the ventricles (fluid-filled spaces within the brain). Such air pockets cast a dark shadow by X ray and thus give important hints on the position of the parts of the brain. This technique has largely been replaced by computed tomography (see below).

Angiography. Angiography was mentioned in the previous section, "Special Examinations for the Heart," as one of the methods used in studying the heart. Angiography is also useful in studying the brain. By injecting a chemical substance in liquid form into the blood as it moves toward the brain, an X-ray picture will reveal the pattern of the blood vessels serving the brain. Thus it becomes possible to identify an aneurysm (abnormal enlargement of a vessel) or a tumor composed principally of blood vessels. The pattern of blood vessels thus revealed may also show a shift of position when one part of the brain is enlarged at the expense of other parts.

Computed Tomography. A recent and very remarkable aid to diagnosis is

Simply defined, tomography is a technique of diagnosis that uses X-ray photographs.

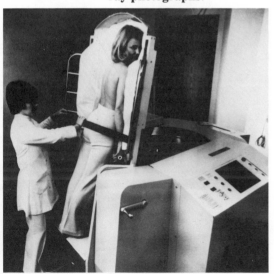

computed tomography (CT), also known as computerized axial tomography (CAT Scanning). Computed tomography gives a remarkable display in two dimensions of structures located within the human body. It is applicable to various parts of the body, but we mention it here because of its great advantage in picturing the structures inside the skull.

The basic equipment for computed tomography consists of a sophisticated X-ray installation plus an associated computer. X rays are passed in various directions through the part of the body being studied, and the thousands of fragments of information thus revealed are organized by the computer, through a series of complex equations, into an image which appears on the screen of an oscilloscope or on a television monitor. This image is then photographed for permanent record. The image thus produced resembles a drawing of the various structures within the body which occur in the particular spatial plane being studied. Many community hospitals now have this equipment, and mobile units are also available.

Endoscopy

Endoscopy is a procedure in which various interior parts of the body are viewed through a slender, highly sophisticated instrument introduced through one of the normal body openings or through a small incision. The instrument used (an endoscope) is essentially a tubular structure which contains telescopic lenses and is associated with a bundle of fiberglass threads which carry light to the end of the instrument. Photographs (even moving pictures) can be taken of what the examiner observes. Tiny samples of tissue can be obtained through the instrument. Small hemorrhages can be controlled by a small cautery device at the end of the instrument. Small areas of tissue can be destroyed, as in the use of the endoscope for performing tubal division (for sterilization) in female patients.

Physicians especially trained in the

YOU AND YOUR HEALTH

use of the endoscope are available in most of the larger medical centers. Endoscopic examinations are useful for exploring the larynx, the esophagus, the stomach, the air passages and lungs, and (through a small abdominal incision) the various organs within the abdominal cavity. Special endoscopic examinations are sometimes made at the time of surgery as in exploring the interior of the kidney or in examining the ducts associated with the liver and gallbladder.

Lives Are Saved by Good Diagnosis

It is quite clear from the information contained in this chapter that medical science has made great advances in the early detection of disease as it affects various parts of the body. Early detection has saved thousands of lives by making it possible to treat disease while still in its early stages.

But in order for you, as the reader of this book, to have the advantages of early detection and lifesaving treatment, you need to cooperate with your family physician whenever you notice evidences that your body is not functioning normally. The various signs and symptoms of disease are listed and briefly discussed in chapter 6, volume 2, and chapter 7, volume 3. By consulting these chapters, you will be informed on the possible meaning of symptoms when they appear.

Do not allow yourself to resort to deceptive reasoning. Some people say, "What I don't know won't hurt me. I do not want to see a doctor because I am afraid of what he might tell me." The Good Book tells us that such a course is unwise. It says, "A prudent man foreseeth the evil, and hideth himself; but the simple pass on, and are punished." Proverbs 27:12.

Why Disease?

Every disease has its cause. As the Scripture says, "The curse causeless shall not come." Only as we understand what causes a disease can we intelligently prevent or treat it.

Many patients who consult a doctor are not so concerned with the cause of their disease. Usually what they want is quick relief. They suffer from a headache or a bad cough, or feel weak and dizzy, and want a remedy. But the doctor must look beyond the symptoms to the cause.

Germs

Ask any high school student what causes disease, and he will doubtless answer, "Germs." But this answer represents a comparatively modern concept. Only during the latter part of the nineteenth century did medical scientists first recognize the important part germs play in infectious diseases.

Parasites and germs are living organisms, many of them belonging to the vegetable kingdom (fungi and their spores). Bacteria are so small that they can be seen only through the microscope. It would take, depending on their size, approximately 8000 to 25,000 placed end to end to make a line an inch long.

Viruses, which are much smaller, have also been found to cause disease. One must use an electron microscope to see them.

About the turn of the century scientists began to catalog germs and the respective diseases caused by them. They learned that when a certain kind of germ invades the body's tissues, a definite disease results. This observation led them to assume that to prevent disease one had only to keep germs from entering the human body. This concept is good as far as it goes.

Some disease-producing germs are breathed into the body—for instance, those carried by the spray of tiny droplets thrown into the air by a cough or sneeze. Some are carried by dust particles in the air—house or street dust.

Then there are the germs of such diseases as malaria, yellow fever, and dengue injected by mosquitoes or other insects. Germs which cause bubonic plague are carried from rat to man by the bite of fleas. The germs of African sleeping sickness are carried by the tsetse fly. The germs of typhus fever are carried by body lice or fleas, and those of relapsing fever and Rocky Mountain spotted fever by ticks.

Other germs are carried by contaminated ice and water and by foods such as salads and milk. The greatest source of danger here is from domestic water supplies contaminated by human excreta. Flies, rats, mice, or unclean hands may carry disease-producing germs and deposit them where they contaminate milk or other food materials. By this means typhoid fever, dysentery, and other gastrointestinal infections are often spread.

The modern science of sanitation is built around a knowledge of the role germs play in producing disease. This science consists essentially of controlling the growth and transmission of germs and of guarding against invasion.

Conditions Under Which Germs Thrive. All germs must have moisture in order to live and multiply. Most of

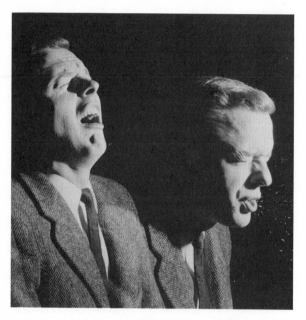

By a cough or sneeze a sick person discharges disease-producing germs into the air around him.

them need air also, but a few can grow without it. The germ which causes tetanus (lockjaw) grows only in the absence of air.

Most germs which produce disease in humans thrive best in about the same temperature as that of the human body (98.6° F. or 37° C.). Very few germs grow at temperatures below 50° F. (10° C.). This fact makes refrigeration of food an effective means of preventing disease. As long as food is kept at low temperatures, any germs it may contain cannot multiply. But some germs remain alive for long periods of time even below the freezing point of water.

On the other end of the scale, the growth of germs is hindered by temperatures above about 115° F. (46° C.). Most germs are killed above 145° F. (63° C.) when these temperatures are maintained for as long as half an hour. On this basis surgical dressings and other such materials are made "sterile" (free from germs) by the use of heat.

Most germs thrive in darkness better than in light. Sunlight is particularly effective in destroying germs.

Certain germs can stop growing and remain dormant for long periods of time, even in spite of dryness and unfavorable temperatures. Then when conditions become favorable again, such germs are revitalized. These dormant forms are called spores.

Chemical Means of Controlling Germs. A great deal of progress has been made in the control of disease-producing germs by the use of chemical disinfectants. Time-honored disinfectants include iodine, phenol solution, potassium permanganate, silver nitrate, and chlorine; but newer and more practical ones are constantly being made available. Care must be exercised in using disinfectants, for almost all are poisonous when taken into the body.

Spores (the dormant form of germs) are difficult to kill. For them it is necessary to use strong disinfectants or high temperatures.

How Germs Harm the Body. Some germs, such as the one that causes tuberculosis, actually destroy certain body tissues. Others produce toxins (poisons) that circulate in the blood and damage organs or tissues apart from those where the germs originate. The diphtheria germ, for example, multiplies best in the tissues of the pharynx (throat), but its toxin can damage heart and nerves. The germs of scarlet fever also grow in the pharynx, but the toxins they produce may damage the kidneys.

The control of germs, important as it is, does not constitute the only means of preventing disease. The human body has ways of altering its resistance to the invasion of germs. Therefore it is important to (1) protect the body, as far as possible, from invasion by germs, and (2) maintain such a high level of general health that the body will be able to combat the germs that may enter.

Some germs, such as diphtheria, are so powerful that once they enter the body they will produce serious illness in spite of the body's defenses. Immunization must be used to combat them.

Heredity

Long before men knew the relationship between germs and disease, they observed that certain maladies such as diabetes and certain forms of anemia tend to run in families. Faulty heredity, however, is usually not the sole cause of a disease that appears to run in a family. Family members often have the same faulty habits. Diet, lack of sanitation, and emotional tensions may render the members more susceptible to illness.

Sex difference also constitutes a factor in the incidence of certain diseases. Men more commonly than women are victims of coronary heart disease, of diseases of the lungs, of liver disease, and of tuberculosis. Women, on the other hand, suffer more frequently from diseases of the thyroid. Even after allowing for the influence of a man's way of life in contrast with a woman's we must still recognize that a man's body is peculiarly more susceptible to certain diseases.

Some persons are inherently more resistant to disease. For example, a heavy smoker runs a much greater risk of contracting cancer than a nonsmoker. Even so, certain smokers do not contract lung cancer. They doubtless inherited such vitality of tissue that they can tolerate the irritating effects of tobacco smoke. Of course, even a person with such natural resistance may still suffer in other ways.

Vaccinia virus particles, or cowpox (here magnified 70,000 times by electron microscope) are used in vaccinations against smallpox.

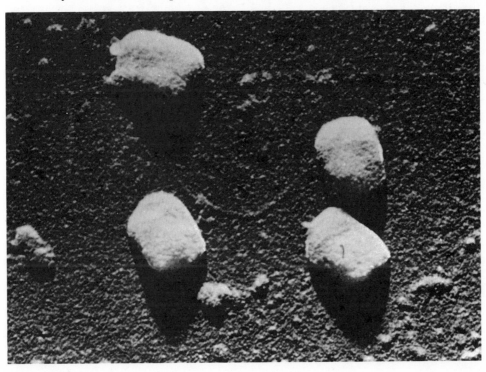

We still cannot order a person's heredity. Everyone must be reconciled to whatever handicaps or assets he may inherit. Especially encouraging then is the fact that heredity is only one of several factors affecting health. Even the person with poor heredity may, by following a plan of healthful living, rise above his inherited weakness. However, the person with a favorable heredity may squander his advantage through careless habits and fall a prey to disease.

Most Diseases Have Multiple Causes

When disease-producing germs were still being discovered and classified, it was easy to assume that a given disease was the direct result of a particular kind of germ. It was then supposed that if a person could remain free from contact with disease-producing germs, he would remain healthy. But if he encountered the germs that produce a given disease, he would fall victim to that disease.

It is now understood, however, that the mere presence of germs in the human body does not always produce disease. Consider tuberculosis for example. The germ *Mycobacterium tuberculosis* is the active agent in causing this illness. This germ is quite widely distributed, however, and even healthy individuals have had many exposures to it. Admittedly, without exposure to the germ, one would not contract tuberculosis. But even when exposed, many people do not contract the disease because of the inhibiting factors of inherent vitality and tissue resistance.

Present evidence indicates that many children, before they reach adulthood, have had contact with *Mycobacterium tuberculosis*. But only a few, proportionately, contract the disease. The factors of personal vitality and tissue resistance figure more prominently in determining whether a person will become ill with tuberculosis than does the factor of exposure to the germ.

Take pneumonia as another example. Any one of several germs may be involved in causing this disease. The most common is pneumococcus *(Streptococcus pneumoniae)*. But simple contact with this germ does not determine that a person will inevitably become sick with pneumonia. This germ is present in the mouth cavities of many healthy individuals. The factors that tend to prevent the development of pneumonia may vary, but in one way or another they make the individual's tissues less vulnerable to the germ or germs which cause pneumonia.

On the other hand, weakening factors contributing to pneumonia could be loss of sleep, fatigue from overwork, undue exposure to cold, or acute alcohol abuse. In addition, possibly a background of unfavorable experiences such as anxiety and worry may have depleted the individual's nervous reserves, thus weakening the brain's usual influence over the body tissues and lessening their ability to function efficiently.

Even in the case of a broken leg a combination of factors may be the cause. It is proverbial among skiers that broken legs occur near the end of the day or, at least, when the persons involved have become weary and careless. Skiers go so far as to predict that a person who says, "I am going down the hill just this once more," is the one most likely to have an accident. Weariness, then, shows up as an important contributing factor to misfortune.

Accidents on the highways typically occur when the drivers concerned are overweary, emotionally upset, or mentally beclouded by the use of alcohol or drugs.

Illnesses occur in "clusters" during a person's lifetime. Extensive studies have been made on the relationship of environmental factors to the incidence of disease, and it has been demonstrated that even unrelated illnesses tend to group themselves in various periods of life. A person may be susceptible to several kinds of illness for a period of several months or years. Then a period of relative freedom from illness can follow, only to be succeeded by another "cluster." On closer study, it may become apparent that these periods of illness came at times when the person was making a poor sociologic adjustment to life. Perhaps he was uncertain over the outcome of a financial undertaking. Maybe tensions within the home robbed him of the vital force necessary to maintain his resistance to disease. Perhaps he was insecure during a period of education or training for future responsibilities. As Lord Lytton once remarked, "Half our diseases come from neglect of the body or overwork of the brain."

Habits of Life

Nutrition. The body's tissues are built from constituents in the diet, and the continued activities of these tissues depend on a constant supply of the food elements they need for energy and repairs. If these elements are adequate both in quality and variety, then the body tissues will be able to carry on their functions properly. But if some are lacking, the body tissues suffer accordingly.

Carefully controlled animal experiments have demonstrated that the outcome of a given infection depends not only on the nature of the germs but also on the quality of the diet—whether or not it promotes the development of tissue resistance to infection. More is said in chapter 53, volume 1, about the means of ensuring an adequate diet.

Excessive intake of food has as detrimental an effect on the state of health as does an inadequate diet. Too great an intake promotes excess body weight; and this, in turn, lays the foundation for diseases of the heart and blood vessels.

A diet which includes too great a proportion of foods with a high content of fats (particularly saturated fats) lays the foundation for degenerative diseases.

Living Conditions. Climate, of course, has its influence on health. Tropical climates pose a particular health hazard. Colder climates introduce elements of fatigue and exposure, poor ventilation, and crowded housing.

Living conditions in the home also have a definite influence on health. The ideal home provides adequate protection from extremes of temperature and also is designed for cleanliness and sanitation. A cheerful atmosphere promotes contentment and optimism, both favorable to good health.

Personal Habits. The laws of health, like the laws of moral conduct, imply a

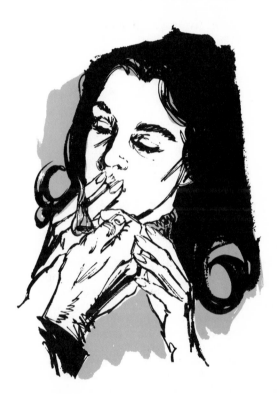

Irritation produced by the use of cigarettes plays a causative role in the development of lung cancer.

promise for obedience as well as a penalty for disobedience. An individual may choose whether he will live in harmony with the principles which favor good health or disregard them and pay the penalty in the form of increased susceptibility to disease. Even a person handicapped by inherited susceptibility to disease may, by compliance with the laws of healthful living, improve his general resistance to illness.

Adequate physical exercise, adequate sleep, recreation in the out-of-doors, regular meals with nothing between, an attitude of optimism—all of these tend to conserve vitality and improve resistance to disease.

Personal habits which deplete one's store of vitality and increase the risk of disease include excesses in eating, irregular hours of sleeping, the use of tobacco and alcohol, unnecessary recourse to drugs, and the use of such stimulants as coffee, tea, and cola drinks.

Attitudes of Mind

A person's thoughts and emotions, when conflicting or out of perspective, interfere with his state of health. We speak here of the mind-body relationship. The branch of medicine which deals with illnesses caused by unhappy thoughts and distorted emotions is called psychosomatic medicine, and such illnesses are called psychosomatic illnesses, psychogenic illnesses, or functional illnesses.

Every person has his limit of tolerance when it comes to distressing thoughts and antagonistic emotions. Some persons have a wide margin of safety in these matters, and others break more easily when under stress. The forms of illness that can result from unresolved stresses vary from person to person. When some persons "break" under stress they develop some form of mental illness. But in the majority of cases, breaking under stress causes symptoms relating to the organs of the body.

Psychological factors such as worry, emotional conflict, and a sense of guilt predispose to many of the illnesses in which the heart, the blood vessels, the digestive organs, and the endocrine organs are affected. At least half of the common illnesses from which persons suffer are caused or at least aggravated by unhappy thoughts and uncontrolled emotions.

It is the brain and the nerves which connect it to all parts of the body that have the controlling influence over the manner in which the organs function. A great deal of this control is carried on without conscious thought.

Take the automobile driver who narrowly escapes a collision at an intersection. His conscious thoughts are centered on traffic rules, control of his car, and resentment of the other driver. In the meantime, however, the organs of

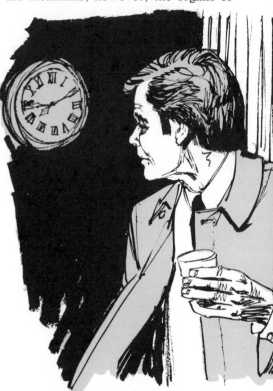

Nervous tension resulting from late hours and overwork weaken vitality and contribute to disease.

his body change their functions. His breathing speeds up. His heart beats faster. His blood pressure rises. His digestive organs discontinue their activity temporarily. More blood sugar is released into the blood, and various other changes make him ready for intense activity, both physical and mental.

With prolonged psychological tensions, the reaction of the organs is about the same as when an emergency arises, except that the readiness for intense activity continues on and on. The body's organs and tissues do not tolerate well this prolonged emergency status, and there finally comes a breakdown in certain organs and tissues.

Many early cases of high blood pressure are still in the "reversible phase," meaning that the blood pressure will return to normal if and when the emotional tension is eliminated. When the response to unwholesome emotions is sustained long enough, however, certain changes occur by which the disturbed functions become chronic. In the "reversible phase" of such an illness we speak of "functional disease." After there has been tissue change, we speak of an "irreversible" situation in which "organic disease" has developed.

An "upset" of the digestive organs can develop into peptic ulcer. Temporary changes in the body's chemistry can predispose to arteriosclerosis. Latent diabetes or asthma or arthritis can be aggravated by psychological tensions.

The Wear-out Diseases

Time has its effect on the tissues of the human body. The average life-span is about 70 years. Some live longer and some not so long. As birthdays come and go, one's tissues become less able to resist disease. Diseases like cancer are therefore more frequent in later life. Some forms of arthritis, some kinds of kidney disease, and many diseases affecting the nervous system are the simple result of the inability of the functioning cells to longer perform their usual activities. Hardening of the arteries (arteriosclerosis), with its dire consequences of heart attack, stroke, and aneurysm, is due to degenerative changes in the walls of the blood vessels.

Inheritance plays a part in determining how fast a person's tissues deteriorate. So also does one's life-style. One who lives conservatively and with due consideration to the laws of health will live longer than another person who, with a comparable heredity, dissipates

his vital forces by careless living and personal indulgence.

What It Means

Sickness is not something that arbitrarily overtakes a person, descending "out of a clear sky" to bring invalidism here and sudden death there. True, some of the causes of disease, such as heredity, are beyond the individual's

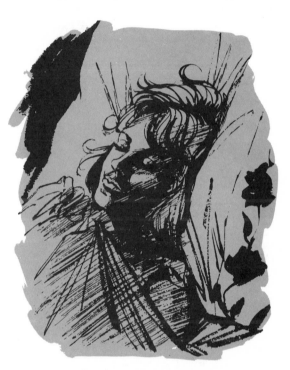

Sleep promotes health, thus increasing resistance to disease.

control. But many illnesses can be prevented—now that we understand better the causes of disease.

The first benefit of this discussion on the causes of disease is to encourage you, the reader, to follow such a life-style as will enable you to avoid as many of the causes as possible and thus prolong your health and usefulness.

The second value is to impress the truth that in order to treat a disease intelligently and effectively, attention must be focused on its fundamental cause. When a person suffers from a

63

disease caused by a dietary deficiency, he accomplishes nothing worthwhile by taking pain relievers or sedative pills. He must discover and correct the cause. And this is where a physician comes into the picture. Any drugstore salesman can suggest medicines that will relieve a person's pain or otherwise make him less aware of his suffering. But only a physician trained in discovering the actual causes of illness can devise and direct a treatment program that will cure by removing the cause.

SECTION **II**

The Body's Defenses; Symptoms

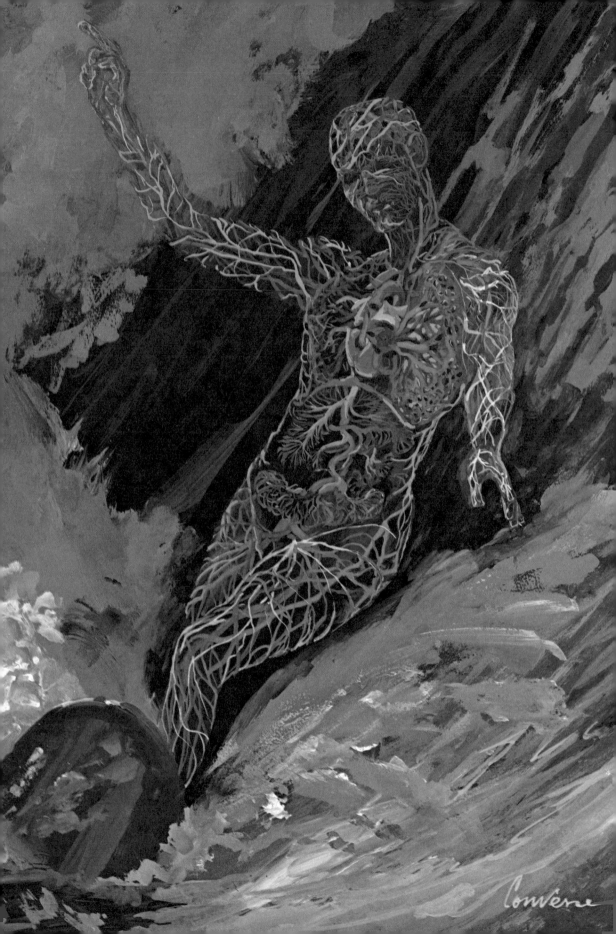

The Marvelous Body and Its Defenses

In this chapter we take an overall look at the human body, noting its plan of structure and the ways in which its various parts coordinate their functions. In particular we will study the marvelous ways in which the body protects itself automatically from the insults of a sometimes hostile environment.

The human body is the masterpiece of God's creation. Plants and animals are remarkably endowed with a capacity for growth, for reproduction, and for carrying on their usual functions and activities; but in creating man, God endowed him with some of His own characteristics. We read in the Scriptures, "God said, Let us make man in our image, after our likeness. . . . So God created man in his own image, in the image of God created he him; male and female created he them." Genesis 1:26, 27.

Man's superior characteristics pertain especially to his personality, to his intellect, and to his ability to choose and to act on the choices made. Man possesses a degree of awareness and consciousness far above that of domestic animals. Through his eyes, his ears, and his other sense organs he perceives all the goings-on around him. So does a horse or a dog. But man can relate his consciousness of the immediate to what has happened in the past and can project it also into the future. He can thus plan ahead and act accordingly.

Man can discipline his imagination, making it a creative force, thus enabling him to produce works of art, to construct bridges and buildings, and to engage in speculative enterprises. He can love and hate; but, more importantly, he can control and adapt his emotions, not allowing them to master him but making them his servants. Man comprehends moral values and thus becomes a responsible individual, properly accountable for his personal philosophy and for what he does to help or hinder other people.

The organs in the body of a human being roughly resemble those in higher animals. True, some differences in structure stand out, but the essential difference is the organization of his brain and the manner in which his brain contributes to his human individuality.

From a physiological standpoint the brain is just another organ, its need for oxygen and food materials supplied by the same blood that flows to other organs. But the human body is organized so that the brain is the master organ. In addition to its providing the basis for individuality, personality, and intellectual interests, the brain influences the function of all the other organs. The other organs serve the brain in one way or another, and the brain serves the other organs. In the present chapter, therefore, we consider the structure and the organization of the entire human body.

The Body's Plan of Organization

Just as a brick house is composed of many bricks, so the body is composed of many structural units called cells. In a brick house, all the bricks are alike. But in the human body the many kinds of cells differ greatly, each kind having its own duty to perform and each located in such a way that it can perform its duty in the best manner.

As an aid to understanding how the body is organized and how different kinds of cells cooperate, let us consider a modern city, with its different kinds of buildings—residences, offices, stores, and factories. The buildings may be compared to the cells in the body. There are various kinds of cells, and it takes the entire number of cells, put together properly, to make up the human body.

In residential areas of a city the houses often look very much alike. We speak of these areas as neighborhoods. So in the human body, the cells in certain places all look alike, and these groups of similar cells we call tissues.

In a large city many districts carry individual names, such as The Bronx or The Rose City District or Chinatown. Each district is composed of many

A typical city like San Francisco illustrates how the human body functions in a coordinated manner.

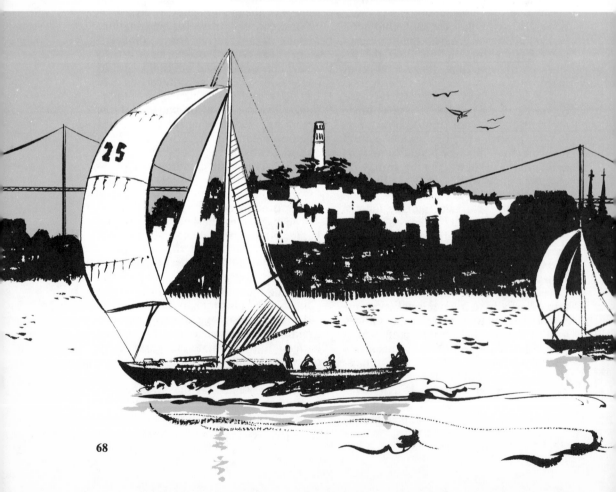

neighborhoods with their look-alike residences, along with some stores and, perhaps, some warehouses and factories. Similarly, in the body we have combinations of tissues that make up organs such as the liver, the stomach, or the spleen. In an organ, several kinds of tissues contribute to the general work of that organ. We will have more to say about cells, tissues, and organs a little later in the chapter.

One of the very important facilities of a city is its water supply and the provision for distributing the water to all parts of the city. In like manner, water is very important to the human body. A little more than half of the adult human body consists of fluid, and water is the solvent in all of the body's fluids. Water is provided through the various fluids taken through the mouth. The body retains what it needs and eliminates the excess through the kidneys and bladder.

Another important city service is food supply. With buildings so close together in the city, crops cannot be raised. Food must therefore be brought in from outside. Likewise, the human body requires a continuous supply of food, which serves as fuel for the body's activities. A person's hunger requires him to take food about three times a day.

The mere bringing of food into a city and into its markets does not satisfy the hunger of the residents. Therefore, in every city we find restaurants where food is made ready to eat. In a similar way, certain organs of the body, particularly the stomach and the intestines, are adapted to the assimilation of food taken through the mouth. These digestive organs prepare the food by chemical processes to be carried by the blood to all parts of the body, where it serves as fuel in each of the body's cells.

Every city has its own disposal system by which trash and the various waste products are carried out of the city and destroyed. In the human body the kidneys and bladder, along with the colon and rectum, constitute the disposal system—the organs of elimination.

Every city must have a transportation system. Taxicabs, busses, trucks, and private cars serve all communities within the city limits. So likewise in the human body, the various organs must be interconnected with supply lines and waste disposal systems. This service is provided very efficiently by the continuous circulation of blood throughout the body. The heart pumps the blood through the lungs, where it receives its quota of oxygen. The heart then pumps this oxygen-laden blood to all other parts of the body. En route the blood receives the nutrient materials provided by the organs of digestion and processed by the liver. As it passes through the outlying tissues, the blood releases its supply of oxygen and food materials in exchange for the carbon dioxide and other waste materials which the cells produce.

Every modern city has its systems of communication by telephone, radio, TV, and messenger service. So in the body a system of communication operates through the nerves and the hormones produced by the endocrine organs, signaling each organ regarding the timing of its activities. Also the sensory nerves make the individual aware of what is happening in the various parts of the body, not only when things operate normally but when injury or disease occurs.

A city maintains a security system for protection against crime, disaster, and tragedy. It has a police force, an organization for fire protection, and persons on duty trained to meet emergencies. Similarly, the human body has defense systems to combat injury, infection, and unfavorable circumstances in the environment. These are described in the latter part of this chapter.

A city has hospitals with emergency rooms and intensive-care units, as well as operatories and quarters for recovery from illness. In a comparable way, the human body possesses marvelous capacities for healing of wounds and recovery from illness. We often think of the doctor and the nurse as the persons responsible for the patient's recovery. Actually, all the doctor and the nurse can do is to facilitate the body's own provisions for healing.

Many cities have manufacturing plants within their boundaries. These produce valuable commodities, many of which are used by persons who live in the city. The human body also is engaged in manufacturing. There are glands located here and there in the body which produce their particular kinds of secretions and hormones. These aid in the activities of the body by promoting chemical processes and by helping to control the body's activities.

In a city institutions engaged in business exert control over activities within the city and outside as well. In a comparable way, large portions of the human body are devoted to activity both within and without. The muscles move various parts of the body and make is possible also for the body to relate itself properly to what takes place outside.

Within a city institutions of learning impart knowledge and develop skills. The body's education department is the brain, which makes it possible for the

A car is more than a collection of parts; so also is a man, the human body being essentially a community of cells.

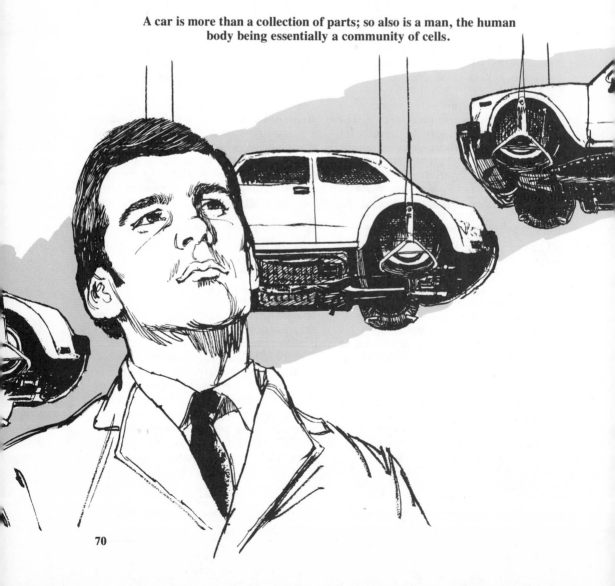

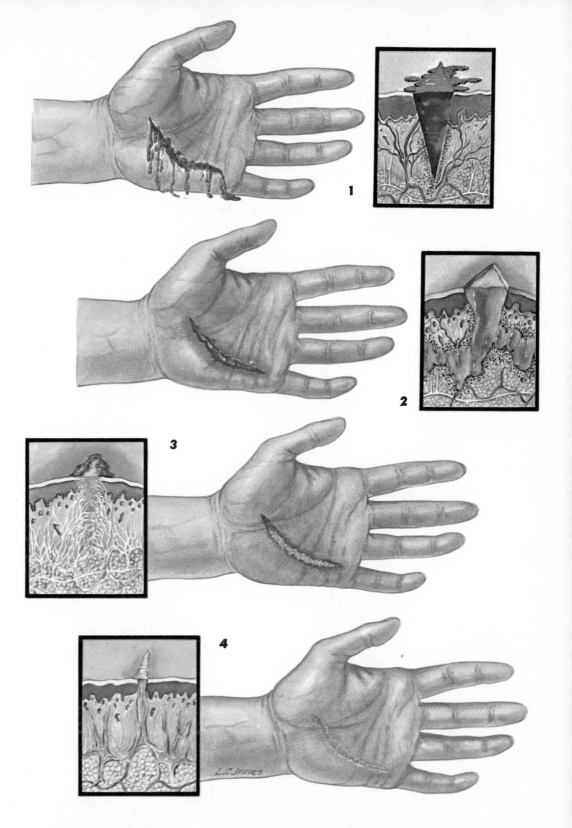

The healing process: 1. A bleeding wound extends deep into skin.
2. Police cells enter and engulf germs and remove tissue debris.
3. New connective tissue repairs wound. 4. New tissue forms scar.

hospital to have new ones put in. "But I am worried," he admits, "because the tissues at the margin of the incision are just about worn out and it's hard for the surgeon to find a place to put new stitches."

"A preposterous story," you say.

And so it is, for a person whose tissues do not heal would soon bleed to death or die of infection. But before we dismiss the illustration, let us ponder long enough to admit that this fictitious man represents you or me except for the miracle of healing.

Again the hypothetical case breaks down, for if human tissues were not capable of self-healing, all mankind would be afflicted and there would be no doctors or nurses able to stitch the lacerations or splint the broken bones of their fellow sufferers.

A surgeon readily admits that his skill is inadequate to bring about the rehabilitation of someone injured. His best efforts would accomplish nothing were it not that healing processes begin where the surgeon leaves off. He sets the stage; the inherent capacity of tissue to accomplish repair produces the final results.

Common Problems and Symptoms

How the Body Says, "I Am Sick"

When something goes wrong with the family car we know it, because the car makes a peculiar noise or it won't start or some of the equipment doesn't operate normally or there is an unusual "feel" about it when it moves. Similarly, the human body, when overtaken by illness, often reveals telltale evidences of something wrong.

How to Use This Chapter

It is not intended that this chapter be read page by page, like a story. Use it as a reference; look up the item that concerns you at the moment. For your convenience, the items are listed in alphabetical order. And don't forget to use the General Index to help you find the information you desire.

Not all of the entries in this chapter are the names of symptoms. Some are the names of parts of the body, with subheadings under each telling what may be troublesome about that part. If you have difficulty in finding a listing that seems to fit the symptom momentarily of concern to you, think of some other word that could apply to this symptom or the same part of the body. Perhaps the list will contain this other word.

For the most part, the names of *diseases* are not listed here. This chapter deals with *symptoms*. So if you want to find out about hay fever, you will find no such listing in this chapter. The General Index at the back of the volume lists *"Hay Fever"* with page numbers indicating where discussions of hay fever are located. But in the present chapter you will find an entry for *"Sneezing,"* with mention that sneezing is one of the prominent symptoms of hay fever.

Some conditions are so troublesome that they deserve care immediately—they constitute an emergency. Emergencies and their remedies are considered in chapter 23, "First Aid for Emergencies," volume 3.

When in doubt on where to find a particular item, consult the General Index at the back of any one of the three volumes.

The List of Symptoms

(Noted: Cross references in this list refer to items in this same chapter unless otherwise stated.)

ABDOMEN, SYMPTOMS
   A. *Cramps in the Abdomen.* See *Cramps: Abdominal Cramps.*

B. *Distension of the Abdomen.* This may be caused by the presence of either gas or fluid in the abdomen. Without realizing it, some people develop the habit of swallowing air. Quantities of air are commonly produced within the stomach and intestine as a result of the fermentation of food in the process of digestion. Usually and normally such accumulated gas is released either by belching or by the passing of flatus through the rectum. This kind of distension we call flatulence.

Certain foods are especially prone to cause flatulence. The list includes cabbage, celery, cucumbers, onions, pears, peppers, beans, and broccoli. Carbonated or alcoholic drinks may have the same effect. Nervousness, anxiety, and the chewing of gum tend to promote air swallowing. Some cases of flatulence are caused by the inherent deficiency of the enzyme lactase, necessary for the digestion and assimilation of milk.

Distension because of gas within the stomach and intestines may also occur in such illnesses as gastritis, intestinal obstruction, celiac disease, sprue, and the serious condition of ileus.

Abdominal distension because of the accumulation of fluid in the peritoneal cavity (ascites) may occur as a complication of such diseases as congestive heart failure, glomerulonephritis, cirrhosis of the liver, and abdominal or thoracic cancer.

C. *Masses in the Abdomen.* Some masses that may be felt within the abdomen are either normal or relatively harmless. In pregnancy, the uterus can be felt in the lower middle area. It increases in size and extends upward as the pregnancy progresses. A bladder very full of urine may be felt as a rather soft mass just above the pubic bone. In a case of constipation in a thin person, firm masses of fecal material may be felt, usually on the left side.

In the course of performing a physical examination, the physician may detect enlargements of the liver, of the spleen, or of the kidneys. There are many possible causes for such enlarge-

Some foods tend to cause flatulence.

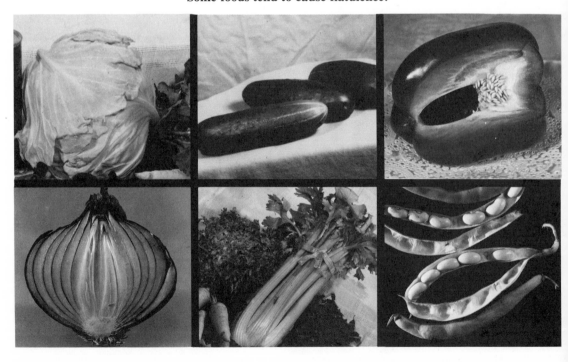

ments, and the physician will take into account the patient's other symptoms and the laboratory findings as he evaluates such enlargements. Cancer of the colon often produces an enlargement that can be detected by the physician. In the female, tumors, cysts, and abscesses associated with the reproductive organs can sometimes be felt through the lower abdominal wall.

D. *Rigidity of the Abdomen.* When the tissues inside the abdomen become inflamed, severe pain develops, together with a protective reflex by which the muscles of the abdominal wall (particularly those overlying the inflamed area) become contracted. This muscle contraction we call rigidity. This condition occurs in acute appendicitis (more apparent on the right side); in perforated peptic ulcer; sometimes in acute inflammation of the gallbladder; in peritonitis from any cause; when there has been bleeding within the abdomen; and, strangely, in cases of bite by black widow spider.

E. *Tenderness in the Abdomen.* In acute abdominal inflammations the abdominal wall overlying the inflamed area becomes sensitive, reinforcing, as it were, the protection afforded by the rigidity of the muscle mentioned in the previous paragraph. Thus, the patient "guards" the internal area of inflammation.

APPETITE

A. *Loss of Appetite.* This problem may be caused by emotional tensions, by reaction to unappetizing food, by unfavorable circumstances at mealtime, as a side effect of certain drugs, or by the use of tobacco. It is also one of the first symptoms to appear in many illnesses and is an important reason for the loss of weight in many chronic, wasting diseases. It is particularly noticeable in cancer of the stomach and in infectious hepatitis.

B. *Increase in Appetite.* Many persons, unhappy with their lot in life, find satisfaction in eating, with the result that they become obese. In such cases the control of appetite consists of solving the basic personality problem. Some persons, during periods of strenuous physical activity or during pregnancy, become accustomed to eating heartily. Then, when their circumstances change, their habit continues on. A voracious appetite commonly occurs in cases in which the thyroid gland is overactive (hyperthyroidism). The thyroid gland controls the rate of the body's metabolism; and when the metabolism is elevated, the individual craves more food in order to provide the extra "fuel" for the accelerated activities of his tissues. In certain tumors of the pancreas an excess of insulin is produced; thus the appetite is increased so as to provide the extra food material now in demand. In tapeworm infestation the appetite may be increased.

BLEEDING (HEMORRHAGE)

A. *Effects of Blood Loss.* Blood accounts for 7 to 9 percent of the body's weight. This means that an adult human body usually contains five or six quarts (approximately the same number of liters) of blood. A person can be suddenly deprived of a pint (half liter) of blood with little adverse effect; but when greater amounts are lost, symptoms develop—the greater the amount, the more serious the symptoms. With severe sudden losses, symptoms will include pallor, thirst, cold sweat, buzzing in the ears, dizziness, blurred vision, restlessness, a rapid and faint pulse, rapid and shallow breathing, and eventual unconsciousness. Such symptoms develop regardless of whether the blood escapes from an external wound or by an internal hemorrhage into one of the body cavities. (*Any severe loss of blood, either apparent or suspected, justifies the immediate attention of a physician.*) For the methods of first aid for loss of blood, see chapter 23 under "Bleeding," volume 3.

B. *Injury, Bleeding as a Result.*

1. Bleeding from the Site of Injury. Blood loss from a crushing injury is not as rapid as from one resulting in a severed artery. In a sharply severed ar-

tery, the blood escapes in spurts, one spurt with each heartbeat. Such severe loss of blood must be controlled promptly by firm pressure directed into the wound.

2. Internal Bleeding from Injury. Internal bleeding may occur whenever a person has received a hard blow, has fallen, has been thrown from a horse or moving vehicle, or has suffered a crushing injury. The development of the symptoms mentioned in "A" above, even though no bleeding is apparent, makes it very urgent to consult a physician.

C. *Bladder, Bleeding From.* Blood appearing in the urine (hematuria) may come from either the bladder or the kidneys. The common causes are cancer, kidney stones, acute nephritis, and infections causing hemorrhagic cystitis.

D. *Lung, Bleeding From.* Inasmuch as blood from the lungs is expelled through the mouth, it may not be easy to tell that the blood is coming from the lungs. Usually, however, blood from the lungs is "coughed up" or "spit up" rather than being vomited. The causes of blood from the lungs include tuberculosis and cancer. Blood-streaked sputum occurs commonly in chronic bronchitis and bronchiectasis.

E. *Mouth, Bleeding From.* The mouth is subject to injuries, ulcers, and tumors, all of which may cause a certain amount of bleeding. Otherwise, it is the gums which bleed most easily. Bleeding when the teeth are brushed is usually caused by peridontal disease (pyorrhea) which calls for examination and care by a dentist. Bleeding from the gums may be caused by a general tendency to bleed, by severe vitamin deficiencies (as in scurvy), or by poor oral hygiene and infection of the tissues of the mouth.

F. *Nosebleed.* See chapter 17, volume 1, and chapter 9, volume 3.

G. *Rectum, Bleeding From.* Any passage of blood through the rectum deserves investigation by a physician. Bleeding from the rectum itself (as in hemorrhoids or anal fissure) is evidenced by a bright-red color. When the site of bleeding is distant (as in a bleeding peptic ulcer), the blood will be almost black in color and tarry in consistency. Bleeding from intermediate points will be correspondingly dark or light, depending upon the distance of the bleeding point from the rectum. Bloody diarrhea is common in ulcerative colitis. Polyps (benign tumors) of the colon may bleed. Bleeding is one of the important symptoms in cancer of the colon and rectum.

H. *Skin, Bleeding From or Into.* Persistent bleeding from minor wounds is characteristic of defects in the blood-clotting mechanism. Small areas of slight hemorrhage into the skin (purpura) may occur in cases of bleeding disorders. See chapter 10, this volume.

I. *Stomach, Blood From.* Blood in the stomach may be expelled by vomiting or by passing it through the intestines. For the latter, see paragraph "G" above. Blood in the stomach may have come from a lesion in the wall of the stomach, such as peptic ulcer, from gastritis, or from cancer, or it may have come from bleeding veins in the wall of the esophagus (as in cirrhosis of the liver), or even from some site of hemorrhage in the pharynx or nose from whence the blood has been swallowed. The appearance of vomited blood gives some clue as to how long it has been in the stomach, dark blood with a "coffee grounds" appearance having been in the stomach long enough to be altered by the digestive action of the gastric juice.

J. *Vagina, Bleeding From.* Periodic bleeding from the vagina occurs normally during menstruation throughout a woman's reproductive time of life. Causes of abnormal vaginal bleeding include polyps of the lining of the uterus or cervix, myoma (fibroid tumor) located in or near the lining of the uterus, inflammation of the lining of the uterus, disturbances of the balance of the hormones that control menstruation, and cancer of the uterine tubes or uterus. Certain serious complications of pregnancy can also cause abnormal bleeding through the vagina.

BLISTERS

A blister is a small collection of fluid in the surface layer of the skin. Blood blisters (in which the fluid is bloody) are caused by bruising or pinching the skin. Water blisters are usually caused by heavy friction against the skin. Damage to the skin by a thermal or chemical burn can cause blisters, as can also such skin diseases as pemphigus. It is best not to puncture a blister; and when a blister does break, care should be taken to avoid infection. In all blisters of unknown origin (usually due to some disease of the skin) a physician should be consulted.

BREAST, SYMPTOMS

Diseases of the breast are considered in chapter 30 of this volume, subdivision ''A. Breast Diseases.'' In the present section we consider the symptoms of lumps and tenderness in the female breast as well as the occasional enlargement of the male breast.

A. *Masses (''Lumps'') in a Woman's Breast.* During the years of a woman's physical prime (from early adolescence until the menopause) her breasts contain glandular tissue capable of producing milk after pregnancy. The presence of this glandular tissue gives the normal breast a nodular consistency. That is, on firm pressure the breast tissue does not feel entirely smooth but composed, rather, of finely alternating firm and soft areas. This normal nodularity of the breast undergoes cyclic changes each month, the nodules becoming most firm and slightly tender, perhaps, just before menstruation is due.

Several conditions can cause abnormal lumps in the breast. These abnormal lumps are to be distinguished from the normal gland nodules mentioned in the paragraph above. The most important of the conditions producing abnormal lumps is cancer. But not all lumps in the breast are caused by cancer. Cancer of the breast is a most serious and deadly disease, tending as it does

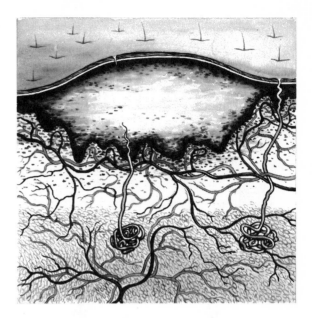

Cross section of skin tissue showing how a blister forms from an accumulation of watery fluid or serum under the epidermis, an elevated spot on the surface of the skin being the typical result.

to spread to other parts of the body.

When a lump develops in the breast, a simple examination by palpation is not always a satisfactory way to tell the difference between a lump caused by cancer and one caused by one of the other less harmful conditions. An X-ray examination of the breast (mammogram) may enable the doctor to determine the nature of the lump. Otherwise the lump should be removed and examined microscopically (biopsy). The safe rule which physicians follow is to consider every lump in the breast cancerous until proven otherwise.

The method of self-examination of the breast which should be performed each month is described in chapter 11, volume 3.

The earlier a cancerous lump in the breast is removed, the better the prospects of saving the patient's life. Therefore it rests with every woman to be alert to the development of a lump in the breast and to report any such to her doctor at once.

B. *Tenderness in the Female Breast.* Normally, a woman's breasts tend to be tender just before the onset of menstruation. The breasts are also tender during pregnancy (beginning about the third week following conception).

Extreme tenderness in the breast occurring during the time a mother is nursing her baby may indicate the development of an infection of the breast (mastitis), which deserves prompt treatment before it progresses to the stage of abscess.

Between the ages of 30 and 50, a woman's breasts may become tender because of the development of cystic mastitis. This is a benign condition, but it requires careful attention by a physician because of the difficulty of distinguishing it from cancer. Pain and tenderness are not usually associated with breast cancer until the late stages.

C. *Enlargement of the Male Breast.* In an occasional case, the breast of an adolescent boy enlarges at the time of his transition from boyhood to manhood. Usually just one breast is affected. This condition is considered in chapter 26, volume 1.

In an older male patient, one or both breasts may enlarge in response to hormone therapy used as part of the treatment for cancer of the prostate, for cirrhosis of the liver, or for tumor of the testes. Also, certain drugs, as Aldactone (a diuretic), or marijuana, may cause this response. Cancer may develop in the adult male breast, but this is a rare occurrence.

BREATH, SHORTNESS OF (DYSPNEA)

In the normal course of events the rate and depth of a person's breathing are automatically controlled in relation to his body's need to receive oxygen and eliminate carbon dioxide. When the tissues are not receiving as much oxygen as they need, breathing is stimulated. Also when carbon dioxide accumulates in the tissues, breathing is stimulated. Either of these situations results in the attempt to breathe deeply and rapidly at the same time—"shortness of breath," commonly called dyspnea.

Shortness of breath occurs normally when a person exercises vigorously and his muscles thus need to exchange oxygen and carbon dioxide at a more rapid rate than usual. The work of the heart increases proportionately because a more rapid exchange of oxygen and carbon dioxide requires a more rapid circulation of blood to carry these gases back and forth from the lungs to the muscles and other tissues.

A. *Obstructive Dyspnea.* Whenever there is an interference with the passage of air to and from the lungs, difficult breathing results. Such interference occurs when a person chokes by inhaling a foreign body that blocks the air passages, when a child suffers from croup in which the tissues of the larynx become swollen and the laryngeal muscles go into spasm, or when a person suffers from asthma in which it is difficult to exhale because the smaller air passages have become partially obstructed.

B. *Pulmonary Dyspnea.* When a disease interferes with the transfer of oxygen and carbon dioxide within the lungs, the body's tissues begin to suffer correspondingly and so signal their need for more adequate breathing. Reflexly, the person goes through the motions of faster and deeper breathing even though the speedup does not remove the fundamental difficulty. This kind of shortness of breath may occur in connection with pneumonia or in fibrosis of the lungs which results from the inhaling of irritating dusts. Most importantly, it is an outstanding symptom of chronic obstructive pulmonary disease (COPD) in which emphysema predominates.

C. *Cardiac Dyspnea.* Dyspnea is a common and significant symptom in serious heart disease. The functions of the heart and lungs are so closely related that when disease of the heart reduces the heart's capacity for pumping blood, difficult breathing (dyspnea) occurs. In the early stages of the heart difficulty, the dyspnea is noticed only at times of strenuous exertion. If the heart disease progresses, the dyspnea occurs with lesser degrees of exertion until, finally, it occurs even when the patient is resting.

D. *Dyspnea of Anemia.* There are various kinds of anemia, but in all kinds there is a deficiency in the blood's ability to convey oxygen. When the tissues demand additional oxygen, as when the individual climbs stairs or otherwise exercises vigorously, there develops a shortage and the organs of breathing react to this shortage just as they do in any other condition in which there is a dearth of oxygen—the individual tries to breathe faster and more deeply.

E. *Functional Hyperventilation.* There is a so-called "hyperventilation syndrome" in which the individual, even though his organs of breathing and his heart are perfectly normal, experiences an episode of rapid and deep breathing. Such an attack occurs typically when the person is at rest and is actually not in need of additional oxygen. His hyperactive breathing is prompted by a subconscious compulsion to breathe deeply or an unwarranted assumption that he is "short of breath." His excess breathing causes him to lose so much carbon dioxide from his body that he becomes lightheaded and may have the feeling that he is somewhat out of touch with what is going on about him.

Such attacks may be caused by bad breathing habits, but, more commonly, they result from anxiety.

CHILLS

A chill, with its paleness of the skin, its sense of coldness, and its shivering, is part of the body's provision for conserving and producing heat. Chills occur both when a person is in an environment of low temperature and when his body temperature rises suddenly. Chills, for example, occur typically in the early stages of pneumonia when the body is reacting to a severe infection and fever develops.

CHILLS AND FEVER

The term "chills and fever" is used to describe the condition in which body temperature is rising and the person feels chilly while the fever is developing. Chills and fever occur in the early phase of many systemic infections. They also occur typically in each of the repeating episodes of malaria. When fever declines sharply, sweating occurs.

COATED TONGUE

The appearance of the tongue's surface may vary according to one's condition of general health. In simple anemia, the tongue may appear pale and small; in pernicious anemia, abnormally smooth. The user of alcohol commonly has a heavily coated tongue. This same appearance, however, may suggest nothing more than poor oral hygiene. The tongue commonly appears heavily coated in cases of high fever or dehydration. Deficient diet and allergic sensitivity to drugs or cosmetics may influence the appearance of the tongue.

COMPLEXION, RUDDY

A conspicuous ruddiness is caused by an increased flow of blood through the skin because of a dilitation of the capillaries. It occurs in fever, in alcoholic intoxication, in the emotion of anger, and when the skin tissues are inflamed as in sunburn. Ruddiness also occurs in one of the forms of heart disease (mitral stenosis). Bluish-redness of the skin occurs in polycythemia, a disease characterized by an excess of red blood cells, and in carbon monoxide poisoning in which the union of part of the hemoglobin with carbon monoxide imparts a cherry-red color.

CONSTIPATION

See the General Index.

COUGH

A cough is a sudden, noisy expulsion of air from the lungs. A person may restrain the urge to cough or, on the other extreme, may force a cough when it would not occur otherwise. Usually, however, coughing occurs automatically. Coughing often occurs under conditions of good health to remove the mucus and foreign materials that have accumulated in the upper air passages.

Coughing occurs when fluid, food, or some foreign object accidentally finds its way into the air passages. It occurs when inhaled smoke or irritating gases cause local irritation of the lining of the air passages. This factor explains the smoker's cough. Coughing also occurs

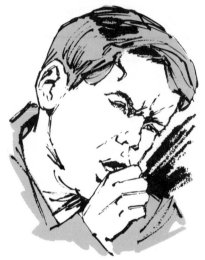

Coughing, generally a normal bodily function, is sometimes a symptom of disease.

when there is local inflammation of the air passages, as in laryngitis, tracheitis, and bronchitis. Coughing accompanies such respiratory disorders as the common cold and influenza.

Coughing is usually a prominent symptom of diseases involving the tissues of the lungs, including pneumonia, pulmonary tuberculosis, emphysema, bronchiectasis, fungal infections of the lung, parasitic diseases of the lung, and lung abscess. Cough also occurs in cancer of the lung, of the pleura, or of the mediastinum. Bronchiogenic carcinoma (the kind of lung cancer associated with cigarette smoking) usually becomes well established before it produces symptoms. But among its important symptoms, when they do occur, are coughing and the spitting of blood.

At first mention it may seem strange that heart failure can cause coughing. When the left side of the heart, for any one of various reasons, becomes unable to propel the blood at its normal rate and pressure, the blood tends to stagnate in the lung tissues. The blood plasma then seeps into the tiny air spaces of the lungs and interferes with the normal exchange of oxygen. Coughing then occurs as a means of clearing out the air spaces.

Sometimes an aneurysm of the thoracic aorta (enlargement of the body's largest artery) causes coughing by producing pressure against the trachea.

Certain contagious diseases, by an inflammatory involvement of the lung tissue, produce coughing. Common among these are whooping cough, certain kinds of influenza, and measles.

Coughing may occur in leukemia. This is produced by an enlargement of the lymph nodes at the center of the chest, bringing pressure against the trachea.

Coughing is sometimes produced by tricks of the mind rather than by organic disease. "Psychogenic cough" may occur as one of the manifestations of a neurosis or merely as a nervous habit.

For the treatment of cough, see chapter 13, this volume.

CRAMPS

Abdominal Cramps. Cramping pain in the abdomen may come from indulgence in alcohol, "intestinal flu," food poisoning, an overdose of some cathartic, poisoning by certain drugs or metallic poisons, typhoid fever, dysentery, or cholera. Abdominal cramps are an important symptom in intestinal obstruction.

Transient abdominal cramps occur commonly in normal pregnancy, but forceful contractions during pregnancy may indicate the onset of premature labor.

For information on other kinds of cramps, consult the General Index.

CYANOSIS

Cyanosis is a condition in which the skin and internal membranes appear bluish or purplish in contrast to their normal pink color. To detect cyanosis in a person with brown or black skin, look inside the mouth or examine the lining of the eyelids. The coloration of the skin and membranes, with its variations from person to person, depends on two factors: (1) the amount and quality of the pigment present in the tissues and (2) the color of the hemoglobin within the red blood cells. When hemoglobin is combined with oxygen, as in blood which has just passed through the lungs, its color is bright red. Hemoglobin which is not attached to oxygen (reduced hemoglobin) is dark, bluish-red. When for any cause there is a marked increase in the amount of reduced hemoglobin (not attached to oxygen), the skin color becomes bluish.

The skin of a "blue baby" appears blue because the infant has congenital heart disease. The defect in the heart permits the two bloodstreams to mix: (1) that coming from the lungs, laden with oxygen, and (2) that on its way to the lungs after having delivered its oxygen to the tissues. This mixture of "fresh" blood and "used" blood contains less oxygen than normal, and thus the infant's skin appears blue.

In high altitudes where oxygen is in short supply, even normal persons become somewhat cyanotic, particularly when they use up their limited supply of oxygen by exercise. Exposure to cold can cause cyanosis in the exposed parts of the body (fingers, toes, nose, and ears) because the blood to these parts has been curtailed by an automatic constriction of the vessels as a means of saving body heat. Even nervous tension or intense emotion can bring about a similar reduction of the flow of blood to certain parts of the skin, thus producing cyanosis in these parts—along with cold, clammy skin.

Pneumonia and certain chronic lung diseases which interfere with the normal function of the lungs in delivering oxygen to the blood may cause generalized cyanosis.

The various forms of heart failure, by failing to keep the circulation of blood at its normal pace, permit the oxygen which the blood carries to be used up more completely than usual so that a blue color is imparted to the skin. Interference with the flow of blood to any part of the body (by obstruction of either the arteries or the veins) will cause a slowing of the circulation in the part supplied and thus a blue coloration of the skin of this part.

DEAFNESS

See General Index.

DIARRHEA

See General Index.

DISCHARGE, MUCOUS

Mucus is a slippery, semifluid secretion produced by small glands located in the membranes that line many of the body's tubes and hollow organs. Mucus serves to keep the membranes moist and to lubricate them, and thus to protect them from injury. In response to irritation of a membrane, mucus is produced in larger quantities than usual. When we speak of a mucous discharge, we refer to an excess of mucus being eliminated from some part of the body.

A. *From the Trachea and Bronchial Tubes*. Mucus is produced at all times by the membranes lining the air passages, but under usual circumstances there is very little excess to be eliminated. When the membranes are irritated or inflamed, as in bronchitis, an excess of mucus is produced, which is then coughed up and expectorated. When the membranes become seriously inflamed in an infection, pus cells will be contained in the mucous discharge.

B. *From the Colon*. When the lining membrane of the colon is irritated or becomes involved in an inflammatory process, as in colitis, the excess of mucus produced is eliminated with the stools at the time of defecation. In severe cases of mucous colitis, some of the stools are composed largely of mucus.

C. *From the Nose.* A mucous discharge from the nose, often watery at first and more viscid later, is characteristic of the early stages of the common cold and also of an attack of hay fever. The nasal sinuses, opening as they do into the nasal cavities, are often involved and add to the mucus already being produced by the membranes lining the nose.

DISCHARGE, PURULENT (CONTAINING PUS)

In chapter 15, volume 3, it is explained that in the conflict between germs and the body's defenses there often occurs some actual destruction of tissue to form ulcers, abscesses, or inflamed surfaces. Dead cells, together with tissue debris and tissue fluid, constitute pus, which then escapes, if and when it can, from the area of destruction. Escaping pus is called a purulent discharge.

The parts of the body from which a purulent discharge may escape include

Exhaustion not traceable to organic causes may stem from debilitating emotional problems.

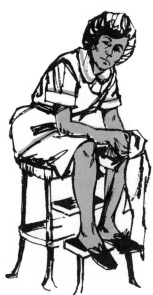

the bowel (at the anal outlet), the ears, the eyes, the lungs (by coughing and expectorating), the nose, the urethra, the vagina, and any part of the body where an abscess has ruptured. The occurrence of a purulent discharge is evidence of a serious infection which deserves attention. See the General Index under such items as *Discharge* and *Pus* for further information on such infections in various parts of the body.

DIZZINESS
See the General Index.

DYSPEPSIA
See the General Index.

EARS, SYMPTOMS
See under *Ear* in the General Index.

EDEMA
See the General Index.

ENERGY, LOSS OF

Loss of energy involves a feeling or a state of exhaustion. Loss of energy may come as the natural consequence of continued activity. After performing either mental or physical work for a prolonged period, a person's capacity for the work involved is reduced. In the case of muscle activity, loss of energy results from a reduction in the amount of oxygen and other vital elements available in the muscle, plus an accumulation of the chemical waste products of muscle activity.

Disease states in which loss of energy occurs include the following: (1) conditions in which the body's tissues do not receive a normal quota of oxygen, as in lung disease and heart disease; (2) conditions in which the tissues do not receive as much glucose (fuel food) as their degree of activity requires, as in malnutrition; (3) conditions in which the body's general rate of metabolism is reduced, as in hypothyroidism; and (4) conditions of profound malaise, or in such systemic illnesses as pneumonia.

Loss of energy is also common with patients who have experienced intolerable life situations or who are troubled by emotional tensions and conflicts. Even though in such cases the symptom is of a functional nature, the patient is sincere in his feeling of physical handicap.

See also *Weakness*.

EYES, SYMPTOMS

See Under *Eye, Eyes*, and *Eyelids* in the General Index.

FEAR

Fear occurs in the experience of every human being—an emotion involving dread of possible unpleasant consequences. Normally it serves a protective purpose by making a person cautious. For a child, a frightening situation may easily become associated with a specific harmless situation so that conditioning results and afterward the harmless situation alone will provoke a fear reaction. See two other related conditions, *Anxiety* and *Phobia*, in the General Index.

FEVER

Fever is an elevation of body temperature above the normal. Body temperature is usually measured by a clinical thermometer held for a minute or two under the tongue. Normally the reading will be about 98.6° F. (37° C.). Under conditions of health it is maintained at a surprisingly constant level by the reflex regulation of both heat production and heat elimination. See chapter 23, this volume. It should be noted that for some individuals "normal" body temperature is somewhat below 98.6°.

The body responds to infections and inflammations, as well as to tissue destruction, by an increase in body temperature (fever). When the increase takes place rapidly, the patient may experience chills while the heat regulating mechanism is accommodating to its new, higher level. Sweating is common when fever is receding.

Fever occurs in heatstroke. Here there is a high external temperature coupled with a failure of the body's heat-dissipating mechanism. Also the use of certain drugs causes an elevation of body temperature. Strenuous physical exercise will cause the body temperature to rise temporarily. In infants the temperature rises in response to dehydration (insufficient fluid within the tissues).

HEADACHE

See the General Index.

HEARTBURN

Heartburn consists of a sensation of "burning" in the upper middle part of the abdomen or along the course of the esophagus. It may be caused by a stretching of the esophagus (usually the lower part) either by swallowing too much food or drink in a single swallow or by the regurgitation of stomach contents into the lower part of the esophagus. Heartburn may occur in conditions of esophagitis and hiatus hernia. It may be aggravated by the use of aspirin, coffee, alcohol, or tobacco. It does not necessarily indicate excess acid in the stomach, for it may occur in persons who lack acid in their gastric juice. It occurs commonly in connection with indigestion.

HEAT CRAMPS

This disorder is characterized by sudden occurring cramps in the muscles of the abdomen and the extremities when the person has been doing heavy work in a temperature above 100 ° F. (38° C.) and has been perspiring profusely. It is the least serious of the three disorders caused by excessive heat. The condition results from a loss of salt (sodium chloride) from the body through excessive perspiration. It can be prevented by taking salt tablets and is treated by the administration of salt either in tablet form or by drinks containing salt. For the details of treatment, see chapter 23, volume 3.

HEAT EXHAUSTION OR HEAT PROSTRATION

This type of prostration occurs when persons have been exposed to excessive heat and have perspired freely but have not taken sufficient salt (sodium chloride) or water to replace the losses. The resulting deficiency hampers the circulatory system because the volume of body fluid is reduced to the point where the flow of blood through the small vessels of the skin is not brisk enough to keep the body cool. The skin feels cool and moist even though the patient is dehydrated.

The severity of the symptoms in heat exhaustion varies from case to case. There is usually weakness, dizziness, headache, and stupor. There may or may not be muscle cramps, mental confusion, or a state of shock.

Treatment consists of placing the patient in a cool place and administering abundant water with a moderate amount of salt. For details of the treatments see chapter 23, volume 3.

HEATSTROKE OR SUNSTROKE

This is the most severe of the three disorders caused by excessive heat. Fortunately, true heatstroke is rare. It occurs in susceptible persons who have had a prolonged exposure to excessive heat or to the sun in a situation where the circulation of air is inadequate. It is characterized by a sudden loss of consciousness, very high fever, and absence of sweating. In severe cases there may be convulsions, coma, and even death.

Often there are warning symptoms of weakness, headache, dizzinesss, nausea, and a pain in the vicinity of the heart. The skin becomes dry, hot, and flushed. The body temperature rises rapidly to as much as 105° F. (40.5° C.). The pulse rate may exceed 160 per minute. This increased rate of heartbeat is the automatic attempt of the body to circulate the blood through the skin fast enough to dissipate the excess heat. There may or may not be muscle cramps.

In heatstroke the usual mechanisms for getting rid of body heat are no longer sufficient to hold the body's temperature within normal limits.

Heatstroke requires emergency treatment which consists primarily of an all-out effort to lower the body temperature. For details see chapter 23, volume 3.

HEMMORRHAGE
See *Bleeding*.

HERNIA
See chapter 17, this volume.

HICCUP

A hiccup is a spasmodic occurrence in which air is taken in quickly only to be checked abruptly by an involuntary closure of the airway at the larynx, thus causing a gasping sound. Hiccups usually occur at intervals of several seconds, with an attack lasting a few minutes and causing no harm. The symptom may become very troublesome, however, when it occurs in connection with a serious illness or following surgery. In some such cases the attack of hiccups may last for hours and may weaken the patient, even endangering his life.

For remedies for hiccup, see chapter 23, volume 3.

HOARSENESS
See under *Speech Disturbances: C. Diseases of the Larynx.*

INCONTINENCE
Incontinence is a troublesome symptom characterized by loss of ability to control the passage of urine or feces.

A. *Incontinence of Infancy.* It takes a few months for the nervous system of the infant to develop sufficiently so that the control of the passage of urine and feces is attained. For more on this matter, see the General Index under *Bedwetting* and *Potty Training.*

B. *Urinary Incontinence of Adulthood.* See the item on *Incontinence* in the General Index.

C. *Incontinence of Feces.* Loss of control of the passage of feces occurs commonly in severe diarrhea. Excessive use of cathartics (particularly mineral oil) often causes an involuntary loss of the watery or oily fecal material.

Injury to the muscles that surround the anus, either by trauma or by a tearing of these structures at the time of childbirth, can interfere with the normal control of fecal evacuation. Hemorrhoids and anal fissures can cause the passages of feces to be so painful that the rectal contents are retained until finally the rectum is emptied involuntarily.

Certain injuries to the local nerves that supply the anal region or injury to the spinal cord can cause a permanent loss of control of the sphincter mechanisms which prevent the free passage of feces.

INDIGESTION
See the General Index.

INTERCOURSE, UNSATISFACTORY
Sexual intercourse is a complex and very personal function, with physical, ethical, and moral components. When one or more of these are less than satisfying to the individual, the entire function becomes disappointing. When all three blend in a manner consistent with the individual's codes and personal expectations, the experience of sexual intercourse provides a gratifying reassurance of personal adequacy.

The sexual reflexes which by their response to appropriate stimuli make intercourse possible are powerful and compelling in comparison with other reflex mechanisms. But their activation rests on a delicate balance between affirmative desire and negative repulsion. Normally and naturally the positive factors dominate. But minor rebuffs, incidental prejudices, and subconsciously operating conditionings can easily tip the balance in the negative direction so that intercourse, if accomplished at all, is a disappointment. This background explains, in theory, why in most cases of unsatisfactory intercourse the basic causes are psychological rather than physical.

The terms *frigidity* and *dyspareunia* refer to a wife's inability to experience normal pleasure in sexual intercourse. *Impotence* refers to a man's inability to perform the sex act, a symptom less common in men than frigidity in women. For more complete discussions see the terms just mentioned in the General Index.

INTOXICATION, ALCOHOLIC
Alcoholic intoxication is the condition in which a person manifests physical and mental symptoms as a result of imbibing a beverage containing alcohol. Perceptual capacities are dulled, judgment is impaired, the comprehension of reality is distorted. An intoxicated person's skin becomes flushed, his reflexes sluggish, and his muscular coordination poor. He may experience double vision, ringing in the ears, and numbness. There is an impairment of consciousness, proportional somewhat to the amount of alcohol consumed. The victim's condition may deteriorate to a state of coma.

A problem in dealing with alcoholic intoxication is that it does not always follow the same pattern. One person's reaction to alcohol may differ from that of another. The same drinker may react differently on two successive occasions. There is danger that a person who has indulged in liquor may be or may become ill from some other cause and this other illness may be overlooked on the false assumption that all of his symptoms are caused by the alcohol.

A common symptom of alcoholic intoxication is mental confusion.

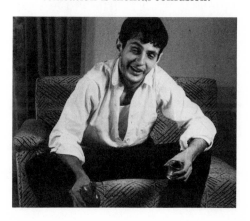

The stupor of alcoholic intoxication is easily confused with that caused by a serious head injury. If a person sustains such an injury while intoxicated, it may be difficult to know how seriously he has been hurt. The rupture or occlusion of a blood vessel within the brain ("stroke") may cause symptoms easily confused with alcoholic intoxication. Uremia resulting from kidney disease causes unconsciousness, which can be mistaken for the stupor of intoxication. The coma which occurs in diabetes, either from lack of insulin or from having taken too much insulin, may be similarly confused.

Alcohol interacts within the body with many drugs, producing effects which greatly exceed the drug's usual actions even to the extent of endangering the person's life. See the item *"Alcohol, Interaction With Drugs"* in the General Index.

Some persons react in an unusual manner when they take even a small amount of liquor. They become mentally confused and disoriented; they experience delusions and hallucinations similar to those suffered by a mentally ill person. A confirmed drinker may develop the complication of delirium tremens, in which there are visual hallucinations such as the false appearance of moving animals of various sizes and colors. In delirium tremens the patient is fearful, irritable, and imaginative beyond reason. Another possible complication of confirmed alcoholism is acute hallucinosis. In this the hallucinations typically pertain to hearing rather than to vision. The patient often "hears voices" accusing him of unmentionable conduct. The mental deterioration of chronic alcoholism must be treated as are the psychoses characterized by loss of intellectual capacity.

For the treatment of alcoholic intoxication, see chapter 23, volume 3.

ITCHING (PRURITUS)

Itching is an uncomfortable sensation which creates the desire to rub or scratch the affected skin area. It may be limited to a small area, or it may be generalized. It is quite normal for various areas of the skin to itch mildly at times. Dryness of the skin often causes itching, as when atmospheric humidity is low or when the skin's oil has been removed by the excessive use of soap. Itching occurs commonly in the latter part of pregnancy and at the time of the menopause.

Itching is the commonest symptom of diseases that affect the skin. It occurs as a symptom of allergy, in response to irritants (including chemicals and drugs), and in emotional states such as anxiety.

Itching of the skin may occur in such internal diseases as those affecting the liver or the bile passages (associated with jaundice), in diabetes, in some forms of kidney disease, in some forms of cancer, and in the excessive use of certain drugs.

Itching is especially troublesome when it occurs in the region of the anus (pruritus ani). In addition to the general causes for itching in other parts of the body, itching at or near the anus may be caused by lack of cleanliness, by local infections, or by the presence of pinworms.

JAUNDICE

Jaundice is a symptom in which bilirubin, a bile pigment, is deposited in certain tissues of the body, giving the skin, the mucous membranes, and the whites of the eyes a yellow color.

To understand the meaning of jaundice we must consider how bilirubin (the substance responsible for the yellow color) happens to be in the body. It occurs normally as a product of the destruction of hemoglobin.

The average life of a red blood cell is about 120 days. As red blood cells reach this approximate age, they are destroyed by the macrophages, large cells occurring in various tissues of the body. As the red blood cells are destroyed, the iron contained in their hemoglobin molecules is salvaged and used again in the manufacture of new hemoglobin. Another part of the hemoglobin molecule is oxidized, while still in the outlying tissues, to produce biliverdin and bilirubin, both of which happen to be colored substances.

We can observe an example, on a small scale, of this transformation of hemoglobin to biliverdin and bilirubin when we notice the color changes that occur in the skin when the underlying tissues have been bruised. Immediately after the injury, the area is "black and blue." Gradually this fades to produce shades of green and yellow, these being the result of the decomposition of hemoglobin as biliverdin and bilirubin are produced.

In the normal course of events, the bilirubin produced by the destruction of red blood cells in the outlying tissues is transported to the liver, where it becomes part of the bile.

It is normal for the blood to contain a certain amount of bilirubin. Only when the amount becomes excessive is some of the bilirubin deposited in the tissues, where it produces the yellow color typical of jaundice. Three general circumstances favor the occurrence of jaundice:

A. *When Red Blood Cell Destruction Is Increased.* Under this circumstance the amount of bilirubin being carried to the liver is so great that some of it seeps into the spaces between the tissue cells, imparting a yellow color. This occurs in certain anemias, collectively called the hemolytic anemias; and occasionally in such diseases as malaria and pneumococcal pneumonia.

B. *When the Liver Becomes Incapacitated.* In certain kinds of liver disease the liver becomes unable to dispose of the usual amount of bilirubin brought to it by the blood. Thus the amount of bilirubin in the blood increases and jaundice appears. Viral hepatitis is the liver disease usually responsible for this type of jaundice. Cirrhosis of the liver sometimes causes jaundice.

C. *When There Is an Obstruction to the Flow of Bile.* There are three possible causes for this type of jaundice: (1) the occasional effect of certain drugs or hormones (including contraceptive pills) in constricting the small bile ducts within the liver, (2) the lodging of a gallstone in the common bile duct, and (3) the development of cancer in the head of the pancreas where it presses against the common bile duct.

For further study see the item *Jaundice* in the General Index.

LUMP IN THE THROAT

This symptom is usually of a functional nature; that is, it is not the result of actual disease but the product of anxiety. Typically the patient with this symptom faces some unsolved problem, and the pent-up emotional tension causes him to be apprehensive about his health. His lump in the throat is the result of a subconscious fear that he may have cancer of the throat or some other life-threatening disease.

We must recognize that sometimes actual (organic) disease develops in the pharynx, larynx, or other parts of the neck. It is wise, therefore, for a person with a "lump in the throat" to consult a physician about the symptom, to determine whether it stems from organic disease or is a functional symptom.

NAUSEA

See under *Vomiting.*

NECK, SWELLINGS IN

Swellings in the neck are commonly caused by an enlargement of the lymph nodes, the thyroid gland, or the salivary glands. Congenital cysts and benign fatty tumors can also produce local enlargements.

Enlargement of the lymph nodes is designated as lymphadenopathy. Enlargements of the thyroid gland occur when this organ becomes inflamed, in certain types of goiter, or in cancer of the thyroid gland. The salivary glands enlarge in mumps and in tumors of these glands.

NECK, STIFFNESS OF

The common type of stiff neck from which a person suffers after sleeping in the wrong position or after being exposed to cold is an example of fibromyositis. The cause is probably persistent muscular tension that reduces the blood supply to the involved muscles. The same malady may cause muscle pain in the shoulder or in the lower back. A more chronic form of stiff neck occurs in torticollis (wryneck) which may last, more or less, throughout life.

Pain in the neck which interferes with the usual motions may occur when the lymph nodes become enlarged in lymphadenopathy. Stiffness and pain in the neck may also occur in some of the forms of arthritis or following some injury which involves the head or neck.

Extreme pain in the neck when the head is flexed forward may indicate an infection or irritation of the meninges (the membranes that cover the brain and the spinal cord).

NERVOUSNESS

Nervousness is an unpleasant feeling of restlessness, often coupled with anxiety, which distracts the attention and makes concentration difficult.

The causes of nervousness may be either psychological or physical. Psychological causes include emotional conflicts, lack of a goal in life, lack of a sense of belonging, thwarted ambition, and mental depression.

Nervousness may be caused by an overactive thyroid gland. It may accompany chronic systemic diseases such as tuberculosis. It commonly occurs in dietary insufficiencies. Nervousness often occurs when the brain is damaged as by encephalitis, brain tumor, or head injury.

NOSE, OBSTRUCTION BY POLYPS AND DEVIATED SEPTUM

In addition to the causes of nasal obstruction mentioned in chapter 9, volume 3, the passage of air through the nose is sometimes hindered by the development of a benign tumor called a polyp. This is an overgrowth of the tissue of the lining membrane. It can be

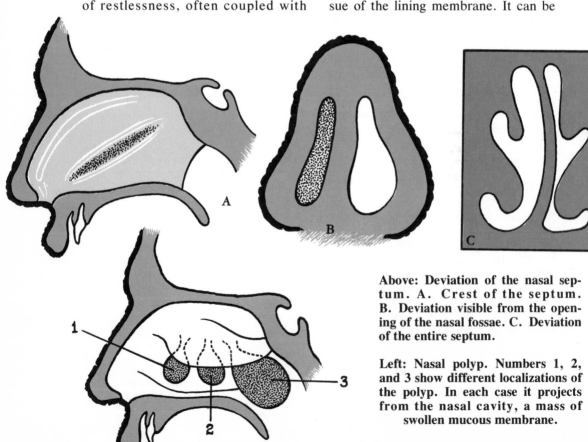

Above: Deviation of the nasal septum. A. Crest of the septum. B. Deviation visible from the opening of the nasal fossae. C. Deviation of the entire septum.

Left: Nasal polyp. Numbers 1, 2, and 3 show different localizations of the polyp. In each case it projects from the nasal cavity, a mass of swollen mucous membrane.

removed by a simple surgical procedure.

The septum separating the right and left nasal cavities is sometimes displaced to one side or the other, and this may interfere with the passage of air. The problem may be the result of a previous fracture.

ODORS, OFFENSIVE

A. *Odors From the Skin*. Odors from a person's skin or clothing may result from lack of cleanliness or may be caused by some skin disease. Sweat—the fluid produced by the sweat glands—is normally odorless. Glands associated with the hair follicles in the skin produce oil. These two products (sweat and oil), particularly when produced in excess, undergo chemical changes as a result of bacterial action; and it is this mixture of decomposed sweat and oil that produces objectionable body odor.

The reasonable way to prevent this type of odor is to bathe frequently and change to clean underclothing after each bath or shower. Antiperspirants, properly used, help to control excess sweating in the armpits. Deodorants serve only to cover up offensive odors but do not attack the problem at its source.

When diseases of the skin cause body odor, it is usually because the skin lesions have become secondarily infected. Obviously, removal of the odor requires proper treatment of the skin disease and infection.

B. *Odors From the Mouth and Nose (Bad Breath, Halitosis)*. The usual cause of "bad breath" is poor oral hygiene. When the mouth is not rinsed after each meal or the teeth brushed regularly, food fragments and tissue debris accumulate between the teeth and in the crevices of the membrane lining the mouth and covering the tongue. By bacterial action, these decompose and give rise to an offensive odor. This situation favors disease of the gums and the teeth, which is an added cause for bad breath, as also are unhealthy conditions in the nose and pharynx such as tonsillitis.

The use of tobacco may taint the breath for many hours after the last cigarette, particularly when the smoker inhales.

An unpleasant odor originating in the organs of respiration may be exhaled as "bad breath." Thus disease of the lungs such as bronchiectasis, lung abscess, or lung cancer can cause offensive breath, particularly when there is cough or expectoration. Volatile substances liberated in the lungs can produce characteristic odors, such as the odor of alcohol from liquor and the odor of onions and garlic from food. In certain systemic diseases volatile substances may be eliminated through the lungs, as in one of the complications of diabetes (sweet, fruity odor of acetone), uremia (odor of urine), or in liver failure (musty odor).

Certain forms of indigestion can also cause "bad breath," particularly when there is eructation (belching) or regurgitating of stomach contents.

Emotional states such as anxiety, nervousness, or irritation may aggravate the problem of "bad breath," presumably by reflex interference with the flow of saliva or by producing indigestion.

C. *Odors From Incontinence*. The patient who loses control of his rectum or bladder requires diligent nursing care; otherwise there will be offensive odors. This is also a problem with patients who have had surgery involving the intestine.

PAIN AS A SYMPTOM

The symptom of pain is so common and so important that an entire chapter, chapter 7, volume 3, is concerned with the descriptions and meaning of the various kinds of pain that occur in many locations throughout the body.

PALLOR

Paleness of the skin and membranes occurs whenever the blood fails to move briskly enough or when it carries less hemoglobin than normal. Blood of a low oxygen content permits the skin and membranes to appear pale, as contrasted with bright-red blood which has just picked up a fresh supply of oxygen from the lungs.

Because complexions vary, it is difficult to judge whether a person is pale by merely looking at his skin. The membrane lining the lower eyelid (observed by pulling down the lower eyelid) serves as a better index of the true color of the blood than does the skin.

Temporary pallor may occur in intense emotional states (fear or anger) or when a person faints.

Pallor occurs in the various forms of anemia, as when blood is lost through hemorrhage, when the body is deficient in iron, when production of red blood cells falls below par, or when red blood cells are destroyed at an abnormally high rate. The type of anemia can be determined only by an examination of the patient's blood in a laboratory.

Pallor occurs in those heart and lung diseases in which there is an inadequate circulation of blood through the tissues. It occurs commonly in cancer and in certain systemic diseases, as scurvy and tuberculosis.

PALPITATION

The heart is an active organ and enlarges and then contracts with each heartbeat. Under usual circumstances a person is hardly aware that his heart is beating, much less that it is moving vigorously within his chest.

The symptom of palpitation consists of an awareness of the heart's action, even when this action is still normal. This awareness that the heart is moving with each heartbeat is common among persons nervously inclined or apprehensive about their condition of health. It occurs also when the heart's action is irregular, unusually rapid, or extremely forceful. The organic diseases with which palpitation may be associated include anemia, disease of the thyroid gland, and certain disorders of the heart.

Of itself, palpitation is not an alarming symptom. But when it occurs otherwise than in connection with extreme exercise or intense emotion, the cause

should be determined by a physician.

PARALYSIS

Paralysis is a condition in which one or more muscles do not respond to the nerve signal for contraction. The usual cause is damage to the nerve or nerve tract which normally activates the muscle or the muscle group. The situation can be compared to that of an electric motor which no longer functions because the wires connecting it to the main line have been severed. Common instances of paralysis are as follows:

A. *Paralysis From Cerebrovascular Accident (Stroke):* Paralysis in this case is caused either by the plugging up of a blood vessel that supplies the brain or by a rupture of such a blood vessel. The plugging up may have been caused by thrombosis (a local blood clot) or by embolism (lodgment of a fragment of blood clot). This so-called "cerebrovascular accident" impairs the nerve fibers in the vicinity and renders them incapable of carrying nervous impulses. The muscles supplied by such disabled nerve fibers cannot, therefore, be controlled by the will and are said to be paralyzed. For further information, see chapter 4, volume 3.

B. *Paralysis From Injury to the Spinal Cord.* See chapter 3, volume 3.

C. *Paralysis in Cerebral Palsy (Congenital Spastic Paralysis).* This affliction stems from damage to the brain tissue which had its origin at or before the time of birth and produces a weakness of the muscles of one or more parts of the body, coupled with spasticity (stiffness) and often involuntary jerking movements. The extent and severity of the body's involvement vary from case to case. The legs are usually more severely involved than the arms. Birth injury, prematurity, or congenital developmental defects are usually responsible.

For further information, see chapter 6, volume 1.

D. *Paralysis in Neuritis.* There are many kinds of neuritis (inflammation of the nerves). Most nerves carry fibers that control muscle action as well as

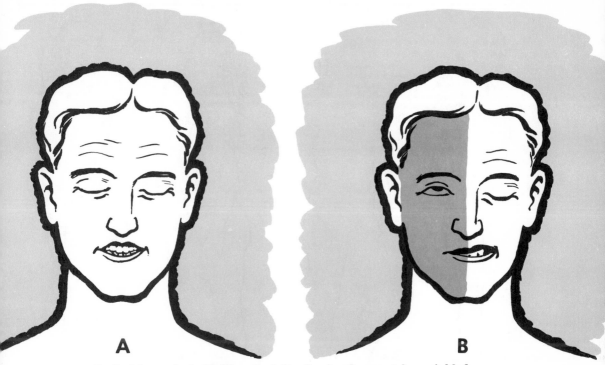

A   B

In facial paralysis (Bell's palsy) the forehead cannot be wrinkled nor the eye closed tightly nor the lips parted to show teeth—all on the affected side. The mouth is drawn toward the good side. A. Normal response to the request, Wrinkle your forehead, close your eyes, and show your teeth. B. Response to the same request in a case of facial paralysis affecting the patient's right side.

those that carry sensory impulses. Hence when a nerve becomes inflamed, there will be a loss of control, or at least a weakness, of the muscles which the nerve supplies. In some cases of polyneuritis (inflammation of many nerves) the loss of muscle function may be so general during the course of the disease that the patient's life can be saved only by the use of a mechanical respirator (to compensate for the paralysis of the muscles of breathing). For further information on the types and manifestations of neuritis, see chapter 4, volume 3.

E. *Facial Paralysis (Bell's Palsy)*. This paralysis involves the nerve that supplies the muscles of facial expression. It occurs on just one side, permitting the mouth to be drawn to the good side and making it difficult to close the eye on the affected side. The onset is usually sudden. In favorable cases, there is a marked improvement within two weeks. The cause remains obscure.

F. *Paralysis in Hysteria*. Paralysis of certain parts of the body is one of the common, even though mysterious, manifestations of hysteria. The paralysis usually involves one whole arm and hand or one whole leg and foot but does not correspond to the exact anatomical pattern of distribution of the nerves. For further information on hysteria, see chapter 5, volume 3.

RASH (SKIN ERUPTION)

A rash is a temporary eruption on the skin, a visible lesion characterized by redness or prominence, or both. Careful observation of the characteristics of

99

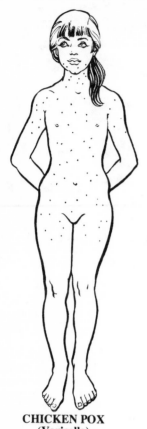

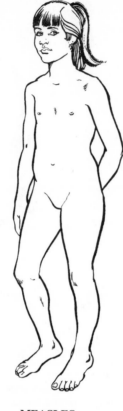

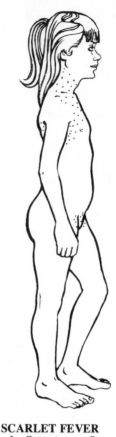

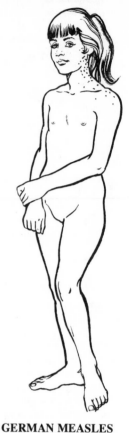

CHICKEN POX
(Varicella)
Early Symptoms: One day of fever, poor appetite, and headache.
Rash: Small red lumps appear first on body. Spread to face and then to limbs. Lumps become small blisters which break and form crusts. All stages of lump-blister-crust are present at the same time.

MEASLES
(Rubeola)
Early Symptoms: Symptoms of a common cold with fever and cough for 3-4 days before rash appears.
Rash: Brick-red spots appear behind ears. These spread from head and neck downward. Persist 5-6 days.

SCARLET FEVER
Early Symptoms: One or two days of severe sore throat, fever, and vomiting.
Rash: Fine "blushing" rash appears under arms, in the groins, on upper chest and neck, and then spreads, usually sparing the face.

GERMAN MEASLES
(Rubella)
Early Symptoms: Practically no warning symptoms.
Rash: Pink spots appear first on head and neck, sparing area around the mouth. These spread to body. Fades in about 3 days.

a rash and of the circumstances under which it appears will help to determine its cause. For descriptions of the various skin lesions that may appear in a skin rash, see chapter 25, this volume.

A. *The Rash of Communicable and Infectious Diseases*. The common communicable and infectious diseases in which rashes appear are as follows:

chicken pox (varicella), German measles (rubella), measles (rubeola), Rocky Mountain spotted fever, scarlet fever, syphilis, typhoid fever, and typhus fever.

B. *The Rash of Pellagra*. Pellagra is a disease caused by dietary deficiency, comparatively rare now since the development of the science of nutrition.

The skin involvement of pellagra begins as an erythema which resembles sunburn and which, in fact, is aggravated by exposure to sunlight. It appears on the parts of the body exposed to light and sun.

C. *Rash in Diseases of the Skin.* Many diseases of the skin are characterized by some form of rash. These usually run a long course, and their relief requires an accurate diagnosis of the skin disease and appropriate treatment. See chapter 25, this volume.

D. *Skin Eruptions Following the Use of Drugs.* Erythema or urticaria may develop as one of the symptoms of drug allergy in susceptible persons following the use of drugs. Some drugs cause these reactions more commonly than others. There is a great individual variation, one person being sensitive to one drug and another person to an entirely different drug. The reaction may occur promptly after the administration of the drug (uncommon) or 6 to 12 days after the start of the medication.

E. *Urticarial Reactions.* Urticaria (hives) may develop under many conditions: allergy to certain foods; sensitivity to an injection of a protein substance; allergy to substances contacting the skin; infestation with parasytic worms or bites by lice, mosquitoes, or bedbugs; endocrine imbalance, as during menstruation or at the time of the menopause; and instances of psychic stress or emotional unrest. See chapter 25, this volume.

F. *Rash in Infants.* For information on the rashes that may affect infants, see *Rash* in the General Index.

RECTUM, PROLAPSE OF

Protrusion of the lining of the rectum occurs chiefly in infants or in elderly persons. The immediate cause is straining at stool or, in the more serious cases, merely coughing or engaging in muscular exertion as lifting. The condition becomes serious if the tissue is allowed to remain in the prolapsed condition long enough for it to be damaged because of reduced blood supply. The immediate remedy consists of returning the tissue to its normal internal location by first lubricating it thoroughly with mineral oil, Vaseline, or mild soap and then exerting gradual pressure through a clean towel. For an infant, this is made easier by lifting the baby by its heels while the replacement is attempted. In an adult, the replacement is facilitated by the patient's taking the knee-chest position.

SLEEPLESSNESS

See the General Index.

SNEEZING

Sneezing is a natural reflex action designed to aid in the expelling of an irritant from the nasal passages. Nasal irritants commonly consist of dust or powders. The membranes lining the nasal passages can also be irritated by anything that causes them to swell. The two most common causes of such sneezing are (1) infection, such as the common cold and (2) allergy—sensitivity to some foreign material that enters the nostrils along with the air, as in hay fever. Chilling of the skin, especially that of the lower extremities, can cause reflex congestion of blood in the membranes of the nasal cavities and thus induce sneezing. For material on the mechanism of sneezing, see chapter 12, this volume.

SORE THROAT

See the General Index.

SPEECH DISTURBANCES

The use of language for transmitting ideas is one of the highest intellectual accomplishments of the human being. It consists in the ability to attach significance to symbols and to select the right symbols to express thoughts. This function, whether performed by speaking or writing, requires a high degree of muscle coordination. It is not surprising, then, that various unhealthy conditions can interfere with the function of speech or, in the broad sense, with the use of language. In the present discussion we are concerned more with conditions that may handicap a person in talking than with those that might interfere with writing, reading, and understanding.

Four components contribute to the expression of ideas by speech. First is the complex activity that takes place in the speech area of the brain by which ideas are organized and symbols (words) are selected to express these ideas. Second is the exercise of control over the muscles that activate the organs of speech. This involves the sending of nervous impulses from the brain to the larynx, the palate, the tongue, the cheeks and lips, and the muscles that control breathing. Third is the production of sound by the larynx. This requires that a stream of air pass through the larynx and the vocal cords be tightened or loosened just enough to produce the desired pitch as they vibrate in the stream of air. And fourth is the modification of the sounds produced in the larynx. This is accomplished by the auxiliary organs of speech (the palate, tongue, cheeks, and lips) in a manner that produces intelligible words. Disturbances of speech may be caused by difficulty in any one of these four components.

A. *Disturbances in the Speech Area of the Brain.* Various parts of the brain are involved in the use of language: the sensory areas of hearing and vision, the area in which memories are recorded, the area in which imagination and creative thinking occur, and the areas in which the muscle actions are initiated and coordinated. These areas are interconnected by many nerve fibers. Collectively they are called the "speech area" of the brain.

Damages to the speech area of the brain cause curtailment in the ability to speak, to write, or to understand words, either spoken or written. Such a handicap in the use of language is called aphasia.

Aphasia may be caused by the curtailment of blood supply resulting from arteriosclerosis, by the development of a blood clot in an artery that supplies this portion of the brain, by the rupture of such an artery, by the lodgment of a fragment of blood clot so as to deprive this portion of the brain of its blood supply, or by the destruction of such portions of brain tissue as by a tumor or an abscess.

The manifestations of aphasia vary all the way from mild limitations in the patient's vocabulary to total inability to express ideas or grasp ideas expressed by others. The patient with aphasia is often humiliated and thwarted by his inability. His organs of speech are not paralyzed, for the words he does use are enunciated normally. Only his capacity for translating thoughts into words and words into thoughts is limited.

B. *Faulty Control of the Organs of Speech.* Damage to any of the nerves that carry impulses from the brain to the organs of speech will, of course, interfere with speech. When the facial nerve which controls the muscles of the cheeks and lips is damaged, the sounds of "b" and "p" are difficult to execute. The hypoglossal nerve controls the tongue; its malfunction makes the sounds of "l" and "t" difficult to produce. The vagus nerve controls the soft palate, the pharynx, and the muscles within the larynx. When the branches to the soft palate are damaged, speech has a nasal sound. When the nerve to one side of the larynx is interrupted, speech is weak and unnatural. When the nerves to both sides of the larynx are incapacitated, the making of normal sounds becomes impossible. When nerves to the diaphragm or to the various other muscles of breathing are damaged, the flow of air through the larynx is diminished and speech may be reduced to a whisper.

In cases of Parkinson's disease or multiple sclerosis, the rhythm of speech is altered because of interference with muscle tone and muscle coordination.

C. *Diseases of the Larynx.* Acute laryngitis, such as may occur with a sore throat or with the common cold, causes the voice to be hoarse. Chronic laryngitis, as in smokers, also produces hoarseness. Benign tumors (as polyps or papillomas) sometimes develop within the larynx and interfere with normal production of sound. Probably the most serious disease affecting the larynx is laryngeal cancer. The first symptom of this condition is usually a persisting unaccounted-for hoarseness. Persistent hoarseness should always be interpreted as a danger signal, for success in treating cancer, when present, depends on how early treatment is begun.

D. *Defects in the Auxiliary Organs of Speech*. Defects of the lip, palate, or other auxiliary organs of speech may be congenital or may result from a mutilating accident or disease. In the congenital group we think of hairlip and cleft palate. These, when taken early in a child's life, can be treated quite satisfactorily by surgery. In tissue losses due to accident or disease, the speech can often be much improved by the wearing of a specially constructed prosthetic device.

E. *Stuttering and Stammering*. Stuttering and stammering, for pratical purposes, are synonymous terms and refer to the same form of speech difficulty. In this condition the flow of speech is interrupted by pauses and by repetition of sounds or syllables. Facial grimaces often accompany the effort to enunciate the desired word.

The problem of stuttering typically appears first sometime between ages 2 and 10. It affects about 1 percent of all school-age children. It is six times more common in boys than in girls. In the usual case, the fault is not with the organs of speech. It occurs as a symptom of some emotional disturbance, such as when a child feels that his personal security or well-being is threatened.

A child's stuttering may be exaggerated by such circumstances as starting to school too soon, being pushed to carry schoolwork scholastically beyond his present stage of development, feeling insecure in the personal relations of home, or being resentful of an older brother's or sister's domination.

The child who stutters should ideally be placed under the professional care of a speech therapist. Parents may do a great deal to help such a child by spending more time in congenial companionship.

STUPOR

In stupor there is a reduction of alertness, a semiconsciousness from which the patient can be partially aroused. Stupor may progress to one of the more severe degrees of coma or shock or to actual unconsciousness. It may occur in a person when under the influence of drugs or when overtaken by an attack of epilepsy. In cases of mental illness, the term stupor describes a condition of reduced responsiveness, as in depression or dementia.

SWALLOWING DIFFICULTY (DYSPHAGIA)

Normal swallowing is a complicated function involving the coordination of muscles of the face, the tongue, the pharynx, and the esophagus. These muscles are under the control of five pairs of nerves and the corresponding integration centers of the brain. The circumstances that cause difficulty in swallowing are listed as follows:

A. *Foreign Body Within the Esophagus*. Large, irregular-shaped objects, if accidentally swallowed, may lodge in the back part of the pharynx. Objects of such shape and size that they enter the upper part of the esophagus will usually pass through its entire length. If they become lodged, it is usually in the upper part of the esophagus. A foreign body lodged in the esophagus naturally interferes with swallowing. If it has sharp edges, it may injure the lining of the esophagus, causing symptoms that persist even after the object is removed. The removal of such a foreign body requires the services of a physician.

B. *Corrosive Injury and Stricture of the Esophagus*. The swallowing of strong acids or alkalis causes serious injury to the lining of the esophagus. In the acute phase of such an injury, the patient may have to be fed by the injection of nutrient solutions into his veins. As the injury heals, there is a gradual shrinking of the tissues with scar formation and narrowing of the lumen of the esophagus. Thus, the swallowing of food or even of liquid may become difficult or impossible. Surgical treatment is often required.

C. *Cancer of the Esophagus.* Cancer of the esophagus occurs most commonly in the lower third (nearer to the stomach than to the pharynx). Difficulty in swallowing is usually the first and continuing symptom of such a development. For this reason the symptom should be reported early to a physician.

D. *Paralysis of the Muscles of Swallowing.*

1. Achalasia or "Cardiospasm." In this condition the waves of contraction that normally propel the food or drink through the esophagus stop short of the stomach, and the food or drink accumulates in the lower part of the esophagus, causing it to stretch. A symptom in addition to difficulty in swallowing may be pain behind the breastbone occurring after eating. The condition seems to be aggravated in many patients by periods of emotional stress.

2. Bulbar Palsy. Bulbar palsy results from damage to nerve cells within the brain stem—cells that would normally control the muscles of swallowing. It can be caused by arteriosclerosis or by toxins produced in such a disease as diphtheria.

E. *Pressure Against the Esophagus.* Structures contained within the chest may press on the esophagus, thus causing difficulty in swallowing. Such pressure can be caused by aneurysm of the aorta, tumor, or diaphragmatic hernia.

F. *Esophagitis.* Inflammation of the tissues of the esophagus may make swallowing painful.

G. *Lesions of Related Structures.* Conditions developing within the mouth, pharynx, or larynx may interfere with swallowing, either because they are painful or because they inter-

fere in a mechanical way. These include cancer of the tongue, cleft palate, inflammation of the lining of the mouth or pharynx (stomatitis or pharyngitis), and cancer of the larynx.

H. *Emotional Conditions.* Fear or acute anxiety may cause an impression of "a lump in the throat" which makes swallowing difficult. A related condition, called globus hystericus, occurs under conditions of emotional conflict and makes it difficult for a person to initiate the process of swallowing.

TENSIONS, EMOTIONAL

Emotional tensions occur in persons ill at ease or baffled by problems seemingly too difficult to solve. In some cases the person knows, at the level of intellect, what he should do, but is deterred by his emotions (fear, love, hate)

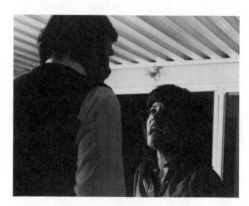

Functional symptoms often stem from emotional tensions.

from acting. In other cases, moving in the sensible direction would require him to forfeit some cherished desire; so emotional pressures build up while the solving of the problem is delayed.

Emotional tensions cause many functional symptoms.

TREMORS

A tremor is a repetitious, involuntary shaking movement produced by the alternate contraction of opposing groups of muscles. Characteristic tremors occur in several forms of disease. Tremors usually disappear during sleep.

In Parkinsonism (paralysis agitans) there is a slow-motion tremor, most noticeable when the muscles are otherwise at rest, which involves the fingers (with a "pill-rolling" gesture), the forearms, the head, and the tongue. A tremor which increases in the part of the body under immediate use is characteristic of multiple sclerosis. Tremor appears in many cases of advanced arteriosclerosis of the vessels of the brain, also in some brain tumors and brain abscesses.

A fine, rapid tremor of the fingers is present in many cases of overactivity of the thyroid gland. Tremor occurs commonly in cases of alcoholism. It often occurs in cases of drug poisoning. Tremor ("the shakes") occurs typically in cases of extremely low blood sugar (hypoglycemia), as when a diabetic patient has taken more insulin than he requires at a given time. Tremor may develop in certain functional disorders, as in anxiety states and hysteria.

Elderly persons sometimes develop a mild tremor, often involving just the head, which persists during most of their waking hours. This tremor has no particular significance except that it constitutes a nuisance.

ULCERS OF THE SKIN
See chapter 25, this volume.

UNCONSCIOUSNESS
Unconsciousness may be caused by many circumstances. Some represent serious ailments which require proper treatment if the patient's life is to be saved.

A. *Unconsciousness From Taking Alcohol, Drugs, or Poisons.* Intoxication by alcohol is the most common cause of unconsciousness among patients admitted to hospitals.

Among drugs that commonly cause unconsciousness when taken in overdoses are sedatives, tranquilizers, the barbiturates, morphine, and other opium derivatives (narcotics).

Among poisons which produce unconsciousness, carbon monoxide gas is probably the most common. This is contained in the exhaust from automobile motors and in fumes from improperly ventilated heating stoves.

If the unconscious person has been working with an insecticide or a weed killer, possible poisoning by such chemicals should be suspected. For specifics on first-aid treatment of the various kinds of poisoning, see chapter 22, volume 3.

B. *Unconsciousness Due to Head Injury.* Unconsciousness is a common accompaniment of severe head injury, such as from a blow, a fall, or an automobile accident. The unconsciousness which immediately follows a head injury results from damage to the brain tissue. The extent of such damage can be measured, roughly, by the length of time the victim remains unconscious.

In some cases of severe head injury with damage to the blood vessels and the membranes which surround the brain, the person may regain consciousness after the injury only to become unconscious again several hours later. This lapse of consciousness after a lucid interval indicates increasing pressure within the skull caused by an expanding blood clot. It threatens the patient's life and requires prompt treatment by surgical intervention.

C. *Unconsciousness Caused by Diseased Blood Vessels Within the Skull.* Blood vessels which supply the brain may become weakened because of arteriosclerosis. Weakened vessels may rupture, producing hemorrhage into the brain, or they may become plugged because of the development of a clot of blood (thrombus) at the site where the vessel is diseased. A piece of blood clot carried by the blood may plug one of the vessels supplying the brain. Such an involvement of the brain and its consequences constitutes what is commonly called a stroke.

D. *Coma in Epilepsy.* Unconsciousness occurs as a part of the usual seizure ("fit") of epilepsy. Duration of the unconsciousness varies from a few seconds (in the milder form of epilepsy) to a few hours.

E. *Coma From Diabetes and Other Metabolic Disorders.*

1. In so-called diabetic coma there is an overabundant supply of blood sugar throughout the body because of an inability of the body to handle it. Toxic products build up that produce unconsciousness. In this type of unconsciousness, the patient's breath has a "fruity" odor.

2. Hypoglycemic coma may occur also in a diabetic patient, but this type of unconsciousness comes from the administration of too much insulin (or oral pills that act similarly), with the result that the available blood sugar falls below the level necessary to maintain the brain's requirements for a continuous source of energy.

Either diabetic coma or hypoglycemic coma may occur in persons with diabetes mellitus. They must be carefully differentiated, however, for emergency treatment in the two situations is opposite: administration of insulin in diabetic coma and administration of sugar (or glucose solution in the vein) in the hypoglycemic variety. See chapter 23, volume 3, for details.

3. Uremic coma occurs in kidney disease because of the accumulation of noxious substances in the blood as a result of the inability of the kidneys to carry on their normal functions of elimination.

4. Hepatic coma may develop in a patient with liver disease (cirrhosis or hepatitis) as a result of the accumulation in the blood of ammonia and related substances normally detoxified by the liver.

F. *Coma Associated With Brain Tumor or Abscess.* In cases with brain tumor or brain abscess, the onset of the unconsciousness is usually gradual but may be sudden when complications develop. The unconsciousness may or may not be associated with paralysis.

G. *Unconsciousness in Meningitis and Encephalitis.* The usual symptoms and signs in meningitis are severe headache and rigidity of the neck, followed by unconsciousness. Loss of consciousness is particularly characteristic of the "lethargic" type of encephalitis.

H. *Fainting; Unconsciousness Caused by Reduced Blood Supply to the Brain.* There are many circumstances, some emotional and some physiological, which can deprive the brain of sufficient blood to cause unconsciousness. For additional information see chapter 9, this volume.

I. *Unconsciousness in Hysteria.* Persons with hysteria may lose consciousness as a functional response to some emotional stress.

For the treatment of the various kinds of unconsciousness, see the appropriate items in chapter 23, volume 3, or consult the General Index for page references.

VOMITING

Vomiting is usually preceded by the unpleasant sensation of being "sick at the stomach" (nausea). The act of vomiting is under the control of a nerve center in the brain stem. Nerve impulses from this center cause a vigorous contraction of the abdominal muscles and the diaphragm, with a relaxation of the muscle fibers at the junction of the esophagus and stomach. This allows the stomach contents to be ejected through the esophagus and mouth.

The causes of nausea and vomiting may be as follows:

1. Psychic Reactions. Emotional shock (as sudden bad news), pain, fright, grief, unpleasant tastes, and offensive smells may trigger the vomiting mechanism.

2. Drugs. Some drugs produce vomiting by irritating the lining of the digestive organs; others, by directly influencing the vomiting center of the brain stem.

3. Poisons. Nausea and vomiting are prominent symptoms in most cases of poisoning, either in food poisoning or in poisoning by chemical substances other than those in offensive food.

4. Disturbances of the Abdominal Organs. Irritation of the organs of digestion, intestinal obstruction, cancer of the digestive organs, inflammation of

the appendix or gallbladder, or gallstones commonly cause nausea and vomiting.

5. Toxicity. Nausea and vomiting occur in uremia and severe liver disease, presumably because of the toxicity which these conditions produce.

6. Increased Pressure Within the Skull. Head injury, brain tumor, brain abscess, and hemorrhage within the skull may cause nausea and vomiting or even vomiting without nausea, probably because of interference with the blood supply to the vomiting center.

7. Excessive Stimulation of the Semicircular Canals. Dizziness or excess stimulation of the sense organs for equilibrium (as in motion sickness) typically cause nausea and vomiting by reflex influence on the vomiting center.

8. Pregnancy. It is typical for an expectant mother, in the early weeks of her pregnancy, to experience nausea and vomiting.

See this item also in the General Index.

WEAKNESS (ASTHENIA)

Weakness involves an actual loss (complete or partial) of the ability to perform in a normal manner.

Gradually progressive weakness may occur in the declining years of old age,

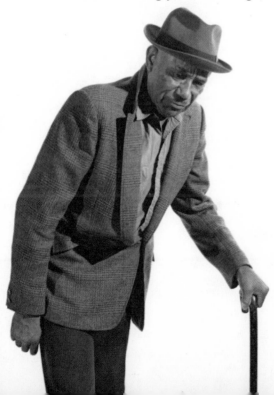

particularly when the elderly person has some chronic illness. It occurs in patients of any age who have been long confined to bed. Even after recovery from an illness the patient will go through a period of "getting his strength back" during which he must increase his activities gradually.

General weakness occurs typically in illnesses associated with fever. It occurs in systemic diseases such as tuberculosis, brucellosis, and malaria.

Weakness is a usual symptom in conditions in which there is an insufficient amount of oxygen available to the tissues, as in anemia and certain forms of congenital heart disease. It occurs in persons who follow fads in diet, particularly when the diet does not contain an adequate amount of protein. In anorexia nervosa, a disease in which the patient has a compulsion to avoid gaining weight, there is weakness because of an inadequate food intake.

Weakness accompanies such disorders of the endocrine organs as Addison's disease, pituitary insufficiency, thyroid disease in which there is either hypo- or hyper-function of the thyroid gland, diabetes mellitus, and hyperparathyroidism.

Weakness is common in viral hepatitis and in some other liver disorders. It occurs commonly in those kidney diseases in which the kidneys become unable to eliminate the necessary amounts of the products resulting from the metabolism of proteins.

Weakness occurs in those diseases of the nervous system in which the nerve centers controlling the actions of the muscles or of the nerve fibers which lead to these muscles are injured or destroyed. Such conditions as "stroke," tumors of the brain or other nervous tissues, and poliomyelitis cause weakness and even paralysis of the muscles which would normally be controlled by the affected nerve structures. Weakness occurs in such muscular disorders as myasthenia gravis, myotonia, and progressive muscular dystrophy.

Weakness even occurs in cases of chronic alcoholism or in persons who have used certain drugs for long periods of time (particularly bromides, barbiturates, cocaine, or morphine and its derivatives).

See also *Energy, Loss of.*

WEIGHT, SUDDEN LOSS OF

Loss of weight is expected when a person goes on a reducing diet. But loss of weight under other circumstances is cause for alarm.

Loss of weight occurs in acute diseases with fever or in any illness where food intake is sharply curtailed. Unexplained loss of weight is one of the signs that should call attention to the possibility of cancer. Loss of weight may not be the first telltale evidence of cancer, however.

Loss of weight in newborn babies may be due to pyloric obstruction, in which little or no food enters the stomach. It occurs also in celiac disease, in exophthalmic goiter, in Hodgkin's disease, and in infestation with hookworm.

The Heart; Circulatory Systems

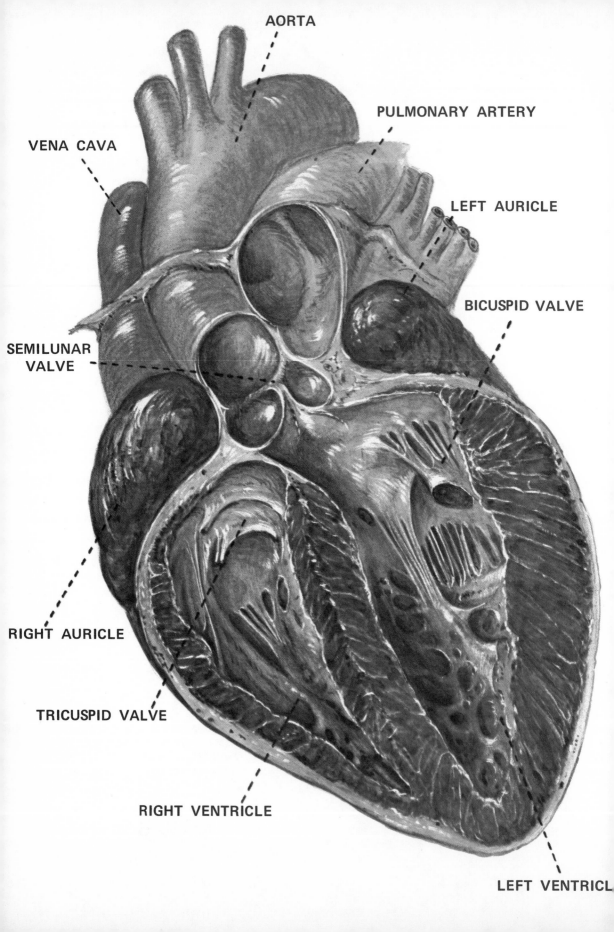

AORTA

PULMONARY ARTERY

VENA CAVA

LEFT AURICLE

BICUSPID VALVE

SEMILUNAR
VALVE

RIGHT AURICLE

TRICUSPID VALVE

RIGHT VENTRICLE

LEFT VENTRICL

The Heart, Blood Vessels, and Blood

In an earlier chapter the body has been called a living machine. It can be compared to a steam or gasoline engine. It uses fuel and produces heat and power, needing oxygen from the air in order to do so. The chief fuel it uses is blood sugar (glucose), which comes from food. Also, somewhat like an engine, the body sometimes needs repair materials. These also come from food. Waste materials results from the activities of the body, just as smoke and ashes or exhaust gases are produced by an engine.

The classes of food needed by the body, both for fuel and for repairs, and how these are changed by the digestive organs and the liver into forms that can be used by the body tissues will be discussed later. But in this chapter we are concerned with two questions: (1) How are the fuel and repair materials and the oxygen carried to the tissues throughout the body where they are needed? (2) How are the waste materials transported from the tissues where produced to the lungs and kidneys to be discharged from the body? Obviously neither the fuel nor the repair materials are produced *where* needed for use. And just as understandably, the wastes, if they were to remain where produced, would soon clog the body

machine and bring it to a dead stop. So both cases require transportation.

The answer to both questions is the same: The job is done mainly by the blood. The blood, the vessels through which it flows, and the heart which propels the blood through the vessels form the main parts of the body's transportation system.

The Heart

The heart is about the size of a clenched fist. In the average man it weighs about ten ounces (400 grams), and in the average woman about eight and a half ounces (350 grams). Its walls are thick and composed almost entirely of heart muscle. As this muscle contracts, it squeezes the blood from inside the heart out into the arteries. The arteries then carry the blood away from the heart to all parts of the body.

The body of an adult man of average size contains about six quarts (5.4 liters) of blood. The blood, pumped by the heart, is constantly on the move. Ordinarily a drop of blood can make one complete trip from the heart to some distant part of the body and back again in about one minute. When a person is exercising, his blood can travel even faster. It is remarkable how the heart keeps on year after year perform-

111

ing the work necessary to keep the blood circulating without wearing out.

The heart does an enormous amount of work. If you were to lift a ten-pound weight three feet off the floor every thirty seconds (about the same as lifting a four-kg. weight to a height of one meter), you would be doing as much work as your heart regularly does. It would be quite an undertaking to lift this weight this high two times a minute for an eight-hour day, but the heart keeps up its work hour after hour and day after day for an entire lifetime. On the average, the heart of an adult pumps more than 4,000 gallons (14,400 liters) of blood each day.

One reason that the heart is able to carry its heavy workload is that it rests briefly between beats. Studies of electrocardiograms (scientific records of the heart's activities) indicate that the organ's rest periods add up to more time than its working periods. Another reason is that the heart's own tissues

have a very excellent blood supply. Weight for weight, the heart's tissues receive about five times as much blood as the average of other tissues in the body. The heart uses about one tenth of all the oxygen used in the body. Still another reason is that this organ has remarkably great reserve power. For a short time in an emergency, it can do ten times as much work as it has to do while the body is at rest.

The arteries which carry blood into the walls of the heart are called *coronary* arteries. It is important to keep all the arteries in as healthy a condition as possible, but especially these. Doing so is largely a matter of proper diet and proper exercise. Diet is discussed in chapter 53, volume 1. But the chief points to mention here are as follows: (1) the advisability of limiting fats, and (2) the advantage of avoiding obesity by moderation in eating. As to exercise, the ideal is to engage in enough brisk exercise *every day* to stimulate

The position and relative size of the heart.

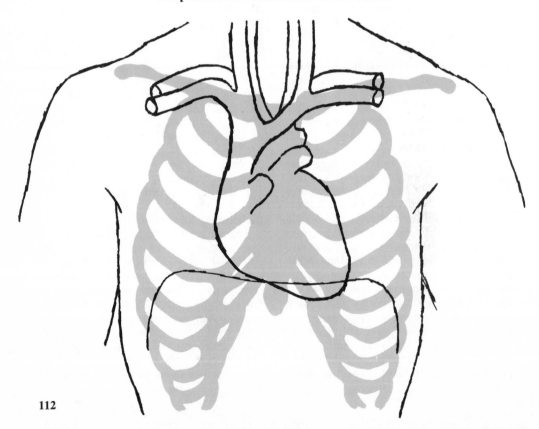

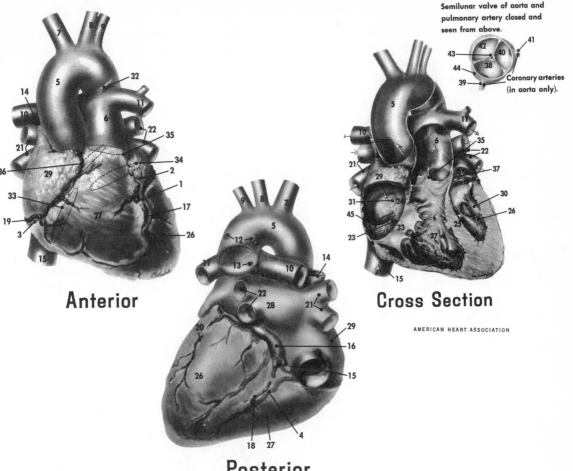

Semilunar valve of aorta and pulmonary artery closed and seen from above.

Coronary arteries (in aorta only).

Anterior

Cross Section

AMERICAN HEART ASSOCIATION

Posterior

Three views of the heart, showing relative position of its parts.

1. Anterior interventricular branch of left coronary artery
2. Circumflex branch of left coronary artery
3. Right coronary artery
4. Posterior interventricular branch of right coronary artery
5. Arch of aorta
6. Pulmonary trunk
7. Brachiocephalic artery
8. Left common carotid artery
9. Left subclavian artery
10. Right pulmonary artery
11. Left pulmonary artery
12. Posterior intercostal arteries
13. Bronchial artery
14. Superior vena cava
15. Inferior vena cava
16. Coronary sinus
17. Great cardiac vein
18. Middle cardiac vein
19. Lesser cardiac vein
20. Posterior vein of left ventricle
21. Right pulmonary veins
22. Left pulmonary veins
23. Opening of coronary sinus
24. Limbus of fossa ovalis
25. Interventricular septum
26. Left ventricle
27. Right ventricle
28. Left atrium
29. Right atrium (shown opened on cross-section drawing)
30. Posterior papillary muscle
31. Fossa ovalis
32. Ligamentum arteriosum
33. Tricuspid valve (anterior cusp of left valve shown on cross-section drawing)
34. Mitral valve
35. Pulmonic valve
36. Aortic valve
37. Left coronary artery
38. Right valvule of aortic valve
39. Right coronary artery
40. Left valvule of aortic valve
41. Left coronary artery
42. Posterior valvule of aortic valve
43. Nodule
44. Aortic sinus
45. Valve of the inferior vena cava

but not to overwork the heart, with due regard to the person's age and previous exercise habits. Exercise is discussed at length in chapter 52, volume 1.

Sometimes in older people the coronary arteries become diseased and unable to carry their usual amount of blood. Such deterioration is serious because it deprives the heart muscle of its quota of blood sugar and oxygen. Sometimes disease of the coronary system causes an artery to become plugged up suddenly. This sudden loss of blood to a part of the heart's wall may cause the heart to lose its efficiency. This is the cause of death in cases of fatal "heart attack."

Each side of the heart contains two chambers. The chambers of the right side receive the blood which comes back from all parts of the body. This blood is brought to the heart by two large veins. One vein, the superior vena cava, brings blood from the head and arms. The other, the inferior vena cava, brings blood from the body and legs. The blood in these veins has already given up most of its supply of oxygen and is loaded with carbon dioxide.

Coming in through the large veins, blood first enters the upper chamber called the right atrium. (See accompanying diagram.) The right atrium sends the blood on into the right ventricle, which has a valve at its inlet and another at its outlet. The inlet valve keeps the blood from flowing backward into the right atrium. The outlet valve keeps the blood from flowing back into the right ventricle after it has been pumped out into the pulmonary artery.

The pulmonary artery and its branches carry the blood from the right side of the heart to both of the lungs. In the lungs, the blood exchanges its load of carbon dioxide for a new supply of oxygen. The blood is then carried by pulmonary veins to the left side of the heart—first to the left atrium, from which it passes to the left ventricle. The left ventricle has more heart muscle in its wall than any of the other chambers of the heart. This is needed

because the left ventricle must pump very forcefully in order to send blood out to all parts of the body. The left ventricle has a valve controlling its inlet and another controlling its outlet, which work much like the corresponding valves of the right ventricle.

The Heart Sounds

When a doctor listens to your heart through a stethoscope, he hears it beating in rhythmic fashion. The heartbeat gives a double sound which is classically described as lubb-*dup*. After this double sound, there is an interval of quiet and then the lubb-*dup* occurs again: lubb-*dup*—lubb-*dup*—lubb-*dup*. The "lubb" sound is produced by the closing of the valves between the atria and the ventricles. That is, when the

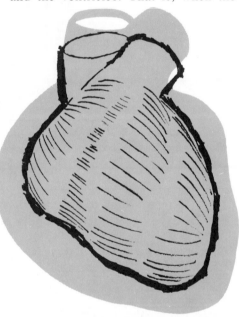

As muscular wall of heart contracts, the size of the heart changes.

ventricles begin to contract, the increased pressure causes the blood in them to back up against their inlet valves and close them. As the ventricles continue to contract, they force the blood in them out into large arteries—the pulmonary artery and the

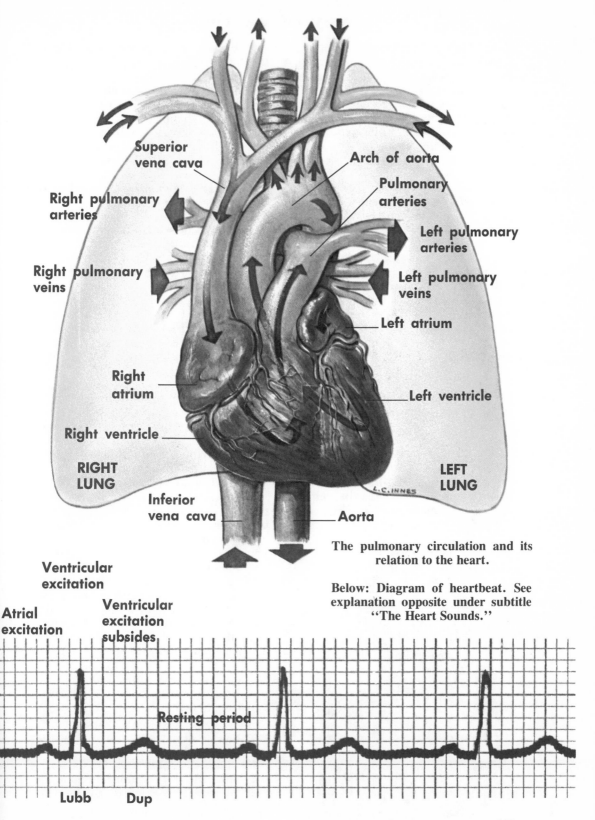

Superior vena cava

Arch of aorta

Pulmonary arteries

Right pulmonary arteries

Left pulmonary arteries

Right pulmonary veins

Left pulmonary veins

Left atrium

Right atrium

Left ventricle

Right ventricle

RIGHT LUNG

LEFT LUNG

Inferior vena cava

Aorta

The pulmonary circulation and its relation to the heart.

Below: Diagram of heartbeat. See explanation opposite under subtitle "The Heart Sounds."

Ventricular excitation

Ventricular excitation subsides

Atrial excitation

Resting period

Lubb   Dup

aorta. Then as the ventricles relax in preparation for their next contraction, the blood which has been forced out into the arteries backs up against the outlet valves, closing them. It is the close of the outlet valves that accounts for the *"dup."* It is during the interval between one lubb-*dup* and the next that the heart rests.

Arteries, Capillaries, and Veins

The left ventricle pumps its blood into the aorta, which is the body's largest artery. The aorta branches so as to carry blood to all parts of the body. The branches of an artery are smaller, of course, than the parent vessel. Finally the branches become so tiny that the blood cells have to pass through them in single file. These very smallest blood vessels are called capillaries. There are many billions of capillaries in one person's body. If they were placed end to end to make a single tube, the capillaries from one adult's body would reach more than twice around the earth.

Cross section of the artery and the small vein. A. Artery. B. Vein. a. Muscular membrane much thicker in artery than in vein. b. Internal membrane. c. External membrane.

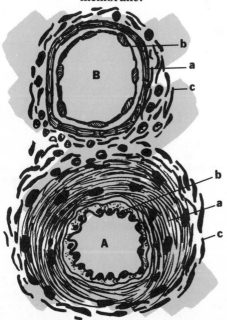

The walls of arteries are composed largely of smooth muscle and elastic connective tissue. This allows for considerable change in the caliber of these blood vessels and, as naturally follows, for considerable change in the amount of blood which can flow through them. The need for such a change will appear more clearly as this discussion continues.

The walls of capillaries are composed mostly of a single layer of endothelial cells. They are so thin that oxygen and food substances pass through easily.

The capillaries do not have either smooth-muscle tissue or elastic fibers in their walls, so they do not change much in caliber. But they can be taken out of, or put back into, service as the needs of the tissue require. The more active the tissue, the greater the number of capillaries in service. When a tissue is relatively inactive, capillaries take turns, in relays, as they care for the tissue's transportation needs. The mechanism of control by which certain capillaries rest while others continue to carry blood is probably by a selective contraction of smooth muscle in the walls of the small arteries at the junction between artery and capillary.

As soon as the blood has passed through the capillaries it starts on its way back to the heart. All vessels that carry blood toward the heart are called veins. The walls of veins are much thinner than the walls of arteries. These walls also have smooth muscle and elastic fibrous tissue in them, but less of it. In a healthy body all the veins are carrying blood all the time, but sometimes they may be almost collapsed and at other times fully distended. Their walls can stretch enough to enable the veins to carry back to the heart all the blood that the arteries and capillaries can bring to them.

Most veins have small valves built into their walls. These valves tend to keep the blood from flowing backward. As you exercise, your muscles squeeze the veins, and the blood inside them is caused to move toward the heart.

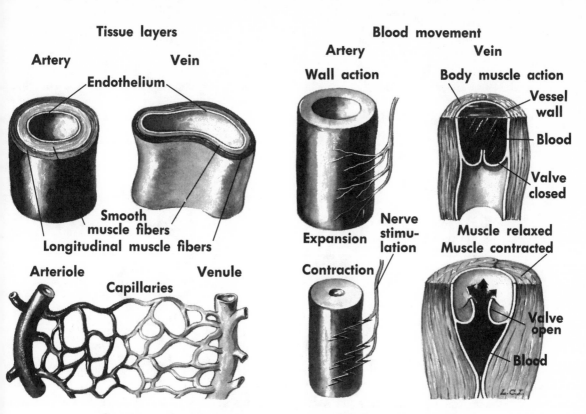

Tissue layers

Artery
Endothelium

Vein

Smooth muscle fibers

Longitudinal muscle fibers

Arteriole

Venule

Capillaries

Blood movement

Artery
Wall action

Expansion

Contraction

Nerve stimulation

Vein
Body muscle action

Vessel wall

Blood

Valve closed

Muscle relaxed
Muscle contracted

Valve open

Blood

L-C.T.

Composite showing three aspects of blood's transportation system: tissue layers of artery and vein; movement of blood through artery and vein; the capillary system.

Then, as your muscles relax, new blood flows in to fill the veins again. This is another reason why it is important to keep your muscles in good condition by taking daily exercise. When your muscles act, they help your blood to move faster on its way toward the heart.

As a barber stands quietly by his chair, the blood in the veins of his legs tends to stagnate. Because he is in a standing position, the blood is not easily lifted back up to the level of his heart. The weight of this column of blood gradually stretches the walls of the veins in his legs until the valves cannot close properly. A vein thus stretched and enlarged is called a varicose vein. (See more on this in chapter 9, volume 2.) Not only barbers but other people whose work requires them to stand for long periods in one location, should make it a point to sit down or lie down occasionally, or to walk about a bit when they can during their working hours, as a means of helping to keep their leg veins in good condition.

Blood Pressure

The arteries of the body have thicker walls than the veins. Larger arteries have thicker walls than small ones. These walls must be thick because the blood as it leaves the heart is under high pressure. The pumping action of the heart is what builds up the pressure of the blood. This pressure is necessary in order to force the blood quickly to all parts of the body. At each beat of the heart, the arteries are stretched a little as they receive a new quantity of blood. You can feel the pulsation caused by each beat of your heart by pressing your finger over the radial artery in your wrist (on the thumb side of the wrist). Counting the pulse at the wrist is the usual means by which a doctor or nurse can tell how fast the

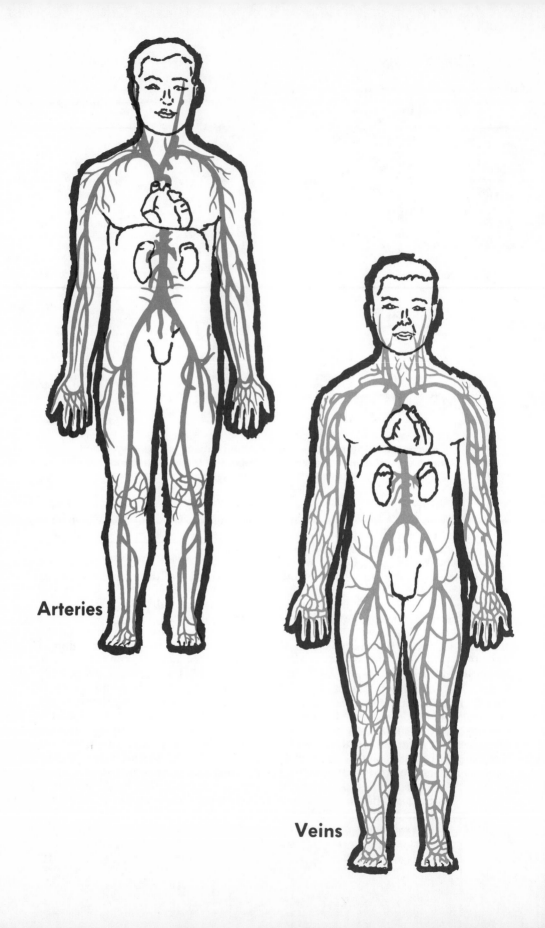

Arteries

Veins

heart is beating. Between beats, the elasticity of the walls of the arteries maintains enough pressure to keep the blood moving.

When a doctor examines a patient, he is interested, among other things in finding out how high his blood pressure is. In order to measure the blood pressure, the doctor places an inflatable cuff around the patient's arm and inflates the cuff with air. As the cuff becomes tighter and tighter, it finally squeezes the arm so tightly that the blood can no longer pass through the artery to reach the forearm. The blood-pressure instrument includes a gauge which tells how much pressure is necessary to keep the blood from coming through the arm's artery. By reading this gauge the doctor determines the patient's blood pressure.

Actually, the doctor takes two readings (the high and the low) when he measures blood pressure. The high pressure is called the systolic pressure and the low reading is called diastolic pressure. The systolic pressure is the highest pressure which the heart produces as it pumps blood into the arteries at the time of a heartbeat. The lowest reading represents the pressure that remains in the arteries just before the next heartbeat takes place.

A normal, healthy young adult whose heart is working properly and whose blood vessels are not diseased usually has a systolic pressure of about 120 and a diastolic pressure of about 80. This is commonly written as 120/80. These figures indicate the height of a column of mercury (measured in millimeters) that this much pressure would support.

By the time the blood reaches the capillaries it is moving slowly. This is fortunate, for the slow movement of blood in the capillaries allows time for the oxygen and food materials to enter the tissues and for the carbon dioxide and other dissolved waste materials to enter the blood. The blood in large arteries may move at a speed of about a hundred feet (30 meters) per minute, which is more than a thousand times as fast as it moves in the capillaries. The blood does not tarry long in the capillaries, for it is due back at its starting point in less than half a minute. A drop of blood takes two seconds or less to pass through its very short capillary pathway at each circuit of the body, the average length of capillaries being about .025 inch (.6 mm.).

As stated before, arteries have smooth muscle in their walls. This makes these walls strong and also provides for change in the size of the arteries. When the smooth muscle in the walls of the arteries contracts, it makes the arteries smaller. When many arteries become smaller, the heart must work harder and the blood pressure therefore rises.

The level of blood pressure throughout the body and the volume of blood flow in local regions of the body are regulated by the precise influence of the autonomic nervous system on the smooth muscle in the walls of the arteries. When need arises for a general increase in blood pressure, the smooth muscle in the arteries throughout the body is contracted. When skeletal muscles are in vigorous use, they require more blood than usual. So the arteries in other parts of the body are constricted, thus directing more blood to the active muscles. During the digestion of food, the digestive organs need more blood. The increase is provided by a reduction of the flow of blood to other parts of the body so that a correspondingly greater volume of blood flows through the digestive organs. When a person is engaged actively in thinking, a greater-than-normal volume of blood flows through his brain.

It is normal for a person's blood pressure to increase during emergencies. This automatic response to an emergency is also brought about by the nerves which go to the smooth muscles in the walls of the arteries. When you become frightened, your blood pressure increases and your heart works harder and more rapidly. This is nature's way of giving you the strength you need at the time of an emergency.

119

Some people, unfortunately, live in a state of emergency most of the time. These are the people who are nervous, anxious, and fearful. The muscles in the walls of their arteries remain contracted most of the time, as if they were facing constant danger. Such people tend to maintain a high blood pressure, which makes their hearts work harder than they should.

Rather frequently in later life the arteries become diseased so that their normal elasticity is decreased, causing what is called arteriosclerosis. This problem involves a partial replacement of muscle tissue by fibrous tissue. It is often combined with a deposit of a fatlike substance called cholesterol on the inner surface of the walls of the arteries. Arteriosclerosis is usually associated with high blood pressure, with a consequent increase in the amount of work the heart must perform.

Under normal resting conditions, the heart of the average adult beats about 72 times per minute, though the rate varies widely in different individuals. During vigorous exercise the rate may increase to as much as 180 beats per minute.

Some of our modern plans for systematic exercise use the heart rate as an index of how much exertion a person's heart can properly tolerate. A formula used by the Cardiac Rehabilitation Center in Quebec specifies that at the beginning of his progressive exercise program a person may safely engage in exercise strenuous enough to increase the number of heartbeats per minute up to 170 minus his age. That is, a person 30 years of age can bring his heart rate by exercise to 140 beats per minute. As tolerance by exercise increases over a period of three months of systematic, daily exercise, the formula changes to 200 minus one's age so that the 30-year-old person may now safely exercise to increase his heart rate to 170 beats per minute. The formula applies in the case of older persons as well as to those in young adulthood.

A person whose heart is not acting normally should avoid excessive exercise, because this increases the work which his heart must do. In a normal person, it is not hard work which damages his heart so much as it is sudden exertion without "warming up." One unaccustomed to vigorous exercise can easily strain his heart by sudden hard work or play. But when he builds up his muscular activity gradually, his heart accommodates well to the increased work load.

The Blood

The blood consists of blood cells and plasma. The plasma is the liquid portion of the blood in which the cells float.

There are two kinds of blood cells— red and white. The red blood cells differ radically from the white cells. In the first place, the red cells are much more numerous. It is estimated that the average adult man has between twenty-five and thirty trillion red cells in his blood. They outnumber the white cells by about seven hundred times. A second difference is that the red cells contain hemoglobin—that marvelous, red, iron-containing substance that carries oxygen to the tissues and aids in the transport of carbon dioxide from the tissues back to the lungs. It is the large number of red cells, each containing hemoglobin, which gives the blood its red color. A third difference is that the red cells have already lost their nuclei by the time they are found in the blood, while the white cells still have their nuclei.

Red blood cells are produced in the bone marrow. More than 200 billion new red cells must be produced daily in order to replace those that wear out. And to ensure that they will be in good working condition, an adequate supply of iron must be available. The figure 200 billion is easy to say or write, but it is hard to comprehend, especially when it refers to work done in the seemingly quiet bone marrow. Figure it out for yourself and you will see that 200 billion per day means about two and a half million every second. This and many

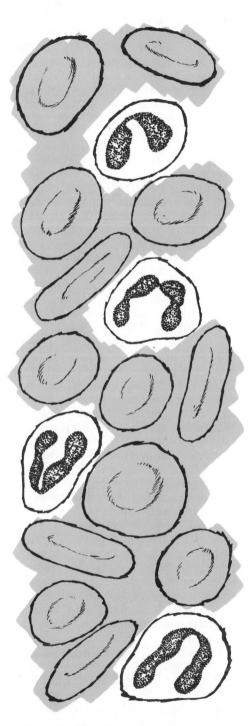

other known facts about the activities of living bodies are almost incredible when we first learn of them, and we ought never to let them be taken just for granted.

Some of the white cells are produced in the bone marrow, and some are made in the lymph nodes or other lymphoid tissue. Their life is shorter than that of red cells. They constitute part of the body's police force. They go to all parts of the body hunting for trouble, and they often die fighting. In cases of infection or injury to the tissues, the white cells gather in large numbers to help prevent the spread of the infection or to aid in the process of healing.

In addition to its red and white cells, the blood contains many small fragments of cells, called platelets. These too are produced in the marrow of the bones. The function of platelets is to help in blood clotting. When a blood vessel is broken or injured, permitting the loss of blood, the platelets accumulate at the site of the damage. Many of them break apart and release a special chemical substance which they contain. This stimulates the formation of tiny threads of fibrin, which is a protein material in the blood. The tangled mass of fibrin threads entraps blood cells in its meshes, and together with them forms the clot, which then prevents further loss of blood from the broken vessel.

The red blood cells are small, but not as small as the platelets. Red blood cells are so small that a row of 65 of them could hide behind the period at the end of this sentence. It would take 3,500 red cells lying side by side to make a line one inch (2.5 cm.) long. The white cells average somewhat larger, so that about 2,500 white cells side by side would extend this same distance. Red cells are disc-shaped; white cells are roughly spherical.

Red cells live from 100 to 125 days after they are produced by the bone marrow. Some of them apparently break down while floating in the bloodstream. Others are removed by the

Interspersed among the red blood cells are four white blood cells with their typically odd-shaped nuclei.

121

spleen. This organ is located beneath the diaphragm, close under the edge of the ribs on the left side. It is a mystery how the spleen can separate the worn-out red blood cells from those in good condition and dispose of them while keeping about 85 percent of the iron which they contain from being lost.

The spleen can act as a part of the body's transportation system in still another way. It is a fairly large organ and contains a considerable amount of blood at any one time. In case of loss of blood, as in severe hemorrhage, the outer covering of the spleen contracts strongly and forces extra blood into general circulation to help take the place of what has been lost. In this sense, the spleen acts as an emergency organ.

The reader can probably remember a childhood experience of getting a "side ache" when running or otherwise exercising violently, or at least he can remember hearing others complain of getting one. In such a case, the pain is caused by the contraction of the outer covering of the spleen to force out blood to help the muscles presently working so hard. Usually the tendency to have such side aches decreases as adult years arrive.

Sometimes there are not enough red cells to carry sufficient oxygen to the tissues, or perhaps the red cells are low in hemoglobin. Such a condition is called anemia. One kind of anemia occurs when a person loses much blood.

The time required for the blood-forming tissues to replace the lost blood cells depends, of course, on the amount of blood that was lost.

Another kind of anemia results when a person does not have enough iron in his body. Iron is required to build hemoglobin. When short of hemoglobin, red cells are not able to carry as much oxygen as they should. A balanced diet contains enough iron to meet the body's requirements. Egg yolk is a good source of iron. So are dried fruits, leafy vegetables, dried peas and beans, and whole-grain cereals.

Still another kind of anemia is called pernicious anemia. This kind results when the bone marrow does not have a sufficient supply of vitamin B_{12}. When this happens, the marrow does not produce enough red cells to meet the body's needs. Also, many of those which are produced have peculiar shape and odd sizes.

The natural sources of vitamin B_{12} are the foods of animal origin, including whole milk and eggs. Pernicious anemia is not caused by a dietary deficiency, however, but by an inherited defect in the ability to absorb vitamin B_{12} from the intestine. The treatment and continued prevention of pernicious anemia, once the disease is established, requires the administration of large doses of vitamin B_{12} by intramuscular injection. Two or three injections per week are usually given until the disease is controlled and then at least once a month for the remainder of life.

Thus far, we have said more about the cells of the blood than we have about the plasma—the fluid part of the blood. The plasma by itself is straw-colored. It contains many chemical substances needed by the tissues. It is the plasma that carries glucose to the muscles to help them produce energy. It carries fat and protein substances needed for tissue building. It carries waste products from the tissues to the skin and kidneys. It carries the minerals, hormones, and enzymes needed both for tissue building and for regulation of the vital processes. It carries disease-fighting antibodies, some of which—perhaps most—are produced in the lymphoid tissues of the body. It carries some of the chemical substances which, in addition to the blood platelets, are important in blood clotting.

When blood is drawn from a person's vein and placed in a test tube or other container, the blood soon clots. Presently this clot shrinks and there escapes from the clot a straw-color fluid called serum. Blood serum differs from blood plasma only in that the serum does not contain those substances present in plasma which contribute to the formation of a blood clot.

Blood Types

Even though the blood from one person looks just like that from any other person, there are some differences. Persons of the same race or even of the same family may have different "types" of blood. The type of your blood can be determined only by a careful examination in the laboratory.

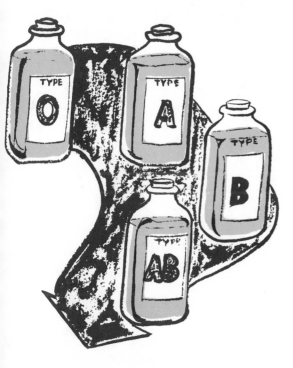

Blood is commonly classified according to four types.

The four common blood types are named by using letters of the alphabet: type A, type B, type AB, and type O. Every person should know the type of his own blood so that in case of emergency he can receive the proper type of blood by transfusion or can safely give blood to someone else who needs it. Doctors know which types of blood can safely be mixed when transfusions are given. Receiving the wrong type of blood may even be fatal.

Most people's blood contains a factor which scientists call the "Rh factor." About 85 percent of the people in the United States have this factor in their blood and are therefore said to be "Rh positive." The Rh factor occurs in about this percentage of all persons of all four blood types. This means that about 15 percent of the people are Rh negative because their blood does not contain this particular factor.

A person who is Rh negative cannot tolerate Rh positive blood, should it be given to him as a transfusion. If such a mistake should be made, much damage to the kidneys would result, with possible death. The reason an Rh negative person cannot tolerate Rh positive blood is that the Rh negative person builds up in his body antibodies which destroy the cells of the Rh positive blood.

A serious complication may develop when a woman with Rh negative blood becomes pregnant with a child who happens to have Rh positive blood. See chapter 3, volume 1, and chapter 10, this volume.

Hemotherapy (Blood Transfusion)

In case of severe hemorrhage or injury with great loss of blood, the lost blood must be restored if the patient's life is to be saved. With the loss of a large volume of blood sufficient number of red blood cells might not be left to carry the amount of oxygen which the patient's tissues require. The doctor then orders a transfusion of blood. This procedure calls for taking blood drawn from some healthy person and introducing it into a vein of the patient.

Often the situation doesn't allow time enough to find a person with just the type of blood that the patient requires. So most cities have blood banks with a supply of the various types of blood. The type needed for a blood transfusion in any particular case can be quickly supplied.

Human blood cannot be manufactured outside the human body. Healthy people interested in helping to save lives therefore donate blood to be

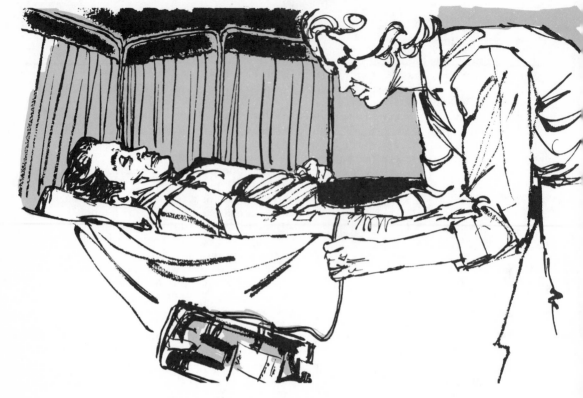

**Human donors are the only source of blood for
patients needing transfusions.**

stored in blood banks for emergencies. The average adult can give about one pint (450 ml.) of blood at a time without endangering his health, provided he does not do so too often.

Conclusion

Having given so much attention to the fluid part of the body's transportation system, let us briefly reconsider where this fluid goes, what it picks up or unloads at each station, and what happens to the cargo. Parts of this story have already been told in this chapter. That is, blood comes to the right side of the heart through two large veins: one from the upper part of the body and the other from the lower part. Next it goes to the lungs, and then comes back again to the heart, but this time to its left side. Then it goes through the aorta and its branches to all parts of the body,

and back again through the two large veins to the right side of the heart.

When the blood arrives at the right side of the heart, it is carrying carbon dioxide and other wastes which it has picked up in the tissues. When it arrives in the lungs, it unloads its carbon dioxide and picks up oxygen, but keeps its other wastes. When it leaves the left side of the heart and arrives at the tissues, it unloads the oxygen and picks up a new load of carbon dioxide, and also picks up more of the other wastes.

So far as carbon dioxide and oxygen are concerned, this is all of the transportation story. But think a moment. What about other wastes? And what about the food materials that the tissues need? During every circuit, part of the blood goes through the skin and part of it through the kidneys. The skin throws off a small part of the wastes in the sweat. The kidneys take off a much larger part and get rid of it in the urine.

During every circuit, part of the blood goes through the digestive organs and the liver. When food is being digested, the blood picks up simple food elements as it passes through the digestive organs. These elementary food elements include glucose (from digested carbohydrate), fatty acids (from digested fat), and amino acids (from digested protein). The blood carries these to the liver where some are reconstituted in harmony with the body's needs, some are passed on to other organs and tissues. When there is an excess of glucose beyond the body's present needs for energy fuel, this is converted to fat and stored as such in various outlying tissues.

Diseases of the Heart

More people suffer and die from heart disease than from any other ailment. One out of every eight adults in the United States has some form of heart ailment. Some forms of heart disease strike suddenly, causing premature death or invalidism. Others allow their victims to linger for years with reduced vitality.

It is coronary heart disease—the one that causes the typical "heart attack"—that accounts for the greatest number of deaths from heart disease. We will give coronary heart disease its proper emphasis later in the chapter.

CONGENITAL HEART DISEASE

The heart develops very early in the life history of a human being. At about three weeks after conception, the heart consists of a single tube which pulsates. It is during the next five weeks (weeks 3 to 8 following conception) that the heart becomes a four-chambered organ. The wonder of it is that it is able to continue pumping blood while still undergoing the marvelous transformation from a simple tube to a four-chambered organ.

Considering its complex plan of development, it is not surprising that mishaps occur from time to time which result in malformations of various features of the heart and of the large blood vessels. About nine out of every thousand babies born have some deformity of the heart or the large vessels adjacent to it.

There are many types of congenital heart disease, and the degree of handicap from these varies from person to person. Many cases can be greatly improved and lives extended by modern heart surgery.

For a more complete discussion of congenital heart disease see chapter 17, volume 1.

RHEUMATIC HEART DISEASE

Rheumatic heart disease is a serious complication of rheumatic fever. As discussed in chapter 17, volume 1, rheumatic fever often follows an attack of streptococcic sore throat or some other form of streptococcal infection. Once a child has had rheumatic fever, the probability exists that he will have other attacks from time to time. Suitable preparations of antibiotics help to prevent these recurring attacks.

During an attack of rheumatic fever there is a strong possibility that the heart will become inflamed. This may take the form of (1) *endocarditis* (inflammation of the lining of the heart or of the valves), (2) *pericarditis* inflammation of the covering of the heart), or (3) *myocarditis* (inflammation of the heart muscle).

A streptococcic infection such as

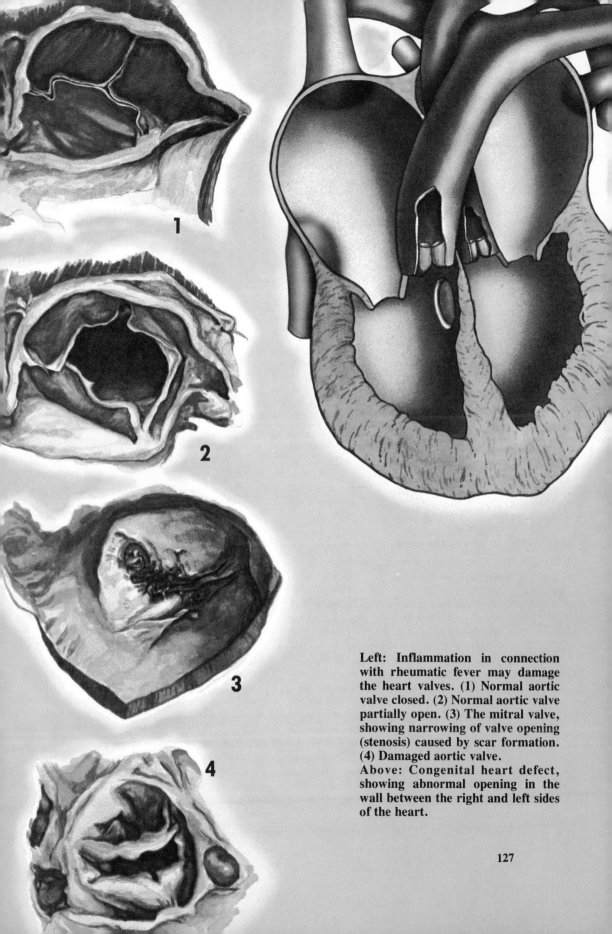

Left: Inflammation in connection with rheumatic fever may damage the heart valves. (1) Normal aortic valve closed. (2) Normal aortic valve partially open. (3) The mitral valve, showing narrowing of valve opening (stenosis) caused by scar formation. (4) Damaged aortic valve.

Above: Congenital heart defect, showing abnormal opening in the wall between the right and left sides of the heart.

127

streptococcal sore throat does not always produce a typical case of rheumatic fever. Such an infection may cause damage to the heart without passing through the stage of rheumatic fever. Thus, the prevention of rheumatic heart disease requires prompt and adequate treatment of all streptococcal infections when they occur. Once the heart becomes thus involved, there is danger of permanent damage to its tissues.

The valves of the heart are delicate structures covered on each surface with the heart's lining membrane. The inflammation of endocarditis typically causes ulcerations of the valves. As the acute stage gradually passes and the ulcerations heal, two defects may result: (1) a narrowing of the valve opening caused by scar formation and (2) an incompetency of the valve because its leaflets no longer fit perfectly when they contact each other. A narrowing of the valve opening is called stenosis. An incomplete closing of the valve, which permits some of the blood to flow in reverse direction, constitutes insufficiency. The valve more frequently affected by rheumatic heart disease is the inlet valve of the left ventricle (the mitral valve).

Care and Treatment

Once the valves of the heart have become damaged, the heart's efficiency may be so reduced that it can no longer keep up with the demands upon it. This deficiency may result in disturbed functions of the heart such as atrial fibrillation or in so-called congestive heart failure, both discussed later in this chapter.

Inasmuch as rheumatic heart disease is a complication of rheumatic fever and inasmuch as rheumatic fever is caused by an infection by the streptococcus germ, the treatment consists essentially of combating the streptococcal infection. This requires the aggressive and continuing use of antibiotic medications as prescribed in chapter 17, volume 1.

In the chronic phase of rheumatic heart disease, which may continue into adulthood, it is advisable to consider surgical repair or even the replacement of a damaged heart valve. Physicians specializing in diseases of the heart and in heart surgery should be consulted.

INFECTIVE ENDOCARDITIS (BACTERIAL ENDOCARDITIS)

Infective endocarditis is a serious disease which, if untreated, is uniformly fatal. The essential feature of the disease is the establishment of a colony of germs in some area of the lining of the heart. The disease was formerly called bacterial endocarditis because the colony of germs that becomes established within the heart was thought to consist always of bacteria. It is now recognized that in occasional cases the infection may be caused by fungi or other disease-producing germs.

There are two types of infective endocarditis, acute and subacute. The acute type is caused by more aggressive, more virulent germs and, if untreated, will run a course of not more than six weeks before causing death. The subacute type is caused by organisms which are more leisurely in producing tissue damage, which cause milder symptoms, but which are just as deadly in the long run as those which cause the acute form of the disease.

Predisposing Circumstances. In order for infective endocarditis to develop, there must first be germs in the blood (bacteremia). The germs then lodge in the delicate tissue which lines the heart (the endocardium). If, for any reason, the endocardium is already blemished, the germs establish at the blemished sites. Such blemishes may consist of (1) congenital defects, (2) heart valves that were damaged by some previous illness (as rheumatic fever), or (3) scars from previous heart surgery. But there are cases of infective endocarditis in which the heart's lining was normal and still a colony of germs lodged there. These are cases (as in drug addicts who use the needle) in which the germs are especially virulent or in which the individual's resistance to infection is at low ebb.

What causes bacteremia? In the normal course of events germs that find their way into the body's tissues are filtered out by the lymph nodes before they have opportunity to enter the circulating blood. But even when a few germs find their way into the blood, there are provisions for destroying or removing them. This is one of the functions of the spleen, where part of the blood filters through this organ continuously. There are also specialized cells belonging to the body's systems of defense located in such organs as the liver that serve to entrap or engulf germs that may be present in the blood as it circulates. But under occasional circumstances germs enter the blood in such large numbers as to temporarily overwhelm the body's provision for eliminating them. It is then that germs may colonize in the lining of the heart.

The type of pneumonia caused by the pneumococcus germ allows large numbers of this germ to be discharged into the blood as it circulates through the lungs. Dental procedures such as the extraction of teeth or the "scaling" of teeth in which the gum margins are partially separated from the teeth, may permit germs already present in the mouth to enter directly into the bloodstream. Surgical procedures such as tonsillectomy, surgery involving the digestive organs, rectal surgery, and the surgical removal of the prostate gland carry the possibility of introducing germs into the blood. Childbirth occasions the same possibility. Victims of drug abuse are particularly susceptible to bacteremia because of their careless use of the hypodermic needle for injection directly into a vein. Inadequate treatment of pimples and boils may permit germs to enter the blood.

Precaution to prevent infective endocarditis. With respect to prevention we have three questions to answer: (a) Who should take precaution? (b) When should precaution be taken? and (c) Of what does the precaution consist?

a. *Who should take precaution?*— Those who have had any form of congenital heart disease; those who have had previous heart surgery; and those who have had a previous streptococcal infection such as streptococcal sore throat or rheumatic fever by which the heart's lining or the heart valves may have been damaged.

b. *When should the precaution be taken?*—Whenever there is the possibility of the release of germs into the blood, as at the time of dental procedures such as extractions and dental prophylaxis ("scaling"); at the time of such surgical procedures as tonsillectomy, rectal surgery, surgery on the digestive organs, or removal of the prostate gland; at the time of childbirth; during an attack of pneumococcal pneumonia; when there are penetrating injuries as caused by accidents; and when there are skin infections, such as boils or carbuncles.

c. *Of what does the precaution consist?*—The administration of an antibiotic medication, under a doctor's direction, throughout the period of time that germs may be released into the blood.

Symptoms of infective endocarditis. The symptoms of acute and subacute infective endocarditis are similar, except that the onset of the acute form is abrupt with severe symptoms as contrasted with the gradual onset of vague symptoms resembling "flu" in the subacute form of the disease. In both forms there is fever, with a higher fever (up to 105° F. [40.6° C.]) in the acute form. This high fever often remits and then returns. The high fever is often accompanied by sweating. Many petechiae develop in the skin in both forms of the disease. These are small, round, purplish-red spots in the skin and the membranes, caused by the leakage of small amounts of blood into the tissue spaces.

In many cases of infective endocarditis the colony of germs responsible for the disease is located at one of the heart valves. Then the physician, as he listens to the heart through his stethoscope, may hear an altered sound described as a "heart murmur."

When a heart valve is the site of an infection there usually develops at this site a modified blood clot called a "vegetation." A vegetation is fragile, and portions may break away and be carried by the blood to distant parts of the body. These vegetations contain germs, and when the broken fragment (called an embolus) lodges, it not only plugs the vessel in which it is lodged, but it also propagates the infection at this new location. An embolus may lodge in most any part of the body, and so the symptoms of this complication vary, depending on whether the embolus lodges in the brain or in the kidneys, in the vessels supplying the intestine, in the spleen, in the lung, or in some of the arteries supplying the extremities. For example, when the kidneys are thus involved, blood may appear in the urine. When the brain is involved, symptoms may resemble those of stroke.

Care and Treatment

Both types of infective endocarditis are uniformly fatal if not treated. The treatment must therefore be prompt, intensive, and continued for four to six weeks. This is one of the diseases in which the use of proper antibiotic medications has proved to be truly lifesaving. But the choice of the particular antibiotic medicine to be used depends on determining first the exact kind of germ responsible for the illness. Inasmuch as the infection is being carried by the blood, samples of blood must be cultured in the laboratory to determine the exact nature of the infection. With this information at hand, the doctor then chooses the antibiotic best suited to combat the infection. Usually the fever begins to disappear within three to seven days after the start of the treatment. If the intensive treatment is stopped too soon, there is danger of recurrence.

ISCHEMIC HEART DISEASE AND ANGINA PECTORIS

The heart's continuous activity requires that its own tissues receive an adequate supply of fresh blood. This is provided through the coronary arteries which branch and rebranch on the external surface of the heart, with the terminal branches penetrating the heart's wall to supply the muscle which contracts with each heartbeat. When a person exercises vigorously, the volume of blood supplied to the heart's own tissues may be as much as five times as great as when the person is at rest.

The muscle composing the wall of the heart is a special kind of muscle (cardiac muscle). It differs from the skeletal muscle such as moves the arms and legs in that the cardiac muscle is not capable of storing energy for future use. The heart muscle must receive its quota of oxygen and food materials moment by moment. This situation calls for mention of the problems that develop when the blood supply to the heart is curtailed:

The term ischemic heart disease has been coined for those conditions in which the blood supply to the heart is in short supply, the word *ischemia* meaning a condition of reduced blood supply.

The usual cause of ischemia in the heart is the development of arteriosclerosis in the coronary arteries which supply the heart. Arteriosclerosis reduces the caliber of these vessels so that they cannot transmit as great a volume of blood as normally. Such vessels can satisfy the heart's needs when the individual is at rest. But when he exercises, the heart muscle is deprived of the amount of oxygen and food materials which it then requires. This is when symptoms develop.

In some cases the reduction in blood supply to the heart's muscle is caused by a spasm of the coronary arteries rather than by arteriosclerosis in these vessels. Time was when medical scientists expressed doubt that temporary constriction of the coronary arteries

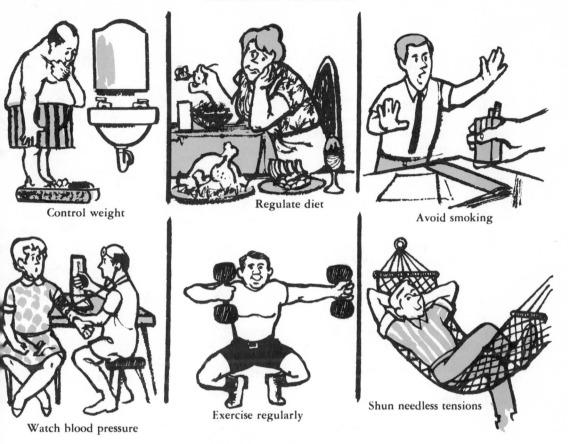

Control weight

Regulate diet

Avoid smoking

Watch blood pressure

Exercise regularly

Shun needless tensions

Safeguards against heart trouble.

occurred. Modern methods of examining the coronary arteries have indicated, however, that spasm does actually occur, even to the extent of reducing significantly the amount of blood carried to the heart muscle. There may be several causes for these attacks of spasm of the coronary arteries, among them being the psychological stress of unsolved problems and the use of cigarettes.

We have mentioned that when the heart muscle does not receive its necessary quota of blood, symptoms develop. The symptoms consist of varying degrees of discomfort, sometimes extreme discomfort, in the central chest, in the arm (most often the left arm), and sometimes in other parts of the body. It is this type of discomfort that constitutes angina pectoris. The reader should note that we have not used the word *pain* in describing this symptom of distress. Some patients with this type of discomfort use the word *pain*, but others describe it as a feeling of pressure. At any rate, in a typical case, the discomfort is extreme and causes the patient to discontinue whatever physical activity has caused the heart to be in short supply of blood.

The symptoms of angina pectoris may be brought on by emotional shock or even by a bad dream in which the person's body reacts as to some sudden emergency. It is in such cases that the basic cause of the discomfort is probably a spasm of the coronary arteries rather than a narrowing because of arteriosclerosis.

Angina pectoris may be mistaken for a genuine heart attack. However, the

Cardiovascular Disorders; Blood Vessel Diseases

A. Cardiovascular Diseases

When we speak of cardiovascular disorders we refer to those conditions in which the heart and/or the blood vessels function abnormally, with the result that the circulation of blood is altered in some unfavorable way. We use the word *cardiovascular* in describing these disorders because the heart (cardio) and the blood vessels (vascular) work together as a functioning unit.

COLD EXTREMITIES (POOR CIRCULATION)

Normal warmth in the hands and feet depends on an adequate circulation of blood through the extremities. A decrease in the flow of blood through these parts may be caused automatically by the body's need to conserve heat, by a decline in the heart's ability to pump blood, or by a reduced capacity of the blood vessels to convey blood. A reduction in blood volume to the arms and legs may be brought about by the action of the nerves as they restrict the size of the blood vessels and reduce the flow of blood, as in emotional tension or when a person is

studying intently. Poor circulation of blood to the hands and feet may occur in shock, in heart disease, in advanced arteriosclerosis, in thromboangiitis obliterans (Buerger's disease), or in Reynaud's disease.

EDEMA (SWELLING OF THE TISSUES)

Edema consists of an accumulation of excess fluid in certain of the body's tissues. The extra fluid accumulates outside of the capillaries in the spaces between the cells. Thus the tissues become soggy and swollen.

Normally, a continual exchange of fluid takes place between the blood within the capillaries and the tissue spaces outside the capillaries. The walls of the capillaries permit water and relatively small molecules of other substances to pass through. Larger protein molecules and blood cells do not normally penetrate the capillary wall. A certain amount of fluid in the tissue spaces enters the lymph vessels instead of reentering the blood capillaries.

Four factors control the balance of fluid which enters and leaves the capil-

141

laries: (1) The osmotic pressure of the blood plasma as compared with that of the tissue fluid. This pressure depends in large part upon the presence of protein molecules (primarily albumin) in the blood plasma. The higher osmotic pressure of the plasma retards the escape of fluid from the capillaries. (2) The height of blood pressure within the capillaries. High blood pressure within the capillaries favors the escape of fluid from the capillaries. (3) The condition of the capillary walls. Only an abnormal capillary wall permits the escape of protein molecules. (4) The capacity of the lymph vessels to carry fluid. When these are obstructed, the fluid which would normally follow this route tends to accumulate in the tissue spaces.

1. *Edema in Heart Disease*. When the heart fails to put out as much blood as the body's tissues require, the kidneys respond by decreasing the volume of fluid they excrete. This increases the volume of total body fluid, with a resulting rise of blood pressure within the capillaries. Then, as mentioned in item number two of the preceding paragraph, edema occurs. The edema (swelling of tissues) is noticed first in the ankles of ambulatory patients and in the sacral region of bed patients. The edema is typically more severe at the end of the day.

2. *Edema in Kidney Disease*. Certain forms of kidney disease allow the escape of albumin from the blood plasma into the urine. Albumin is thus lost from the body faster than it can be replenished. The consequent lowering of the blood's osmotic pressure permits an excess of fluid to escape through the capillary walls into the tissue spaces.

3. *Edema in Cirrhosis of the Liver*. In cirrhosis the liver's production of protein declines, with a consequent lowering of the blood's osmotic pressure. This favors the development of edema. Also, cirrhosis hinders the flow of blood coming to the liver from other abdominal organs and this causes an increase of blood pressure in the capillaries of these organs. This results in an accumulation of fluid in the abdominal cavity (ascites).

4. *Edema in Malnutrition*. Here, the edema is attributed to damage to the capillary wall and to a reduced intake of protein materials from which the albumin of the blood plasma is normally derived.

5. *Edema in Local Inflammation*. Blood tends to stagnate in an inflamed tissue area. The capillary walls are damaged and local swelling occurs.

6. *Edema in Allergy*. The tissue swelling which occurs in various allergic manifestations (hives, hay fever, angioneurotic edema, etc.) is attributed to the effect of histamine (a chemical liberated in the allergic reaction) on the walls of the capillaries.

7. *Edema in Local Injury*. Local injury, whether by mechanical force, heat, or cold, causes damage to the capillaries, with resulting local swelling.

8. *Edema in Poisoning and Toxemia*. Poisonous substances containing arsenic, lead, antimony, gold, or mercury, as well as the toxins produced in such diseases as diphtheria and scarlet fever, damage the capillaries and thus permit the escape of excess fluid into the tissues.

9. *Edema From Obstruction of the Veins*. When the return of blood through a vein is impeded, the consequent increase of blood pressure within the capillaries results in a swelling of all tissues drained by this particular vein. In some cases tumors compress the large veins which enter the heart, and the resulting edema may involve large portions of the body.

10. *Edema From Obstruction of the Lymph Vessels*. The lymph vessels may be obstructed when involved in a region of inflammation, when invaded

by a tumor, or when affected by such a disease as filariasis. With lymph drainage obstructed, fluid accumulates in the tissue spaces, causing edema of the involved portion of the body.

11. *Edema in Anemia*. When anemia becomes so severe as to cause the heart to work beyond its capacity, edema may develop.

12. *Edema in Pregnancy*. Swelling of the ankles often occurs during the last three months of pregnancy. Pressure on the veins which pass through the pelvic region is an important causative factor. Also, in pregnancy, the amount of protein in the blood plasma is often lower than usual.

FAINTING (SYNCOPE)

Fainting involves a temporary loss of consciousness. In its common form it results from reduction in the supply of blood to the brain. It may be caused, however, by anything that interferes with the vital functions of the brain cells, such as deprivation of oxygen.

The usual kind of fainting is triggered by an emotional shock, such as the receiving of bad news, panic (fear), being jostled in a crowd of people, or the sight of blood or torn flesh. A general

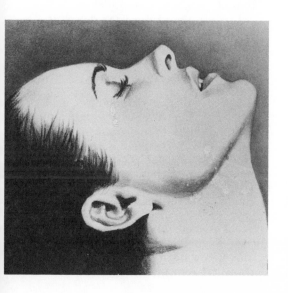

decrease in the volume of circulating blood, such as occurs following a severe hemorrhage, may predispose to fainting. Inadequate action of the heart, as in coronary artery disease, may do the same. Arteriosclerosis of the blood vessels leading to the brain may so reduce the amount of blood to the brain that fainting occurs easily. Reduced capacity of the blood to carry oxygen, as in anemia or carbon monoxide poisoning, may cause fainting. So can also a condition of low blood sugar (as following an overdose of insulin) because of its unfavorable effect on the oxidative processes within the brain cells.

When a person is found unconscious, several other possible conditions in addition to fainting should be considered, because the method of handling the case should be influenced by the real cause. To be differentiated are the unconsciousness of acute alcoholism, of heavy doses of sedatives or tranquilizers, of head injury, of stroke, of an overdose of barbiturates, of epilepsy, of diabetes, and of hysteria.

Care and Treatment

The immediate treatment for the common type of fainting is to put the patient in a horizontal position with the feet elevated slightly above the level of his body, and to apply cold water or a cold compress to the face and head. Tight-fitting clothes at the neck or waist should be loosened. For the first-aid handling of a person who faints, see chapter 23, volume 3.

CIRCULATORY SHOCK

Circulatory shock is a serious condition which develops when the major organs of the body fail to receive an adequate supply of blood. The victim becomes mentally confused or even unconscious. His skin is cold and clammy, his pulse (heartbeat) rapid and weak, and his breathing shallow. He is weak, pale, and restless. If allowed to go untreated the condition of shock becomes progressively more serious until the patient dies from the persisting shock.

The usual circumstances which make it possible for shock to develop are as follows:

1. *Heart failure.* When, for any reason, the heart cannot pump the volume of blood the body needs, shock develops. This problem may occur in connection with a heart attack from coronary heart disease, from functional impairments of the heart itself, or from obstruction (such as pulmonary embolism) of one of the large blood vessels.

2. *Hemorrhage.* In severe injuries so much blood may be lost by hemorrhage that the cells of the body suffer for lack of oxygen, and the victim goes into shock. This deprivation occurs even in internal hemorrhage. A bleeding peptic ulcer, bleeding veins in the esophagus, internal bleeding into the chest cavity, or bleeding from rupture of any of the internal organs causes a reduction of blood in the blood vessels and consequently a reduction in the amount of blood being pumped by the heart. In the case of an internal hemorrhage, the victim may present the same symptoms of shock as though the hemorrhage were external. For further consideration of the first-aid handling of hemorrhage, see chapter 23, volume 3.

3. *Injury.* In some injuries the degree of shock is greater than can be accounted for by the amount of blood lost. In damaged tissue, blood or blood plasma may leak into the tissue spaces as the tissues swell. The amount of circulating blood is thus reduced, and the blood pressure declines.

4. *Infection and Toxemia.* In severe infection the toxins produced by the germs may interfere with the normal control of the caliber of the small blood vessels, allowing them to relax. The blood pressure falls, the rate of blood flow slows down, and the blood supply to the tissues suffers—producing a state of shock. A similar situation obtains in some cases of poisoning.

5. *Burns.* Extensive burns are commonly associated with a condition of shock, because blood volume is reduced by loss of plasma from the burned surfaces. Also, the body's reaction to the tissue damage involved in a burn has the effect of lowering the blood pressure, thus making the victim susceptible to shock.

6. *Psychic Trauma.* Severe emotional shock (as the news of death, fright, severe pain, or unpleasant sights) can make a person so distraught that his autonomic nervous system loses control over the body's smaller vessels. The shock which results compares in some ways to ordinary fainting, except that in this case the condition of shock may persist for a longer time.

Care and Treatment

The definitive treatment for shock from failure of blood circulation consists of treating the underlying condition and, usually, of injecting a blood plasma expander or giving a blood transfusion. Preferably, the patient should be treated by a physician in a hospital. The following suggestions indicate what a first-aider can do until professional help is available:

1. Keep the victim lying down. In order to conserve his strength, all activity must be minimized and even the work of his heart reduced (the reclining position reduces the heart's work load).

2. Elevate the victim's feet and legs. This maneuver encourages the return of blood to the heart.

3. Conserve body heat. Keep the victim warm, particularly in cold weather, by placing him on a blanket or otherwise protecting him from the cold floor or ground. Keep him covered with a blanket or clothing, but avoid overheating him.

4. Keep the victim quiet. Do not move him until the time comes to transport him to the hospital. Avoid

unnecessary conversation.

5. **Administer drinking water cautiously.** If the patient is conscious and vomiting, it is wise to offer him small drinks of water to make up in part for the loss of his body fluids. Give this a sip at a time. Use no alcoholic drinks.

6. **Transport the victim carefully.** Keep him in a reclining position while being transported and avoid all excitement and unnecessary changes in position.

HIGH BLOOD PRESSURE (HYPERTENSION)

High blood pressure is a common disorder, occurring during the lifetime of one out of five Americans. It is not a disease in the sense of being caused by germs or resulting from deterioration of certain of the body's tissues. Rather, it represents the body's response to conditions that trigger a constriction of blood vessels throughout the body and thus increase the heart's work load.

We take high blood pressure so seriously because it sets the stage for certain life-threatening complications such as stroke, heart disease, and kidney failure.

Quite arbitrarily doctors consider blood pressure greater than 160/90 within the range of high blood pressure. To understand these figures we must first consider how blood pressure is measured—the meaning of these two readings, the high and the low. See chapter 7 in this volume.

Average normal blood pressures are lower in children (90/60 at age 6) than in young adults (120/80). The normal range for blood pressure in a healthy young adult is 90 to 140 for the systolic and 60 to 90 for the diastolic. The blood pressure tends to increase slightly as a person becomes older, even though he is in perfectly normal health. Persistent readings above 160 systolic or above 90 diastolic fall into the range of high blood pressure. Notice that we said *persistent* readings above these figures. A single blood pressure reading may not indicate truly a person's actual level of blood pressure. Momentary ex-

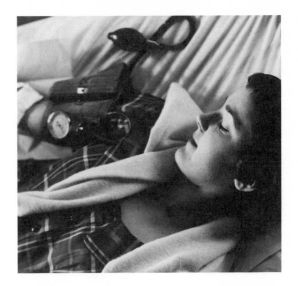

citement or nervousness may shoot the pressure up higher than ordinary. In fact, the temporary elevation of blood pressures is one of the body's normal reactions to stress, excitement, or any emergency. Therefore, a series of at least three blood pressure readings should be taken at different times when the individual is at rest in order to determine his real, average blood pressure.

Many factors may cause a person's blood pressure to remain high, any one of which or any combination of which may be to blame in a given case. Overeating with resultant obesity is a common causative factor. The use of large amounts of salt in the food is a contributing factor, as indicated by the observation that in countries where persons use relatively little salt the incidence of high blood pressure is low. Stress—physical, social, and business—is a factor in producing high blood pressure. The smoking of a single cigarette may temporarily raise the systolic blood pressure between 5 and 10 points. Persistent smoking is a contributing factor to the development of high blood pressure.

Acute infections, such as tonsillitis, sometimes lead to kidney disease, which may bring with it high blood pressure. In some cases the increased pressure is a natural compensatory mechanism to maintain a normal filtration rate through the hardened walls of the small blood vessels in the kidneys. Kidney disease of the slowly progressive type is often accompanied by hardening of the arteries, high blood pressure, and enlargement of the heart. Sudden attacks of convulsions in pregnant women (eclampsia) and other kidney disorders of pregnancy are associated with an increase in blood pressure.

Many cases of high blood pressure are accompanied by practically no telltale symptoms. In fact, blood pressure has been described as the "silent killer." It is therefore wise to make sure that your blood pressure is measured each time you visit the doctor's office.

High blood pressure is typically associated with the development of arteriosclerosis (hardening of the arteries). Therefore the same precautions that a person takes to retard the development of arteriosclerosis are also effective in delaying or preventing the development of high blood pressure. The ideal way of life centers around the maintenance of fitness as described in chapter 52, volume 1.

Care and Treatment

As already stated, the hazard of high blood pressure consists of the risk of life-threatening complications, including stroke, heart disease, and kidney failure. It has been clearly demonstrated that the risk of these complications, even in a person who already has high blood pressure, is greatly reduced when the person follows a care and treatment program that brings his blood pressure into the normal range.

1. First attention should be given to eliminating the conditions that may have contributed to the high blood

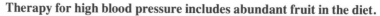

Therapy for high blood pressure includes abundant fruit in the diet.

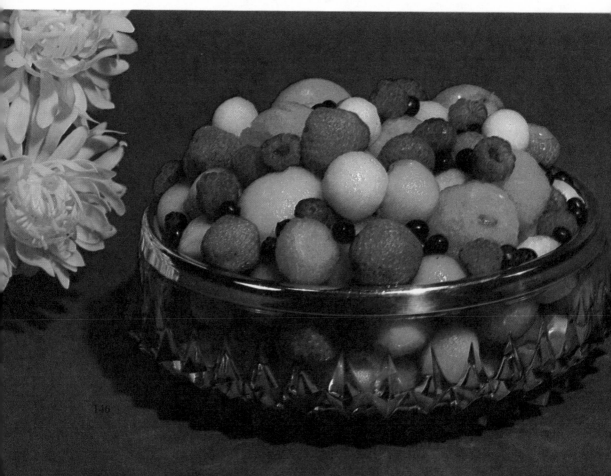

pressure: obesity, excess salt in the diet, the use of foods high in animal fat (which contribute to the development of arteriosclerosis), smoking, lack of physical exercise, and stressful life situations.

2. The person with high blood pressure should place himself under the care of a physician. There are several classes of medications now available that act in one way or another to reduce blood pressure. Success in using them requires that the patient follow the doctor's directions carefully and that he report at frequent intervals so that the doctor can modify his program as may be indicated. Lowering the blood pressure too rapidly should be avoided, for the heart and kidneys have already adjusted themselves to the increased pressure.

3. When taking medications to lower one's blood pressure, it is important that these medications should not be discontinued without the doctor's knowledge. Sudden discontinuance may cause the blood pressure to rebound to its former high level.

LOW BLOOD PRESSURE (HYPOTENSION)

Modest degrees of low blood pressure (with the systolic pressure no lower than 90) occur quite commonly in persons perfectly normal in health. The lives of such persons will not be shortened by their having low blood pressure.

Greater degrees of low blood pressure may be caused by an impoverished diet, by the presence of some chronic wasting disease, by disturbances in the adrenal glands or the pituitary gland, or by problems in which the autonomic nervous control of the blood vessels is defective. Some such cases may exhibit symptoms of weakness, fatigability, headache, shortness of breath, dizziness, inability to concentrate, and digestive disturbances. Of course, such symptoms are not limited to cases with low blood pressure, and therefore it is necessary for a

physician to determine the actual cause of such symptoms.

Care and Treatment

In cases with significant low blood pressure, the treatment consists of removing the cause, once this has been determined by the physician. In mild cases, where no specific cause is known, attention to the development of fitness as mentioned in chapter 52, volume 1, should be of help.

B. Blood Vessel Diseases

The preceding chapter emphasized the dependence of all parts of the body on a continuous flow of blood. It is the circulating blood that brings to all tissues their constant supply of oxygen and food material and removes, as it flows along, the waste products that the body's cells produce.

The heart does not alone perform these important tasks. It takes the blood vessels—arteries, capillaries, and veins—to convey the stream of blood which the heart propels. When an artery is affected by disease, the part of the body which receives the blood conveyed by this vessel will suffer accordingly. We speak of coronary heart disease as a major killer. Recall that the basic cause of this type of heart disease is an inability of the coronary arteries to supply the heart's muscle with a sufficient amount of blood. Any other organ of the body will be similarly handicapped if its supply of blood is reduced.

In the remainder of this chapter we deal with the various kinds of disease that may affect the body's blood vessels.

ARTERIOSCLEROSIS (HARDENING OF THE ARTERIES)

Medical science uses two terms somewhat interchangeably when referring to hardening of the arteries—arteriosclerosis and atherosclerosis. In this set of books we have deliberately chosen to use the term arteriosclerosis because of its broader scope in referring to the degenerative changes that occur in the body's arteries.

Atherosclerosis, the more limited term, refers particularly to the changes that occur in the innermost layer of the arteries—the layer next to the flowing blood.

In order to understand the impairment that takes place in arteriosclerosis we must understand the structure of the artery. The normal, healthy artery is lined by a single layer of flattened cells so smooth on the surface next to the flowing blood that the bloodstream flows along without turbulence. This lining layer of cells (called endothelium) normaly forms a fluid-tight seal so that even the blood plasma does nost pass through it, this in contrast to the condition in the capillaries, where the fluid portion of the blood can pass between the cells that line the capillaries. A layer of delicate muscle (smooth muscle) immediately surrounds the lining layer of endothelium.

Presumably the first thing that hap-pens in a previously normal artery as arteriosclerosis develops is some form of damage to the lining cells, or endothelium, such as high blood pressure may inflict. Once damaged, the endothelial lining cells permit the fluid portion of the blood to penetrate into the surrounding layer of delicate muscle cells. The blood platelets, the tiny packages of chemical substances always found in the circulating blood, are attracted to these sites of damage, and there they liberate a chemical substance that reacts with cholesterol (a normal constituent of the blood plasma). This chemical reaction stimulates the muscle cells, which then begin to increase in number and bulge into the lumen of the artery. Some of the cholesterol is deposited among these newly formed muscle cells to form plaques (hard thickenings of the lining of the artery). It is these firm plaques that are responsible for the condition called hardening of the arteries.

The increase in the number of muscle

An arteriosclerotic plaque developing within an artery. (a) Early stage of development. (b) The plaque enlarges and a blood clot (thrombus) forms on its surface. The lumen of the artery is narrowed. (c) A portion of the thrombus may break away forming an embolus which will then lodge in one of the artery's branches causing an embolism of the tissue served by this branch.

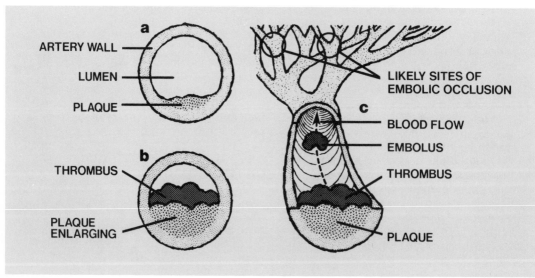

cells, along with the formation of the cholesterol-filled plaques, encroaches on the lumen of the artery, making it smaller. The wall of the artery is weakened by this development. Its lining is no longer smooth, and we now have the basis for complications to develop: (1) a reduction in the volume of blood which the artery transmits, (2) the possibility of small blood clots forming within the lumen of the artery, (3) the possibility of the artery's wall weakening to the extent that it bulges to form an aneurysm, and (4) the possibility that the artery wall may rupture, permitting the escape of blood (hemorrhage). A still further possibility is that the blood clot (thrombus) which forms at the site of a plaque may break apart, allowing a portion of it (an embolus) to be carried by the flowing blood until it lodges in one of the artery's branches. The resultant plugging of the branch causes an embolism, with death of tissue in the area served by this branch.

Consequences of Arteriosclerosis

In the previous chapter it was noted that the blood supply to the heart may be reduced gradually as arteriosclerosis develops in the coronary arteries, causing ischemic heart disease; or it may be cut off suddenly in one of the branches of the coronary arteries to cause a heart attack. Similarly, in other parts of the body, such as the brain, the kidneys, and the legs, the blood supply may be reduced gradually as arteriosclerosis develops in the arteries supplying these parts. And, particularly in the brain, it may be reduced suddenly at the time of a stroke.

A gradual reduction in the blood supply to the kidneys sets the stage for kidney disease, which becomes a serious complication. A gradual reduction in the blood supply to the legs causes a symptom called claudication, which consists of intense pain in the muscles in the calf of the leg when the muscles are used actively.

Persons with diabetes are particularly susceptible to arteriosclerosis. In these cases it is usually the tissues of

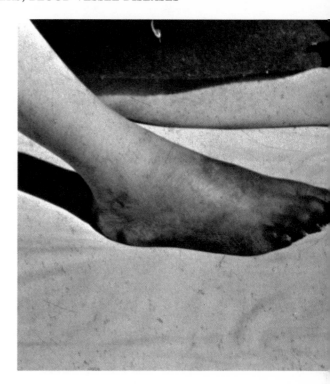

Gangrene in the extremities may result from arteriosclerosis.

the lower extremities, particularly the feet, that suffer first as the blood supply to these parts is gradually reduced. Typically, there develop ulcers on the skin of the legs which tend to persist in spite of efforts to cause them to heal. Often there develop cracks in the skin between the toes. These breaks in the skin become infected, and because of the reduction in blood supply to these parts the infection persists, and the ulcers and fissures refuse to heal. As the condition worsens, the tissues actually die for lack of sufficient oxygen and food materials. We then speak of the condition as gangrene, a serious complication that threatens the patient's life. The only effective treatment is to amputate the part that has become gangrenous, and even then the site of the amputation heals slowly.

Prevention of Arteriosclerosis

Just as with coronary heart disease,

concise but are designed to be informative. Understandably, diagnosis of these conditions requires the facilities available in modern hospitals and clinical laboratories, and treatment demands the services of a physician.

The first part of our discussion of blood diseases pertains to the several conditions in which the red blood cells are affected in one way or another. As a preliminary, then, let us consider briefly the normal role of the red cells and the ways in which the body's functions become handicapped when the red cells are abnormal in composition or in number.

The primary function of red cells is to carry oxygen from the lungs to the tissues. Each red cell (erythrocyte) is essentially a small elastic package of hemoglobin—a red, iron-containing substance capable of transporting oxygen from the lungs to the tissues.

All living tissues require a continuous supply of oxygen. The more active the tissue, the greater its need for oxygen. Three factors help to determine the amount of oxygen which the blood can bring to a tissue: (1) the amount of hemoglobin in each red blood cell, (2) the relative number of red blood cells in the bloodstream, and (3) the speed with which the red blood cells arrive in the tissue under consideration.

In anemia there is either a reduced amount of hemoglobin in each of the red blood cells or else the total number of red cells is less than usual. In either case the oxygen-carrying capacity of the blood is reduced and the tissues suffer on this account. Strangely, however, in the opposite condition of polycythemia, in which there is an excess of red blood cells, the tissues may also suffer for lack of oxygen. In this case the difficulty lies in the fact that with a high population of red cells the blood becomes syrupy and moves so slowly that it cannot deliver its oxygen as fast as necessary for tissue health.

Of all the tissues, brain tissue has about the greatest and most continuous need for oxygen. Headache is one of the symptoms that may herald the brain's need for more oxygen. (This is only one of the many possible causes of headache.) In the light of the explanation given above we can see that this kind of headache can occur either when the number of red blood cells is below normal (in anemia) or when the number is above normal (in polycythemia).

With this as an example, it becomes clear that the symptoms of blood diseases depend on what effects these diseases produce on the body's tissues rather than on what changes can be observed in the blood itself.

Now for a consideration of the various blood diseases:

ANEMIA

The term anemia applies to conditions in which the amount of hemoglobin or the number of red cells in a specified volume of blood is below normal. Normal blood is 40 to 45 percent red cells and 55 to 60 percent plasma. On the average there are 12.5 to 15.5 grams of hemoglobin per 100 milliliters of blood. The normal red-cell count is 4.5 to 5.5 million cells per cubic millimeter. All these values tend to be 10 percent lower in women. A person is considered anemic if his blood values are less than the lowest figures mentioned here.

Anemia may be the result of inadequate or improper formation of red blood cells by the bone marrow. A small amount of vitamin B_{12} is necessary for the cells to mature, and an adequate amount of iron combined with a proper arrangement of protein is needed so that each cell may receive its full supply of hemoglobin. Anemias resulting from failure of this system are called anemias of production. Other anemias occur when fully formed adult red blood cells are destroyed prematurely. These are called hemolytic anemias. When red blood cells are lost because of bleeding, the resulting anemia is called anemia of hemorrhage, or secondary anemia. Finally, anemias due to bone marrow damage are called aplastic anemia, the separate section discussing this problem to be found

159

later in this chapter under *Bone-marrow Failure*.

A. *Iron-deficiency Anemia (Microcytic Hypochromic Anemia)*. Iron, an integral part of hemoglobin, is vitally important in the transport of oxygen from the lungs to the tissues and of carbon dioxide from tissues to lungs. When a deficiency of iron occurs, the production of red cells is less affected than is the formation of hemoglobin. But the deficiency causes the bone marrow to produce small cells. Then as lack of iron becomes more severe, red cells with less than optimal hemoglobin content are formed. Thus the red blood cells in this condition are both small (microcytic) and pale (hypochromic). In severe iron deficiency, the rate of red cell formation is curtailed, causing a low red cell count.

The most common cause of iron deficiency is blood loss, such as in prolonged bleeding. Women have iron-deficiency anemia more than men, one reason being that excessive menstrual bleeding may bring about the loss of more iron from the body each month than can be replaced by the iron contained in the usual diet. Pregnancy and loss of blood during delivery cause a tremendous drain on the iron reserves in women, and frequent pregnancies impose demands which the present-day American diet cannot supply. Hence a physician usually prescribes iron-containing medicine for pregnant patients.

Iron-deficiency anemia may be the result of unsuspected bleeding from the intestine. Often considerable blood loss can go on for a long time without the patient's suspecting anything wrong. Special chemical tests of the stool are often used to determine whether blood is present. Gastrointestinal bleeding can occur with ulcers, hemorrhoids, or small growths in the colon. Often the development of anemia is the first indication of a cancer of the colon. Intestinal parasites, particularly hookworm, can also cause severe iron-deficiency anemia.

Another cause of iron-deficiency anemia is lack of hydrochloric acid in the stomach, a lack which reduces the absorption of iron from food. Cancer of

There are three times in a woman's life when she is most susceptible to anemia: adolescence, time of pregnancy, old age.

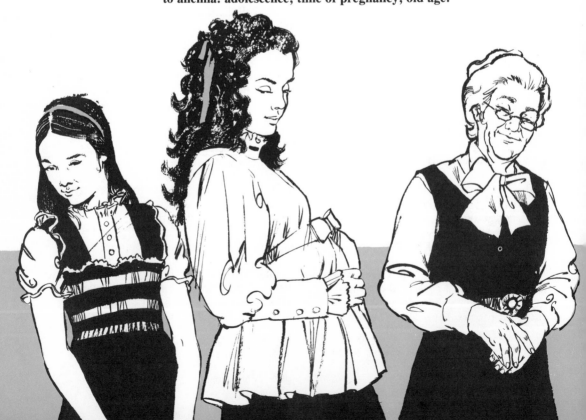

the stomach or the intestine, severe diarrhea from intestinal infections, and the surgical removal of most or all of the stomach or of the small intestine may also interfere with the absorption of iron. Certain vitamin deficiencies, such as that of pyridoxine (vitamin B_6), and the prolonged consumption of such poisons as lead, arsenic, or mercury prevent the efficient incorporation of iron into hemoglobin when red blood cells are being developed. Prolonged infections such as tuberculosis or prolonged inflammations such as rheumatoid arthritis prevent the movement of iron to the bone marrow where hemoglobin is formed.

Some of the common symptoms and signs of iron-deficiency anemia are fatigability, faintness, palpitation, shortness of breath with exercise, headache, pallor, and—in severe cases—deformed fingernails.

Care and Treatment

1. Iron-deficiency anemia always has a cause. This must be discovered before any corrective treatment is begun. The patient can help the physician by taking special note of changes in the color of the bowel movements, by making a diet inventory list, or (in a woman) by noting a change in the amount of menstrual flow.

2. A pregnant woman should be under the care of a physician.

3. Women whose menstrual flow is excessive should seek medical help. Anemia may be corrected easily, but the underlying cause of the excess flow may be something serious. Abnormal bleeding is one of the seven danger signals of cancer. (See chapter 10, volume 3, for complete list.)

4. A well-balanced diet is important.

5. The choice of which medicinal iron or iron tonic to take should be guided by the doctor.

B. *Macrocytic Anemia (Pernicious Anemia and Others).* Macrocytic anemias are characterized by red cells which are larger than normal. These anemias are caused by a deficiency of vitamin B_{12} or of folic acid. About 90 percent of macrocytic anemias in temperate climate countries are pernicious anemias. The rest are due to other causes of vitamin B_{12} deficiency or to lack of folic acid, a close cousin to B_{12} and also a member of the B vitamin group.

A lack of vitamin B_{12} may occur in several ways, one being failure of the stomach to aid in absorbing it. The main site of absorption is the ileum. In order to absorb B_{12} properly, the stomach must secrete a substance called intrinsic factor, which serves as a transfer agent locking itself to B_{12} and guiding it across the intestinal lining to enter the bloodstream. Without the intrinsic factor, vitamine B_{12} is absorbed poorly. Pernicious anemia refers to that anemia which occurs when the stomach is unable to secrete the intrinsic factor.

Macrocytic anemias may also be caused by insufficient B_{12} in the diet, or when certain germs living in the intestinal tract use up B_{12} before it can be absorbed. Vitamin B_{12} deficiency can develop in individuals on restricted diets, in persons who have had all the stomach removed, in persons whose stomach lining has degenerated so that it no longer produces sufficient intrinsic factor, or in special situations when certain tapeworm or bacterial infections in the intestines compete for and deprive the body of vitamin B_{12} before it can be absorbed.

Vitamin B_{12} and folic acid are necessary to form and mature the red blood cells, granulocytes, and platelets. Vitamin B_{12} is required also for the maintenance of nervous tissue. When the combination of anemia, nervousness, and peculiar sensations such as numbness and tingling in the hands and feet occurs, pernicious anemia may be present.

Folic acid is extremely important in the proper development of all rapidly growing tissue. It exists in abundant quantities in fresh vegetables. Folic acid deficiency is found most commonly in food faddism, alcoholism, chronic diarrheal states, and the later stages of pregnancy. In the latter condition, the mother needs especially large amounts of folic acid in order to supply adequately the baby's needs for its rapidly developing body tissues.

The pernicious anemia patient is usually over thirty. Typically he is of the Caucasian (white) race and likely of English, Irish, or Northern European descent. The onset of the disease is often subtle, the first likely symptoms being merely weakness, fatigue, pallor, and palpitation or breathlessness on exertion. Typically the patient has snowy white hair, a yellowish waxy complexion, and a smooth tongue. There is often a poor appetite, though weight loss is not frequent. Symptoms of indigestion are usually present. A striking change in behavior, and nervousness, numbness, and tingling of the hands and feet are commonly experienced. A peculiar inability to coordinate the feet when walking, especially in the dark, is characteristic.

Laboratory tests will show the patient to have a moderate to severe anemia, red blood cells extremely varied in size, shape, and color, no free acid in his stomach, and a low level of vitamin B_{12} in his blood. The average red cell size is greater than normal, hence the term macrocytic anemia. The white-cell count and platelet count are usually below normal.

The inability of the person with pernicious anemia to absorb vitamin B_{12} because of a lack of the intrinsic factor can be tested by administering an oral dose of vitamin B_{12} which has been marked with a tiny amount of radioactive cobalt. If no trace of this labeled B_{12} can be detected in the bloodstream or the urine, detectable with special instruments, the suspicion that the patient makes no intrinsic factor of his own is confirmed.

Care and Treatment

1. Vitamin B_{12}, a specific remedy for pernicious anemia, must be given by injection at no greater than monthly intervals. If the diagnosis of pernicious anemia is confirmed, the injections must be continued for the remainder of the patient's life. When properly instructed, some member of the household can give the injections, but a physician must supervise the treatment program and arrange periodic physical examinations and laboratory tests.

2. The elderly patient under treatment for pernicious anemia should be

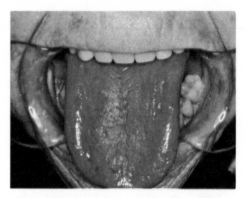

Condition of the tongue figures in diagnosis of pernicious anemia.

advised to limit his activity until the hemoglobin level reaches 8 to 9 grams per 100 ml. of blood or higher depending on the general condition of his health.

3. Physiotherapy consisting of exercises to improve muscle strength and coordination should be instituted in patients with involvement of the nervous system. Patients with serious nervous system degeneration require expert nursing care to prevent bedsores and bladder infections. Progressive improvement of nerve dysfunctions may continue for a year or more after adequate treatment has been started.

4. Blood transfusions are rarely necessary except in the severely ill patient. With vitamin B_{12} injections and plenty of nutritious food the blood should return to normal within six weeks.

5. Folic acid deficiency may be treated by oral or injectable medication; but for the expectant mother, a special emphasis on fresh leafy vegetables in the diet will protect her unborn child in most cases.

6. "Blood tonics" by mouth without a doctor's advice should be avoided because some will correct the anemia but permit progressive, occasionally irreversible, degeneration of the nervous system.

C. *Hemolytic Anemia*. The destruction of red blood cells while they are in circulation is called hemolysis. Causes of destruction may be severe burns, chemicals of various kinds, or complications of certain infections or malignancies.

Red cells that normally "wear out" are removed from circulation in the spleen, the liver, and the bone marrow. Iron and protein from destroyed red blood cells are retained by the tissues and reused in the production of new hemoglobin. That component of the old hemoglobin which imparts the red color (pigment) undergoes chemical changes in the liver and is normally eliminated in the form of bile pigments, which pass through the bile ducts, gallbladder, and intestinal tract as part of the bile.

In the hemolytic anemias, in which there is an increased rate of red-cell destruction, the provision for eliminating the pigments derived from old hemoglobin may be overwhelmed, with the result that the bile pigments accumulate in the tissues, causing jaundice. This type of jaundice can be recognized by the yellow coloration of the skin and of the whites of the eyes.

D. *Congenital Types of Hemolytic Anemia*. Some persons inherit a condition by which red blood cells of poor quality are produced by the bone marrow. In some cases the red cells do not contain the right amount of enzymes. This may permit the cells to be destroyed by the spleen before they reach their usual life-span of 120 days. Or it

may make the red cells more susceptible than normal to the damaging effects of certain drugs. The associated anemia is designated as congenital nonspherocytic hemolytic anemia.

In other situations, the walls or envelopes of the red cells are defective, resulting in peculiar shapes which appear to be more vulnerable to the incessant pummeling they receive as they pass through small blood vessels. Hemolytic anemias of this type may be recognized by observing the red cells on a blood smear and by discovering a family tendency to anemia and jaundice. One such disorder is chronic familial jaundice, or hereditary spherocytosis. In this particular difficulty, surgical removal of the spleen retards the rate of red-blood-cell destruction but does not improve the quality of the red cells produced by the bone marrow.

Care and Treatment

1. The patient with congenital nonspherocytic hemolytic anemia should obtain from his physician a list of the drugs which may cause him to have a flare-up of severe anemia. He also must make sure that the physician in attendance during each hospitalization knows of his problem and avoids prescribing drugs that may be harmful. The wearing of some identification with a mention of his disorder is advisable.

2. Congenital spherocytic anemia is best treated by removal of the spleen. This surgical procedure is usually postponed until the child reaches his early teens.

3. Tranfusions may have to be given during a severe anemia phase of both kinds of hemolytic anemia.

E. *Hemoglobinopathic Hemolytic Anemias (Sickle-cell Disease)*. A common disorder occurring frequently in blacks and also in a few Caucasians of Mediterranean origin, is sickle-cell anemia. This hereditary disease causes the production of an abnormal type of hemoglobin by the bone marrow. This abnormal hemoglobin differs from the normal by a small change in the structure of the molecule.

Sickle-cell hemoglobin has peculiar sensitivity to a lowered oxygen supply such as occurs when climbing a high mountain, taking an automobile trip over high mountain passes, flying in an aircraft with an unpressurized cabin, or when suffering from pneumonia. Red cells with this type of hemoglobin form sickle or crescent shapes when subjected to lowered oxygen concentrations. These peculiarly shaped cells do not pass through the small blood vessels readily, and consequently may block the blood supply to vital areas.

There are all degrees of sickle-cell disease. Many persons become aware of the defect in connection with a routine physical examination. Others develop their first symptoms when they drive over a high mountain pass. Still others are severely handicapped from the time of birth.

Among the first symptoms to be encountered in sickle-cell disease is sudden, severe, abdominal pain, followed by the appearance of dark-colored urine. Also associated with it may be severe leg cramps, acute pain in the left side, and a yellowish discoloration to the eyes (jaundice). In the severest cases slight exercise may bring on the pain, there may be severe anemia, a huge liver, repeated fevers, recurrent bone pain, and chronic ulcers of the legs. Patients with sickle-cell disease show a marked susceptibility to infections. When patients with this disorder develop a cold or pneumonia they should seek medical help early.

Care and Treatment

1. A person who suspects that he has sickle-cell anemia should present himself to the physician for examination.

2. If diagnosis is confirmed, the patient should place himself under a physician's care early in the course of any infection and follow his instructions.

3. Avoid situations where a lowered concentration of oxygen may be present, such as trips over high mountain passes, flights in unpressurized aircraft, skin diving without breathing equipment, and strenuous exercise.

4. In a crisis the patient should seek medical attention at once; but until help comes he may also obtain and breathe oxygen temporarily, lie down to conserve energy, and breathe deeply.

5. Obtain a highly nutritious diet rich in proteins and folic acid. Folic acid is found mainly in leafy green vegetables.

6. Blood transfusions, other intravenous fluids and intensive pain-control medications are sometimes necessary.

F. *Mediterranean Anemia (Thalassemia).* Certain aberrations of hemoglobin formation may occur because of inherited tendencies. They have all the earmarks of a hemolytic disorder. Most of these are uncommon and beyond the scope of this chapter, but one disorder, Mediterranean anemia (thalassemia), an inherited defect, appears most commonly among people who have originated from around the Mediterranean Sea, *e.g.,* Italians, Greeks, Turks, and southern Spanish. Patients with this disorder are unable to form enough normal adult type hemoglobin and consequently suffer from the continuous production of a fetal type of hemoglobin.

The cells filled with this fetal hemoglobin die much sooner than normal cells. The bone marrow responds to this low oxygen and rapid cell death by vigorously making more red cells. Patients will have large thick spongy bones filled with red bone marrow. They have large livers and spleens, are perpetually jaundiced, and continue to pass dark-colored urine.

Severely affected children often die before their tenth year. Many others die as young adults because of iron overload due to many transfusions. However, all degrees of severity, as with sickle-cell diseases, may exist.

Care and Treatment

1. Physicians can do relatively little for Mediterranean anemia except to keep the patient comfortable. The degree of severity will determine the outcome. A few have responded remarkably to surgical removal of the spleen.

2. It is important to avoid infections and to take in plenty of nutritious food, particularly green leafy vegetables because of their folic acid content.

3. Blood transfusions may have to be used over an extended period of time.

G. *Autoimmune Hemolytic Anemia.* This anemia, the least understood type, may develop with amazing suddenness or with gradual progression. In some cases it appears spontaneously. In others it follows viral pneumonia. It may appear in association with other infections, with cancer, or with leukemia. It is similar to the reaction observed when the wrong type of blood is transfused inadvertently.

The body has a unique way of identifying its own tissues and defending them from invasion by foreign cells. This peculiar characteristic develops early, even while the child is still in its mother's womb. This defense mechanism may be set in motion when biologically active tissues are transplanted from one person to another, *e.g.*, kidney, heart, or liver. The simpler the transplant, the greater the prospect of success. Blood, being in this sense a simple tissue, is often transferred successfully in blood transfusions.

At times, under conditions not well understood, the body suddenly starts rejecting its own red blood cells, a situation brought about by the formation of a special type of protein which destroys red cells or makes them susceptible to destruction by the spleen. This protein is similar to gamma globulin which the body produces to fight infections. Autoimmune hemolytic anemia is such an example of a self-destroying disease.

Autoimmune hemolytic anemia can be ushered in with a chill, fever, vomiting, pain in the back or abdomen, and the production of yellow to reddish-brown urine. The spleen may enlarge rapidly, thereby aggravating the condition. Often other cells of the blood are affected.

The diagnosis depends on being able to demonstrate the abnormal gamma globulin attached to the red cells. This requires specialized laboratory tests. The treatment is first directed toward the associated disease, if present, which may have triggered the hemolysis. Then drugs may be prescribed which suppress the body's ability to produce anti-red-cell globulin. Finally the spleen may have to be removed. The treatment program may of necessity be conducted in a different order.

Care and Treatment

This complicated disease requires expert medical care. To place oneself in the care of a good physician is most prudent. Cortisone in large doses is often required, or the doctor may elect to remove the spleen.

H. *Hemolytic Disease of the Newborn (Erythroblastosis Fetalis).* Much publicity has been given the Rh factor in human blood. Actually there are at least twenty different blood groups which have been positively identified, and more may yet be discovered. Of these, the ABO and Rh groups are of most significance in hemolytic disease of the newborn. The ABO group (blood belonging to this group is either A, O, B, or AB) is the most important when transfusion is considered; but for several reasons it is of less importance in the "baby and mother" disease.

If blood from a person with type A is transfused into a type B person, it will likely be destroyed because the type B person has antibodies (certain protecting proteins) antagonistic to type A red cells. In the Rh system antibodies do not develop until the foreign cells have once stimulated the recipient's defense mechanism. The first time Rh positive blood cells are introduced into the bloodstream of an Rh negative recipient, they will doubtless be tolerated. By a second time, antibodies will have developed which promptly destroy the foreign cells.

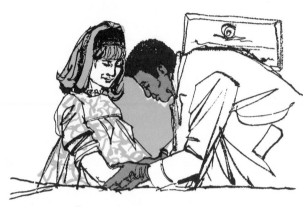

Prenatal consultation reduces risks.

Identification of a blood group is done in a blood bank by mixing cells or plasma of known type with cells or plasma of the unknown type on clean glass slides or paper and observing whether "clumping" occurs. Anti-A plasma will agglutinate (clump) A cells, and anti-Rh positive plasma will agglutinate Rh positive cells.

Hemolytic disease of the newborn occurs when red blood cells from a baby with blood of a type different from that of the mother seeps across the membrane of the placenta and enters the mother's bloodstream. If the mother is Rh negative and the baby also Rh negative, their blood is compatible and nothing will happen, providing the ABO group is compatible also. But if the baby is Rh positive and the mother is Rh negative, anti-Rh antibodies which can easily cross the membrane back into the baby's bloodstream begin destroying the baby's Rh positive red cells before the baby is even born.

For a further explanation of the problem of Rh incompatibility, for a discussion of the means of preventing consequent damage to the baby, and for a discussion of the nature and treatment of hemolytic disease of the newborn when it occurs, see chapters 3 and 6 of volume 1.

POLYCYTHEMIA

Polycythemia, either primary or secondary, is a condition in which there is an abnormally large number of red blood cells in the circulating blood.

The fundamental cause of primary polycythemia (polycythemia rubra vera) is not known. The immediate reason for the abnormally large number of red blood cells is that excess quantities are produced by the bone marrow. The total amount of hemoglobin is also increased, accounting for the deeply flushed appearance of the patient's face. With the excessive number of red blood cells the blood becomes "thick" and small vessels may be obstructed, producing corresponding symptoms of partial blindness and small strokes. The lips may appear purple because of the lessened speed of blood flow, and regional lack of oxygen.

Secondary polycythemia occurs in individuals who have damaged lungs or who are born with false chambers or passages in the heart or large blood vessels. In these situations, the blood may become as thick as in patients with polycythemia rubra vera, but in secondary polycythemia the bone marrow keeps making red cells because the body tissues are suffering for lack of oxygen. A substance called erythropoietin, made by the kidney, is responsible for driving the bone marrow to make more red cells. When mountain climbers ascend to high altitudes, their total hemoglobin and the number of their red blood cells increases, in this case a normal provision by nature, to make it possible for more oxygen to be captured from the thin air and supplied to the tissues. Another form of polycythemia may result from the production of erythropoieticlike substances by tumors, *e.g.,* cancer of the kidney.

The signs and symptoms of polycythemia are headache, dizziness, fainting spells, unusual itching after bath, a feeling of fullness in the head, frequent nosebleeds, and sometimes ankle swelling.

Care and Treatment

Various forms of treatment are acceptable for primary polycythemia, the simplest being repeated phlebotomy (bloodletting). Many individuals go on for years giving up about six pints of blood a year and feeling quite well. Certain powerful drugs can be given to control the production of red cells. So far there is no known cure.

Treatment for the usual case of secondary polycythemia requires the correcting of the underlying defect of the heart or lungs, if that is possible, or the removal of the tumor.

Bleeding Disorders

Blood circulates throughout the body through blood vessels. Since these are tubes made of tissue, any disruption of the tube will permit the escape of blood into the surrounding structures or to the outside in a never-ending stream were it not for an amazing mechanism which constantly seals tiny leaks or large breaks. It is hard to appreciate the value of this self-sealing mechanism until a person afflicted with bleeding problems is observed.

Hemostasis (the prevention of bleeding) is a cooperative effort on the part of tissues, blood vessels, platelets, and the clotting mechanism. The pressure of surrounding tissues acts to stop bleeding from puncture-type wounds. Cut ends of blood vessels retract like elastic bands, causing mechanical pressure to close the open ends. Substances released from injured vessels and tissues and from platelets stimulate the vessels to constrict and the blood to form clots. This amazing piece of jellied blood plugs vessel openings and pulls the ends of the broken vessel together. It hangs on until the vessel heals; then it disappears, often without a trace.

Platelets, previously mentioned, are formed in the bone marrow. The prime function of these little chemical packages of tremendous potency is constantly to plug the millions of tiny holes in the walls of blood vessels so as to constantly prevent blood from seeping into the tissues. When breaks appear, the platelets plaster themselves over the defect and quickly form a patch over the hole. Platelets also release chemicals which initiate blood clotting.

The process of blood clotting must surely be one of the most unusual mechanisms in nature. Of particular interest is the delicate balance between clotting at all and clotting too much; for if no clotting took place, man would die of hemorrhage, and if too much took place, he would become one big clot on the day of his birth. Defects in blood clotting do occur, and some of the most common will now be discussed.

THE PURPURAS

Purpura is a condition in which numerous small hemorrhages develop within the skin. These small discolored spots may appear spontaneously or they may appear in areas in which there has been mild trauma, as when bumping the arm against a door. Purpura results from toxic or chemical injury to blood vessels or from blood seepage due to a low platelet count. Sometimes changes in tissues from poor nutrition, hormonal imbalance, advancing age, or certain drugs may cause purpura.

A. *Nonthrombocytopenic Purpura.* Nonthrombocytopenic purpura (purpura in the presence of normal platelet levels) occurs most commonly in elderly people. A high percent of individuals over eighty have purplish patches over the backs of their hands and arms. This is called senile purpura and is due to the loss of supporting tissue, through aging, around small blood vessels. It is not a serious condition, and no treatment is necessary.

Purpura also appears with vitamin C deficiency, following the administration of certain medicines, particularly cortisone, and in the presence of diabe-

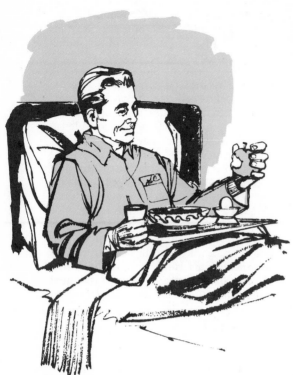

A patient with severe purpura must have strict bed rest.

tes mellitus or chronic kidney failure. It accompanies severe infections such as erysipelas, plague, and sometimes measles and chicken pox. This is the cause of "black measles," "black pox," or "black plague."

Care and Treatment

1. There is no effective remedy for nonthrombocytopenic purpura. The maintenance of the best state of health possible is advisable. Vitamin C in large doses produces no obvious benefits.

2. Purpura which accompanies measles or other infections is a serious disorder and requires a physician's attention immediately.

B. *Thrombocytopenic Purpuras*. Thrombocytopenic purpuras result from reduced platelets and occur most commonly as the result of drugs, chemicals, infections, or malignancies.

These agents may depress the formation of platelets by the marrow, may destroy platelets, or may cause them to be used up excessively. Some degree of thrombocytopenia is present in all pancytopenias due to marrow damage, and purpura is often seen.

Idiopathic thrombocytopenic purpura, for which no cause is found, may occur at any age, but it is most common in children and young adults. In children the condition is often temporary and disappears after a few weeks or months. Spontaneous cures in adults are less likely. Even though the disease is self-limited, it may be deadly and should not be taken lightly. The onset of thrombocytopenia in children is often preceded by an infection which occurred several weeks previously. The greatest danger is not the bleeding into the skin or the nosebleeds but the possibility of hemorrhage into vital structures such as the brain.

Thrombocytopenia may come in repeated attacks. It is characterized by fever, often by nausea, vomiting, abdominal and joint pains, prostration, bleeding from the bowel, the mouth, or the bladder, as well as by the development of a crop of skin hemorrhages. Or it may appear without any associated feeling of ill health. The skin hemorrhages can be distinguished from tiny superficial varicose veins by the fact that purpura does not disappear when pressure is applied.

Care and Treatment

1. In a severe case of purpura, strict bed rest may be advisable as a precaution to prevent hemorrhages into vital areas. Even in moderate cases strenuous activity should be avoided.

2. All purpuras should be under the care of a physician, both for diagnosis and appropriate treatment.

3. Patients with severe purpura should be prevented from straining at stool and from coughing.

CLOTTING DEFECTS

Blood clotting depends on a complex

168

series of chemical reactions involving proteins and enzymes in blood plasma and in tissues. In addition, calcium and phosphorus and perhaps other minerals must be present.

Many of the clotting proteins and enzymes are made in the liver from ingredients derived from the diet. If liver damage is present, as in cirrhosis or hepatitis, or if the liver is too young as in some premature babies, clotting factors may not be synthesized in adequate amounts to prevent bleeding. Some individuals are born with an inability to produce one or more of the clotting factors.

Clotting factors can be deliberately lowered by "blood thinners," better known as anticoagulants. These are used with patients who have suffered a heart attack or who have developed thrombophlebitis. The aim is to decrease the clotting tendency in order to prevent a recurrence of the heart attack or to prevent extension of the clot in thrombophlebitis. The taking of too much medicine can cause serious hemorrhage. Anyone taking anticoagulants should strictly obey the instructions of his physician and report to him the first sign of spontaneous bleeding.

A. *Hemophilia*. Persons with hemophilia are known as "bleeders." These may have all degrees of bleeding. In a child who has severe hemophilia, death can occur early in life as a consequence of some minor injury. With a less severe case there is a tendency to bleed slowly for prolonged periods from even minor cuts or scratches. Sometimes bleeding into the tissues begins without apparent tissue injury. A favorite site for large bleeds is in the large muscles of the back and buttocks. However, any part of the body may become involved. Bleeding into the joints is common in the severely affected cases. Following a joint hemorrhage there will be inflammation, redness, and stiffness; and each hemorrhage causes more and more joint dysfunction until finally the whole joint may become useless. The shoulder, elbow, knee, and hip joints are the ones most commonly involved.

Hemophilia usually results from an individual's inability to make factor VIII (antihemophiliac factor, AHF). A congenital defect, it is passed on from father to daughter to son, but girls are rarely affected by the actual manifestations of the disease. It cannot be transmitted directly from father to son but must always come to the son from the mother. This means that a man who is a bleeder of this type will have sons and daughters who are not bleeders unless the mother also has a family background of bleeders of the same type. The sons of his daughters, however, could be bleeders.

Great advances in the last few years have been made in handling cuts, wounds, accidents, or surgery in persons with hemophilia. It has become possible to concentrate factor VIII (AHF) so that 10 c.c., when injected will have the potency of a whole unit of fresh blood, and now hemophiliacs may look forward to the prospect of normal living.

Care and Treatment

1. Prevention of bleeding is of the first importance. The afflicted person should protect himself as far as possible from any injury. No dental extractions or surgical operations should be attempted without careful preparatory treatment.

2. Hemophiliacs should acquaint themselves with centers stocking factor VIII (AHF) concentrates where they may be taken in case of an accident.

3. If bleeding occurs from a surface wound, pressure should be applied and retained until a pressure dressing can be applied. There is a tendency for the hemophiliac to bleed for about eight to ten days after a wound is inflicted.

4. If bleeding persists or if bleeding has occurred into the tissues, a physician should be called at once. He may advise giving fresh frozen plasma or a factor VIII (AHF) concentrate.

5. It is wise for the hemophiliac to wear an identification tag or bracelet so that in case of an emergency where quick action may be necessary and when unconsciousness occurs, those administering care may institute quick and appropriate treatment.

B. *Vitamin K Deficiency.* Vitamin K is the parent substance from which the liver produces four of the blood clotting factors. Vitamin K is present in small quantities in leafy green vegetables, but most of the body's supply is made by bacteria in the bowel from other food material. Bile salts promote the absorption of vitamin K. Body stores of this vitamin are so small that complete deprivation may result in bleeding within a week or two. Bleeding may appear from the nose, gums, throat, kidneys, bladder, or bowel.

Numerous clinical situations may cause vitamin K deficiency. When the bile duct is obstructed with gallstones or scar tissue, bile salts cannot get into the intestine and little absorption of vitamin K can take place. In severe prolonged diarrheas, changes in the intestinal lining and the rapid onward movement of the intestinal contents decreases the amount of absorption. When strong modern antibiotics are prescribed for a week or more, enough of the bacteria in the intestine may be destroyed to stop or retard formation of vitamin K and therefore only that obtained from the diet is available.

Care and Treatment

1. A thorough medical examination should reveal the problem. A generous intake of leafy green vegetables or vitamin K supplement administered by a physician will help to correct the difficulty.

2. Any non-induced bleeding condition of a serious nature should be referred to a physician immediately for treatment. The blood pressure, and thus the bleeding, decreases if the afflicted person lies down and rests quietly until help arrives or until he can be taken to a physician.

Bone Marrow Failure

In order that the body may produce an adequate number of blood cells of all types, it needs a healthy marrow bed in which parent types of each cell may grow. There must be an adequate circulation of blood to the marrow to provide nutrients so that each kind of cell can mature properly. There must exist an adequate stimulus to accelerate cell growth and maturation when there is an increased need as in anemia. The young cells must have a place to grow and must be able to develop into normal adult cells. There must be enough stored food material for use during the most rapid growth phase. Parent cells in the marrow must be able to respond to a message of blood loss by increasing their production of young cells. They must also reduce their rate of productivity at the right time lest the blood become too thick and clog up the circulation.

Obviously this is a complicated system, wonderfully devised, delicately balanced with automatic controls of many types. This balance can be influenced by many factors.

PANCYTOPENIA

When there has been damage to the bone marrow bed or the parent cell types or when their ability to produce new cells has been drastically reduced, pancytopenia develops. This term designates a decreased number of all types of blood cells.

Pancytopenia exists when bone marrow fails to produce the various blood cells customarily originating here, *e.g.*, red cells, granulocytes, and platelets. It is a serious disorder carrying a high mortality rate. Many patients with pancytopenia give no history of exposure to X-ray radiation, toxic drugs, or the industrial chemicals known to cause this disease—chemicals such as chloramphenical, benzene, certain hair dyes, some insecticides, and some plant sprays. Still damage may have come from this source, certain people being peculiarly susceptible to ordinarily harmless concentrations of certain drugs or chemicals.

Symptoms of pancytopenia will depend on which cell type is most affected. The resulting anemia will cause lack of energy, a high pulse rate, and all the symptoms of anemia previously described. The depression of granulocytes (one kind of white cells), whose function is to combat infection, will of course leave the patient comparatively unprotected from germ invasion. Since the skin, the gums, the throat, the lungs, and the intestine are the first lines of defense against infections, a person with low concentration of granulocytes can be expected to develop repeated and protracted infections of these areas. Platelets are important in plugging tiny leaks in blood vessels. They prevent minor bumps from becoming big bruises and small cuts from becoming major bleeding problems. Platelet depression or absence will be characterized by bleeding gums, repeated or prolonged nosebleeds, easy bruisability, and the development of a fine reddish rash—minor hemorrhages into the skin. In women, there is usually a sharp increase in the amount and duration of menstrual flow.

A person afflicted with pancytopenia may not recognize the true nature of his ailment, but he is usually aware that something is seriously wrong. He should consult his physician at once. The doctor can by appropriate examinations and tests discover the offending agent so that it may be avoided in the future. The recovery rate from pancytopenia is less than 50 percent, and much less when the patient experiences repeated exposure to the original insulting agent. Outlook for a cure depends on how severely the bone marrow bed or the parent cells have been damaged.

Care and Treatment

1. When infections recur time after time, a physician should be consulted.

2. All use of solvents, headache remedies, or prescription drugs not recently prescribed should be halted. No further use of pesticides or garden sprays should be made.

3. It is especially important to protect against lacerations of the skin which may become infected and to avoid contact with persons who have colds, sore throat, or cough. It is best to stay out of crowds.

4. The maximum state of good health should be maintained with plenty of rest, good wholesome food, liberal amounts of water, and moderate exercise.

APLASTIC ANEMIA

Aplastic anemia is caused by the complete failure of bone marrow to produce red blood cells. Commonly, the bone marrow deficiency is partial rather than absolute. It is then called hypoplastic anemia. This more com-

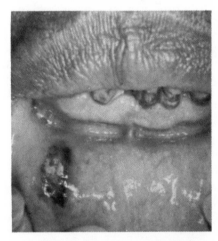

A symptom of aplastic anemia is canker sores on the lips or tongue.

mon type is nearly always a temporary condition, while the aplastic anemia is likely to be of irreversible nature.

The symptoms of aplastic anemia are those of any severe anemia: easy fatigability, palpitation of the heart, pallor, shortness of breath on exertion, ankle swelling, and canker sores on lips or tongue. Commonly, the term "aplastic

171

anemia" is used synonymously with pancytopenia, the condition described in the preceding section. If used in this sense, the symptoms will be those described under pancytopenia.

When no recovery of the bone marrow's ability to make red cells occurs, the patient will be dependent on repeated blood transfusions. He will need anywhere from two to four units per month to keep the red-cell concentration up. The level at which the physician elects to keep the red count or hemoglobin will depend on the activity needs of the patient. For example, a retired man can get along well on less than 50 percent of the normal red-cell count, whereas a workingman may need 75 percent. Additional treatment may be required if other cell types are also depressed.

Care and Treatment

1. No attempt at self-treatment with iron or blood tonics should be attempted, because one of the problems in aplastic anemia is that the patient accumulates too much iron. Your physician should decide what medicines are needed.

2. A concerted attempt should be made to reduce excess activity, but regular light exercise should be taken.

3. All further exposure to cleaning solvents, pesticides, weed killers, or patent medicines should be stopped and strictly avoided. In some cases recovery has been prevented by a mild second exposure to the injurious agent.

4. A few medical centers are now prepared to treat selected cases of irreversible aplastic anemia by a procedure known as "bone marrow transplant." It involves taking marrow from a compatible donor (usually a brother, sister, parent, daughter, or son) and injecting such marrow into the afflicted person. With very close and careful medical management, the implanted marrow will grow and supply the cells which have been in short supply.

AGRANULOCYTOSIS

Agranulocytosis is another blood condition resulting from marrow injury, known or unknown. Specifically, it is an absence in the bloodstream of granulocytes (often also referred to as neuterophiles), which is that variety of white cell most concerned with fighting disease germs. Granulocytopenia or neutropenia is a similar condition but of less severity. The terms agranulocytosis, granulocytopenia, and neutropenia are often used interchangeably. Granulocytopenia implies a reduction rather than an absence of the white cells. This condition is always present in pancytopenia also and may be present with aplastic anemia, or it may exist by itself.

Agranulocytosis may come as a single attack and rapidly progress to a fatal termination if not promptly and vigorously treated. It may also occur as a series of attacks with none severe enough to cause death, or it may develop a long-drawn-out course, with frequency and severity of symptoms proportionate to the degree of the reduction of the white cells below the normal level.

In the typical acute attack—always serious—the onset is abrupt, with chills, fever, headache, severe sore throat, and prostration coming on in rapid succession. Early delirium is common. Fortunately however, in the more common and less serious granulocytopenia, there is only a mild to moderate depression of granulocytes. The patient may then have only a slightly more than normal susceptibility to infection and may be able to lead a near-normal life. Still, any infection contracted by the patient is serious and should be promptly treated with appropriate antibiotics.

The cause of agranulocytosis is not always clear, but the drugs and chemicals likely to cause pancytopenia or aplastic anemia are also likely to cause agranulocytosis. Many more drugs have been incriminated as causal agents in granulocytopenia than in aplastic anemia, outstanding among them being some of the most valuable drugs for treating infections and heart, kidney and glandular conditions. Many tranquilizers cause trouble for a few people peculiarly sensitive to doses ordinarily harmless. Pharmaceutical companies and physicians have worked together to remove from use those drugs which can cause harm and for which other drugs can be used. However, no replacements have been found for some medicines valuable in the treatment of particular disease states. The possibility of developing such a serious disease as agranulocytosis is one of the reasons that taking drugs without a physician's supervision is a perilous practice.

Care and Treatment

1. Whenever a rise in the frequency and severity of skin, throat, or lung infections is experienced, a physician should be consulted. He will likely order a complete blood count and tell you quickly whether agranulocytosis is the problem. If it is, he can identify the offending agent, start suitable treatment early, and prescribe precautionary measures against future infections.

2. As far as possible, avoid infections and exposure to infectious diseases by avoiding large crowds or public gatherings.

3. Take no drugs of any kind, including herbs, without the express permission of the physician.

4. Visit your physician regularly and have a blood count taken each time.

5. Keep the general state of your health at the best possible level by abundant rest, daily moderate exercise, and good wholesome food.

6. Promptly cleanse all open wounds with soap and water, and protect them from contamination.

LEUKEMIA

Some forms of leukemia are among the most feared of all diseases, perhaps because nearly everyone remembers a child who died within a few weeks after becoming ill with leukemia, despite all that physicians could do. However, not all types have such a poor outlook.

Several different diseases which affect the white blood cells are grouped under the general term leukemia. They range in manifestation from vicious killers of children and adults to milder forms which permit older people, if afflicted by them, to carry on full activity without discomfort or treatment for ten to fifteen years. Nevertheless all are considered malignant. They are named according to the degree of cell change produced or according to the course of the illness and to the kind of cell involved. Leukemia therefore may be designated as acute or chronic, and then as lymphocytic, granulocytic (myelocytic), or monocytic; *e.g.*, acute granulocytic (myelocytic) leukemia.

In the normal course of events, parent cells (also called stem cells), located in the bone marrow or in the lymphoid organs, constantly produce younger cells destined to become mature and circulate in the blood. This continuous production is necessary in order that cells which wear out in the circulation may be constantly replaced. This multiplication of cells is accomplished by cell division—a biological process in which one cell is squeezed in two in the middle, thus producing two cells. In the early stages of their development, these young blood cells have the ability to divide again and again, each time producing offspring of the same order as themselves. As they mature they develop the capacity to carry out the function for which they were designed. For example, the mature granulocyte becomes able to combat infections caused by germs. Also they eventually lose the ability to multiply by dividing.

In leukemia, the parent or stem cells, or their immediate offspring, lose the ability to mature. In a sense they become "juvenile delinquents," as a famous leukemia expert describes them, retaining the ability to divide and thus go on forming many cells like themselves but being unable to take up their

173

adult duties. The more immature the cells remain, the more acute the leukemia, the more serious the disease, and the less likely that the treatment will be effective.

The continuous division of daughter cells, all paying no attention to the usual controls effective on normal blood-forming tissue, may produce a fantastic number of cells in a very short time. This "runaway" cell growth uses up the nutrients and the space required by the remaining normal parent cells, and they die or do not proliferate. Often the abnormal young cells break out into the bloodstream and circulate as immature blood cells. The behavior of leukemia and its classification depend on the degree of maturity that the involved cells achieve. Acute leukemias have predominantly very young cells, while the chronic leukemias sometimes have cells almost normal in appearance.

Infection of the mouth and bleeding gums may be symptoms indicating acute leukemia.

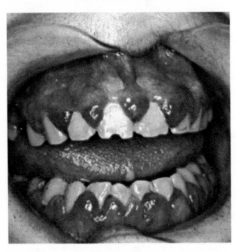

A. *Acute Leukemias.* Acute leukemia occurs as commonly in an adult as in a child. In children it strikes more frequently below the age of six than above; and in children, too, it is more

likely to be acute lymphocytic leukemia, while in the adult acute leukemia tends to be of granulocytic cell type. No race has been found to be exempt and no predilection of one sex over the other is seen.

The symptoms of either acute lymphocytic or acute granulocytic leukemia are indistinguishable except that lymph node enlargement is more common in the lymphocytic variety. The disease may begin suddenly, anemia being the first indication. Bleeding tendencies, infection of the mouth or throat accompanied by fever, extreme weakness, and headache are common. A white-cell count less than normal is the usual case in acute leukemia. In children there is often a history of an infection preceding the main attack by several weeks. Bleeding from the nose, gums, or rectum or excessive bleeding following tonsillectomy or a tooth extraction is common, indicating that the blood platelets are in short supply. At times, in the later stages of the disease, bleeding into vital areas such as the brain occurs. The spleen is enlarged more than the liver. Pain and tenderness in the bones and joints is common, probably because of the pressure of growing cells inside of the marrow cavity. Symptoms of anemia are usually present and may be severe.

A physician makes the preliminary diagnosis on the basis of a blood test. He sees young cells normally not present in the peripheral blood. He then performs or arranges for a bone marrow puncture so that a sample of marrow cells may be studied under the microscope. If he sees a disorganization of white-cell elements, he confirms the diagnosis of leukemia.

Treatment depends on the type of leukemia and the age of the patient. In some situations, one of the cortisones works best. In others, medicines designed to deprive cells of their ability to divide are given. Additional treatment, such as antibiotics for infections and transfusions for severe anemias, are used commonly. Great progress has been made in recent years in the development of drugs which relieve symptoms and in some cases cure the disease. The use of these powerful drugs deserves the best attention of a specially trained physician. The object of these medicines is to retard the growth of the abnormal cells without injuring the normal ones.

Cancer treatment is plagued by faddism more than all other areas of medical practice combined, except perhaps the "keep young" area. In spite of what some people would lead the patient to believe, physicians are as anxious as anyone can be to find a cure for leukemia. They have seen too many beautiful, talented children cut down at the threshold of life, to hold back on any medicines offering a cure, but they are equally anxious that the medicines used will do more good than harm. Do not trust individuals who promise cures in other countries or offer to sell medicines not handled by authorized drugstores.

Care and Treatment

1. The parents of a child suspected of having leukemia should consult their family doctor, who will likely direct them to a specially qualified physician for the evaluation and initial treatment of such a disorder.

2. During the periods of well-being, no favors should be shown to the child that the other children of the family do not enjoy.

3. It may be necessary to afford the afflicted child particular protection against physical injury because of his bleeding tendency.

4. A regular healthful diet and liberal rest are in order.

5. It is especially important that appointments with physicians be kept. Regular blood counts must be made.

B. *Chronic Leukemias.* Chronic leukemias always have an insidious onset, symptoms appearing commonly after several years of disease have elapsed. The same basic mechanism as occurs in acute leukemias is operative also in the chronic leukemias—an inability of the cells to mature, hence uncontrolled division of the cells and unimpeded accumulation. Since the process is slower and the abnormal cells more normal than in acute leukemia, higher counts of cells are seen in the bloodstream. Sometimes an abnormally high white-cell count is the only indication that something is wrong. After several months a person may have accumulated more than 100 times the normal number of leukocytes in his body. This extra tissue growth causes a drain on the body for nutrients and results in lassitude, weakness, and unexplained fatigue. These extra cells may infiltrate various organs and, depending on the degree of infiltration, may reduce that organ's function and efficiency. This is the cause of the enlarged liver and spleen.

Chronic granulocytic leukemia and chronic lymphocytic leukemia occur in the older age group, average age of onset for the former being forty-five and for the latter fifty-five. There is usually a larger spleen with chronic granulocytic leukemia and larger lymph nodes with chronic lymphocytic leukemia. Autoimmune hemolytic anemia is sometimes associated with chronic lymphocytic leukemia.

A person with chronic leukemia may experience the symptoms of anemia, may develop unusual lumps, may be unable to cope with infections as in agranulocytosis, or may have a bleeding tendency because of a low concenteration of platelets. Enlargement of the liver and spleen is an expected development. Nearly always a blood test shows an elevated white-cell count. At times, particularly with chronic granulocytic leukemia, there are nearly as many white cells as there are red cells, hence the term "leukemia" (white blood).

Treatment of chronic leukemia may involve the use of drugs or X-ray irradiation. No attempt is made to cure the patient, only to lessen the symptoms and treat complications as they develop. Chronic granulocytic leukemia

175

more often than not changes to acute leukemia after about five years.

Care and Treatment

1. Any patient with symptoms of a leukemia should be examined by a physician.

2. If diagnosis of leukemia is confirmed, the patient should accept the treatment program recommended and not seek so-called "cures."

3. He should follow the same precautions and instructions noted under agranulocytosis above.

The Lymphoid System and Related Diseases

In order to understand the structure of the lymphoid tissues of the body and how they provide a filtering system, we must begin with a simple description of the tissue fluid and the passages through which this fluid moves.

Tissue Fluid

As blood flows through the capillaries, part of the blood plasma escapes into the small spaces between the cells that make up the body's tissues. The blood cells are too large to escape. Only a small part of the plasma's protein escapes. Part of the substances in the plasma, such as minerals and food materials, move along with the fluid that escapes. As soon as this fluid enters the tissue spaces, it is called tissue fluid. In composition it is very much like blood plasma, except that it does not contain as much protein.

Tissue fluid moves slowly. Most of it seeps back into the blood capillaries and again becomes a part of the circulating blood. But part of it (about three liters a day in an average-sized adult) enters a special system of capillaries called lymph capillaries. Unlike the blood capillaries, the lymph capillaries have open ends which permit the tissue fluid to enter directly from the tissue spaces. As soon as tissue fluid enters a lymph capillary it is called lymph. Lymph and tissue fluid are really the same. The name we use depends upon where the fluid is located.

Lymph capillaries join each other to form small lymph vessels. These join to form larger lymph vessels, very much as small veins combine to form larger veins. Lymph vessels are built very much like veins except that their walls are even thinner. Like veins, lymph vessels have valves which keep the lymph from flowing backward.

Lymph moves in the lymph vessels very much like blood moves in the veins, only more slowly. It does so by action of nearby muscles. As the muscles contract, they press upon the lymph vessels, and this action forces the lymph to move along. It cannot go backward because the valves prevent its backward flow.

The lymph from the right side of the head, from the right arm, and from the right side of the chest, drains into a single lymph vessel which empties into a vein in the right side of the neck. The lymph from all the rest of the body drains into a larger lymph vessel which is called the thoracic duct. This duct pours its lymph into a large vein in the left side of the neck where it mixes with the blood. Thus the lymph from the en-

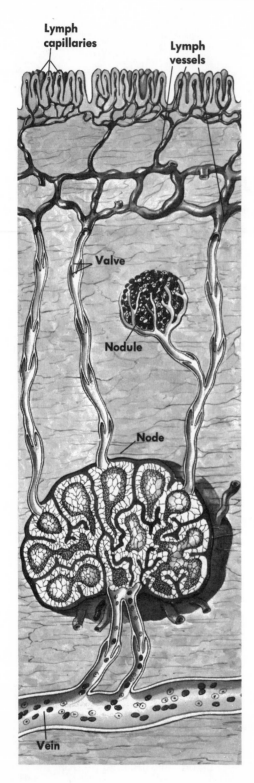

Lymph capillaries

Lymph vessels

Valve

Nodule

Node

Vein

tire body is returned to the bloodstream from which it came.

Lymph Nodes

Along the course of the lymph vessels tiny filtering organs called lymph nodes are interposed, some as small as a pinhead and some as large as a bean. When studied under the microscope, they are found to contain meshworks of delicate connective tissue through which the lymph must percolate as it moves on its way. Located within a lymph node are several kinds of cells which belong to the body's defense system. There are police-duty cells (phagocytes), designed to swallow up and destroy germs that might be carried along by the lymph. The largest number of cells in a lymph node are called lymphocytes, many of which are produced right in the lymph node. Some of these stay in the lymph nodes where they help to combat infection, while others float away in the lymph and constitute one of the major kinds of white blood cells that circulate in the blood. Still another kind of cell in the lymph nodes is the plasma cell.

Now we begin to see the reasons for having a separate system of lymph vessels with their lymph nodes. Sometimes when tissues become infected, germs find their way into the tissue fluid and thus into the lymph. The lymph nodes filter out these germs, and the police-duty cells located there attack the germs as they pass through. When germs enter a lymph node, the lymphocytes there react in such a way as to stimulate the plasma cells to

Diagram showing channels through which the lymph passes on its way from the lymph capillaries to a blood vein. Between these two points the lymph passes through lymph vessels of increasing size which contain valves. Some lymphocytes are added to the lymph by a solitary lymph nodule, and others are added by the lymph node, through which the lymph filters.

produce just the right kind of anti-bodies to protect the body against these particular germs and the toxins which they may produce.

Perhaps you have noticed small, hard lumps (kernels) in the side of your neck when you have had a sore throat, or maybe you have noticed lumps under your arm when you have had an infection in your hand. These hard lumps are enlarged lymph nodes, which have become active in their work of combating an infection. These large nodes are often tender and painful. They are working as actively as they can to prevent the spread of infection to other parts of the body.

In addition to germs, tissue fluid sometimes contains small particles of foreign material which have gained access to the tissues through an injury, through food taken into the body, or through air routinely breathed. This possibility of small particles finding their way into the tissue fluid is especially pronounced in the lungs. When smoke or coal dust is in the air, small particles of carbon enter the air passages as one breathes. These find their way through the walls of the air passages and into the tissue fluid within the tissues of the lungs. As the tissue fluid enters the small lymph vessels, it soon finds its way to lymph nodes located nearby. These nodes filter out the particles of carbon and retain them for the rest of life. Carbon is not soluble, and so it cannot be washed away by any of the body's fluids. When a person has lived in an atmosphere polluted by a great deal of smoke, the lymph nodes inside his chest appear almost black because of the many carbon particles they contain.

The lymph vessels that carry lymph from the breast are of special interest because they provide the usual route by which cancer cells are conveyed from cancer of the breast to other parts of the body. These lymph vessels converge in the axilla (armpit) or in the base of the neck. In these locations many lymph nodes filter lymph that originates in the breast. In a neglected case of cancer of the breast, it is these lymph nodes which become involved first as the cancer begins to spread to other parts of the body. In the surgical treatment of cancer of the breast the surgeon attempts to search out and remove those lymph nodes in the axilla which have become cancerous, leaving, where possible, healthy lymph nodes to continue their warfare against cancer and infections.

The Lymphoid System

Now that we have considered the structure and function of the lymph nodes, we are in a position to broaden our concepts to include the entire lymphoid system, of which the lymph nodes are the simplest example. The human body contains several organs and tissue masses composed of tissue pratically identical to that which composes the lymph nodes. This lymphoid tissue, wherever found, is composed of a meshwork of loose connective tissue containing many cells, mostly lymphocytes. The mature lymphocytes do not remain in any single location. A constant interchange takes place between those located in the lymphoid tissues and those which circulate in the blood. About one third of the total number of white blood cells consists of lymphocytes.

Although all lymphocytes are derived from the same embryological tissue, they are further processed before ending up in the lymphoid tissues. Some migrate to the thymus and become responsible for local or cellular immunity. They are called ''T'' lymphocytes. Others are "processed" in some unknown area of the body and produce antibodies. They are called ''B'' lymphocytes.

The lymphoid system includes the spleen, the thymus, the tonsils, the appendix, and scattered collections of lymphoid tissue in the wall of the lower part of the small intestine called Peyer's patches.

In addition to the functions already listed for lymph nodes, the lymphoid system helps the body reject poisons

179

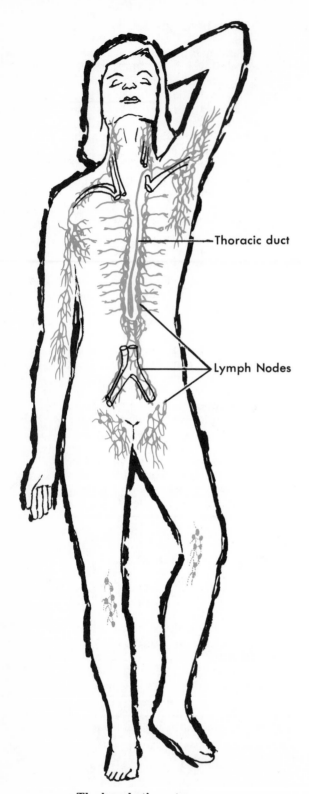

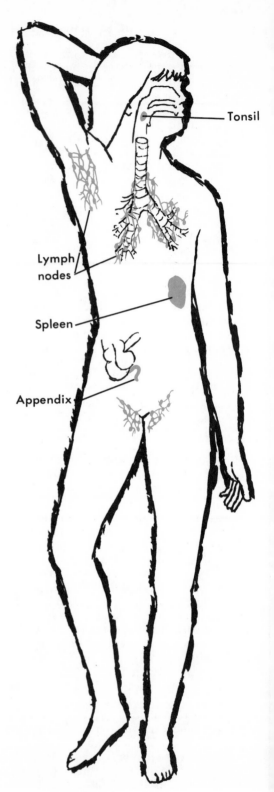

Thoracic duct

Lymph Nodes

Tonsil

Lymph nodes

Spleen

Appendix

The lymphatic system.

The lymphoid organs.

180

and injurious proteins. It probably regulates the healing process. It is the body's lymphoid system that causes transplanted tissues and organs to be rejected. Malfunctions of this system are presumably responsible for diseases such as allergies and certain ailments of the joints, skin, lung, and kidney in the so-called autoimmune category. Since the lymphoid system is widely scattered throughout the body, the physical removal of part of it, if diseased (such as removing the spleen or some of the lymph nodes), appears not to have any major deleterious effect on the body. Certain chemicals, however, can paralyze or destroy the entire lymphoid system.

The Spleen

The spleen is a solid organ, red in appearance, located just under the diaphragm on the left side of the body, where it is protected by the lower ribs. In its internal structure the spleen appears to be a giant lymph node, with one major difference. Lymph nodes are inserted in the course of lymph vessels,

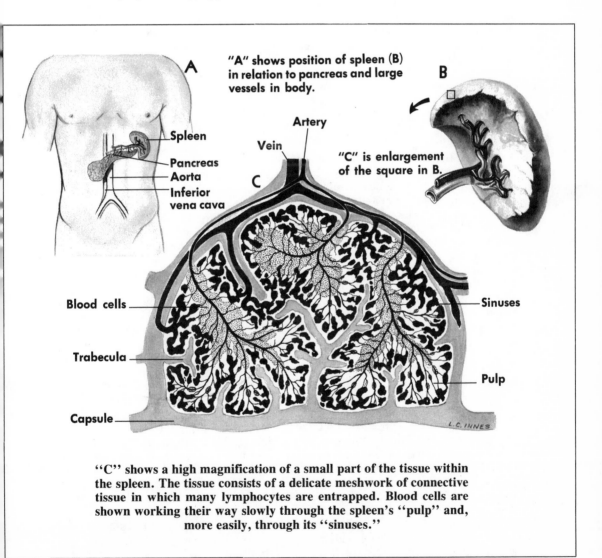

"A" shows position of spleen (B) in relation to pancreas and large vessels in body.

"C" is enlargement of the square in B.

Spleen
Pancreas
Aorta
Inferior vena cava

Artery
Vein

Blood cells
Trabecula
Capsule

Sinuses
Pulp

L.C. INNES

"C" shows a high magnification of a small part of the tissue within the spleen. The tissue consists of a delicate meshwork of connective tissue in which many lymphocytes are entrapped. Blood cells are shown working their way slowly through the spleen's "pulp" and, more easily, through its "sinuses."

and thus they serve as filters for the lymph which moves slowly through the lymph nodes. But the spleen does not filter lymph; it filters blood. Thus it serves as sort of an extra safeguard to filter out germs and particles of foreign substances that may not have been trapped by the lymph nodes and may have actually entered the bloodstream. Because it filters blood, the spleen has a longer list of functions than those of lymph nodes. They include:

1. *Destruction of germs.* The police cells located in the spleen can engulf germs and foreign particles carried by the blood, just as lymph nodes can as they filter objectionable substances carried by the lymph.

2. *Production of blood cells.* In normal adult life the spleen produces lymphocytes just as do the lymph nodes. During fetal life the spleen is capable of producing many kinds of blood cells, even those that in adult life would be produced by the bone marrow. Even in adult life, when some extreme demand for new blood cells arises, as following a severe hemorrhage, the spleen can supplement the work of the bone marrow by producing other types of blood cells.

3. *Storing of blood.* To a certain extent the spleen serves as a reservoir for blood. It is not a very large organ; but, even so, when a severe hemorrhage occurs, the capsule of the spleen contracts, squeezing out the blood which the organ contains so as to increase the amount of circulating blood.

4. *Destruction of old red blood cells.* As mentioned in a previous chapter, the average life of a red blood cell is about 120 days. The spleen serves as a monitor, checking on the red blood cells as they move slowly through its tissues. Those red blood cells that have become decrepit are destroyed as they pass through the spleen, and the hemoglobin which they contain is carried by the blood to the liver. There the iron

portion of the hemoglobin is salvaged for use in the construction of new red blood cells.

5. *Destruction of platelets.* The platelets are tiny packages of chemical substances carried by the blood along with the blood cells. They are normally and primarily concerned with the process of blood clotting. The spleen is capable of destroying worn-out platelets. In a certain disease condition (thrombocytopenia), this function of the spleen becomes overactive to the extent that the number of platelets in the circulating blood is reduced. One of the ways of combating this disease is to remove the spleen by surgery.

6. *Production of antibodies.* Many of the antibodies needed to combat infections are produced here, in the spleen.

The Tonsils

The tonsils belong to the lymphoid system, for they are constructed of the same kind of loose connective tissue impregnated with lymphocytes as found in the lymph nodes and spleen. The tonsils are not primarily concerned, however, with filtering either lymph or blood. They are located, one on either side, at the dividing line between the mouth and the pharynx. The lymphoid tissue which composes the tonsils is located in the substance of the membrane which lines the mouth and pharynx. The surface of the tonsil next to the passageway for food is dotted with many little depressions shaped like test tubes. Under normal conditions the tonsils serve as a testing laboratory for the food being taken into the body. Small portions of food enter these tiny depressions on the surface of the tonsils and come into contact with police cells. If the food is contaminated, these police cells activate the body's mechanism by which antibodies are produced.

Under normal circumstances the tonsils serve very effectively to protect the body from the damage which germs and other harmful agents might cause. There are times, however, when the germs which enter the depressions on the surface of the tonsil are so damaging that they injure the tissue of the tonsil itself, causing the tonsil to become infected. When this infection progesses to the stage of an abscess, we then speak of quinsy, in which an

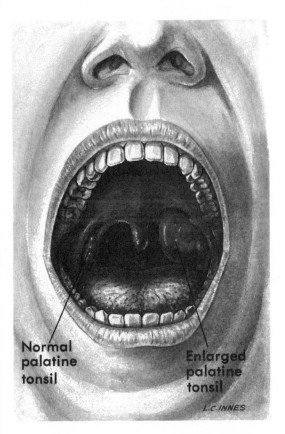

Normal palatine tonsil

Enlarged palatine tonsil

L.C. INNES

infection beginning in the tonsil involves other tissues in the wall of the pharynx. Tonsils which have become seriously damaged cannot hold their own against germ invaders. Small lymph vessels which originate in the tonsils carry this infection to the lymph nodes located nearby in the tissues of the neck. These nodes then become enlarged as they attempt to stem the progress of the infection. This is the usual course in the case of tonsillitis.

In years past, it was assumed that all tonsils once infected should be removed surgically. The present attitude toward removing tonsils is more conservative, for, by the use of antibiotics it is possible to treat many cases of sore throat and avoid the serious development of infections in the tissues of the tonsils. Removal of tonsils (tonsillectomy) is still recommended in extreme cases in which tonsillitis develops repeatedly or in which response to antibiotic medicines is only temporary. Even in such cases the removal of the tonsils should be delayed until such time as the infection of the tonsils subsides.

The pharyngeal tonsils (adenoids) consist of a lymphoid organ located on the back wall of the pharynx, behind the nasal cavity. This small organ functions in about the same manner as the tonsils. It, too, may become infected and enlarged, particularly in early childhood. It sometimes becomes so enlarged that it actually interferes with breathing. The child who has enlarged adenoids tends to breathe through his mouth at night. This tendency to mouth breathing has an unfavorable influence on the development of the bones and soft tissues of the face. Persistent mouth breathing in a child is sufficient reason for surgical removal of the pharyngeal tonsils (adenoids).

For more on diseased tonsils and adenoids, see chapter 9, volume 3.

The Appendix

The appendix is a small, dead-end tube, about the diameter of a pencil and about three inches (7.5 cm) in length, attached to the first portion of the large intestine. The wall of the appendix is composed mostly of lymphoid tissue. For this reason we mention the appendix here. Probably the normal function of the appendix is similar to that of the tonsils—to sample the kind of germs (noxious substances) that may come by and stimulate the body's protective mechanisms.

Just as the tonsils sometimes become overwhelmed by the infections which they are designed to combat, so the ap-

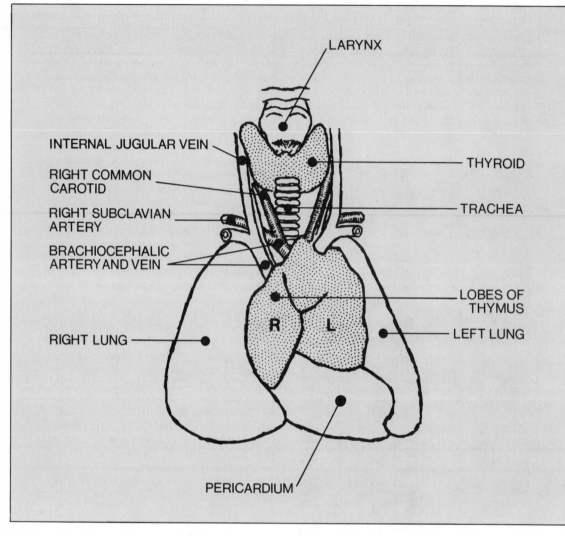

Showing the position of the thymus in the lower neck and upper thorax.

pendix also may become diseased. When this occurs and the appendix becomes actively inflamed, we speak of the condition as appendicitis.

The wall of the appendix is thin and soft. When it becomes infected, danger threatens that the wall will actually rupture, spreading the infection into the general cavity of the abdomen. For this reason an acute case of appendicitis constitutes an emergency. The treatment for appendicitis is the removal of the appendix by surgery. See more

about appendicitis in chapter 17, this volume.

The Thymus

The thymus is a lymphoid organ located in the front of the lower neck and upper chest. It develops early during embryonic life, reaches its maximum phase of development at about 8 years of age, and then slowly decreases in size and regresses in function throughout the remainder of life.

The thymus plays a decisive role in

the development of other organs of the lymphoid system, for it produces a hormone substance (thymosin) which stimulates the lymph nodes and the spleen to produce an important type of lymphocyte concerned with cellular immunity. Without the influence of the thymus, the lymph nodes and spleen could not perform their function of maintaining the body's defense against infection.

The thymus produces a small proportion of the lymphocytes contained in the blood. However, the thymus does not serve as a filter for either lymph or blood.

Complications of Suppressing the Lymphoid System

As indicated earlier in the chapter, the lymphoid system is designed to protect the body against the hazards of infection. It may therefore be properly called the immune system.

It is this same system of organs and the antibodies they produce that cause problems, however, when an effort is made to transplant a tissue or an organ from some other individual. The lymphoid system is triggered to produce antibodies of such nature and such influence as to reject any material foreign to the particular person. It is because of this rejection reaction that surgeons have experienced disappointment in their hope of being able to transplant a healthy heart into a person whose own heart has become unable to perform its usual work. And the same applies to a greater or lesser degree in the attempts to transplant other tissues or organs from one person to another. Under normal circumstances, the lymphoid system performs its intended work well. But the vigilance of this system to reject any foreign substance becomes a handicap in the matter of transplanting tissues and organs.

In their effort to find ways of successfully transplanting tissues and organs, medical scientists have devised ways of suppressing the lymphoid system while the transplantation of a tissue or organ is being accomplished.

Certain chemical medications are used to dampen the activity of the lymphoid system and thus suppress the rejection reaction. These efforts to suppress the lymphoid system have been more successful in the transplantation of kidneys than in the transplantation of hearts.

It happens that most of the chemical medications used in the treatment of cancer by chemotherapy also have the effect of suppressing the lymphoid system. The use of such chemical medications is surely justified both when organ transplantation is being performed and when cancer is being treated. However, this suppression of the lymphoid system reduces the patient's ability to resist infection. Extra precautions must therefore be taken to protect a patient against contact with germs whenever chemical medications are used to suppress the lymphoid system.

Acquired Immune Deficiency Syndrome (AIDS)

Beginning in 1978 there appeared in the United States a mysterious disease in which the lymphoid system (the immune system) becomes unable to perform its usual function of protection against infections. Called acquired immune deficiency syndrome (AIDS), the disease occurs especially among homosexuals and others who are sexually promiscuous and among drug abusers who inject into their veins. The number of cases has been increasing rapidly. Almost half of the cases end fatally. The affected persons suffer from any one of a variety of infections, especially of the lungs, skin, and membranes. As yet, there is no satisfactory treatment.

Lymphadenopathy (Involvements of the Lymph Nodes)

The commonest involvement of lymph nodes is an inflammation in response to a regional or systemic infection. For this condition we use the term *lymphadenitis*.

As explained in the previous section, the lymph nodes serve a protective function by helping to prevent the

185

spread of germs, toxins, and foreign materials throughout the body. It is understandable, then, that when an infection develops in a certain part of the body, the lymph nodes that serve this

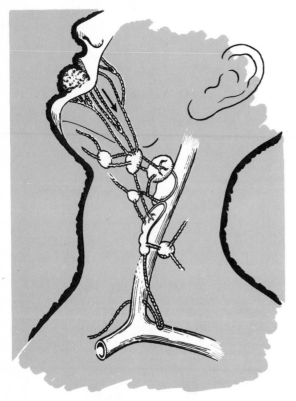

Infections involving the lymph nodes beneath the jaw and in the sides and front of the neck cause enlargement of these nodes, the swellings sometimes being called "kernels."

part become inflamed. Lymph nodes, normally inconspicuous, now become enlarged, tender to the touch, and painful.

Infections in the scalp cause an enlargement of the nodes at the back of the neck. Those of the eyes, ears, teeth, mouth, and pharynx involve the nodes beneath the jaw and in the sides and front of the neck, which can then be felt as tender lumps (kernels). Infections of the hand activate the nodes in the axilla (armpit). Infections of the

breast also affect the nodes in the axilla. Infections of the lower extremities and of the genital organs involve the inguinal nodes located in the groin. Involvements of the internal organs affect the nodes placed deeply in the body cavities.

Infections which affect lymph nodes may be caused by bacteria, viruses, spirochetes, or fungi. Streptococci and staphylococci are the most common offenders. When an infection is generalized, as in such diseases as measles and infectious mononucleosis, the lymph nodes of the entire body are affected accordingly.

Lymph nodes become involved, of course, in the diseases of the lymphatic system like leukemia and Hodgkin's disease. Many types of cancer are carried to other parts of the body by the lymph stream rather than by the blood. This explains why the lymph nodes located in the path of lymph drainage from a cancer often become cancerous. Lymph nodes so involved usually feel more firm than those activated by infection. Removal and microscopic examination of lymph nodes often give the surgeon valuable information on the spread of cancer.

Lymphomas

The lymphomas are a group of diseases that involve serious alterations in the organs of the lymphoid system. They are characterized by an enlargement of some or all of the lymph nodes, plus an involvement of the spleen and often of the bone marrow. The symptoms vary from case to case, occurring late in some cases and early in others. This variation in the timing and intensity of the symptoms often makes the diagnosis difficult. In fact, the diagnosis of lymphomas cannot be made for certain except by the procedure of biopsy, in which a sample of tissue, usually from an involved lymph node, is removed and studied microscopically.

The lymphomas are classed as forms of malignancy, because they progress toward a fatal outcome. Newer, intensive methods of treatment by radiation and/or by chemotherapy bring about remissions and possibly cures in about half the cases.

Because of the progressive course of these illnesses and because some of their characteristics resemble those of leukemia, the lymphomas are often considered to be forms of cancer. They are described here, however, rather than in chapter 11, volume 3, because of their specific involvement of the lymphoid system of organs.

HODGKIN'S DISEASE

Hodgkin's disease is the best known of the lymphomas because it is a discrete disease in which a unique form of cell structure (Reed-Sternberg cells) can be observed by a microscopic study of the affected tissues. An estimated 6000 new cases of Hodgkin's disease develop each year in the United States. And the non-Hodgkin's form of lymphomas are more numerous.

Cases of Hodgkin's disease tend to develop during either one of two age periods: ages 15 to 34 and after 50 years of age. The cases which develop in later life are usually more rapidly progressive in their serious course.

The first evidences of Hodgkin's disease may appear gradually. There is a painless enlargement of lymph nodes, usually in the neck, with a gradual increase in the number of lymph nodes involved. Those located where they can be felt are elastic to the touch. Troublesome itching may accompany this early lymph node enlargement. Some cases progress for a period of months without other symptoms developing. But in other cases there will be persistent fever, night sweats, fatigue, weight loss, and anemia. The disease progresses at a variable rate over a period of months or years. On X-ray examination it can be discovered that the lymph nodes in the chest are usually involved. In addition to the ivolvement of the spleen, the liver is also often affected. Various additional symptoms may develop because of pressure of the enlarging lymph nodes against vital structures within the body.

Care and Treatment

Those physicians who have become skilled in the treatment of Hodgkin's disease have developed a scheme of four stages of the disease. By a careful study of the affected tissues in a given case, plus an observation of the patient's particular symptoms, the case can be assigned to one of these four stages. This preliminary "staging" is important because the plan of treatment most successful for one stage may not benefit the cases which properly belong in other stages.

Radiation therapy and/or combination chemotherapy are the forms of treatment adapted to the individual case. Both of these carry the possibility of serious side effects. Therefore, patients with Hodgkin's disease should preferably be treated at a medical center where the professional staff is skilled in the handling of such cases. With properly administered intensive treatment, the prospect of a ten-year, relapse-free survival is about 50 percent.

NON-HODGKIN'S LYMPHOMAS

The non-Hodgkin's lymphomas constitute a group of several separate forms of illness, distinguished by differences in the cell types which occur in the affected tissues. In none of these do we find the unique cell type characteristic of Hodgkin's disease. Non-Hodgkin's lymphomas may occur at any age, but their frequency of occurrence increases with age.

The signs of these diseases are similar to those of Hodgkin's disease, with weakness, weight loss, fever, night sweats, and anemia being among the usual symptoms. In some cases it is a persisting enlargement of the tonsils that first calls attention to the illness. There is a greater incidence of involvement of the liver, the bone marrow, and the lymph nodes in the vicinity of the spleen and intestines in non-Hodgkin's lymphoma than in Hodgkin's disease.

Care and Treatment

Essentially the same treatment procedures are used for non-Hodgkin's lymphomas as are effective in Hodgkin's disease. Here also the particular manifestations of a case must be evaluated before a choice is made among the treatment possibilities.

Some cases tend to progress so rapidly that intensive treatment must be used. In other cases, particularly in elderly persons, the progress of the disease is slow, and palliative forms of treatment may be justified.

SECTION IV

The Respiratory System

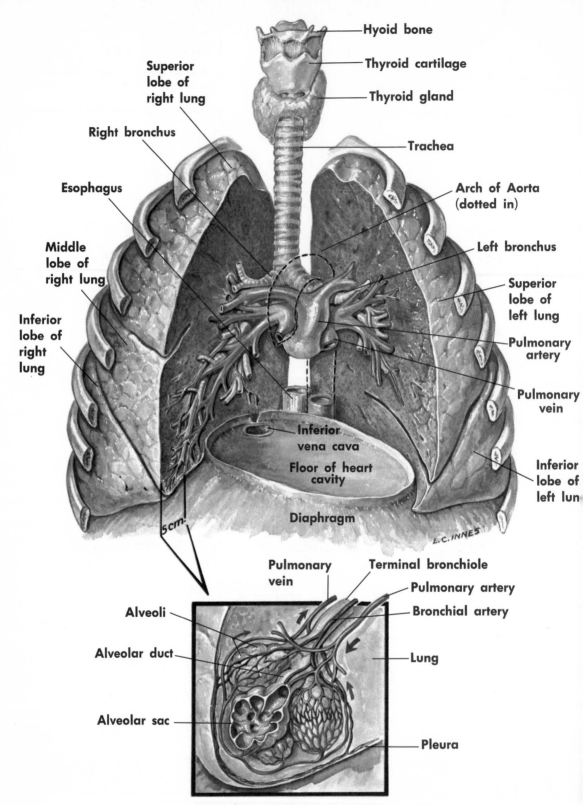

Hyoid bone

Thyroid cartilage

Thyroid gland

Superior lobe of right lung

Right bronchus

Esophagus

Trachea

Arch of Aorta (dotted in)

Middle lobe of right lung

Left bronchus

Superior lobe of left lung

Inferior lobe of right lung

Pulmonary artery

Pulmonary vein

Inferior vena cava

Floor of heart cavity

Inferior lobe of left lun

5 cm.

Diaphragm

L.C. INNES

Pulmonary vein

Terminal bronchiole

Pulmonary artery

Bronchial artery

Alveoli

Alveolar duct

Lung

Alveolar sac

Pleura

View of the lungs and details of their structure.

The Larynx, Air Passages, and Lungs

The human body has more constant need of air and the oxygen which it contains than of any other substance. A person can go for days without food; he can go many hours without water; but he can go only about four minutes without oxygen. At any one time, under ordinary conditions, the body contains 1200 ml. (a little more than one quart) of oxygen—enough to last about four minutes. The body does not store oxygen. Some of the cells in the brain are so dependent on oxygen that they receive permanent damage once their supply of oxygen is cut off.

Oxygen makes up about one fifth of the air of our atmosphere. Most of the remaining portion is nitrogen. As far as the body's needs are concerned, nitrogen simply comes and goes with the air that is breathed only because it is part of the "package" in which oxygen is provided.

In the lungs, oxygen from the air is transferred to the blood. The hemoglobin of the red blood cells serves as a vehicle to carry the oxygen from the lungs to all tissues of the body. Every cell within the body uses oxygen to maintain its vital activities. The oxygen unites with food materials within the cell to produce the cell's energy. As a by-product of this chemical action, carbon dioxide is produced within the cell. This gas is transferred to the blood and carried back to the lungs, where it leaves the blood and enters the air within the lungs. Thus, the air exhaled from the lungs contains more carbon dioxide, and slightly less oxygen than the air taken into the lungs. Under normal circumstances an adult takes air into his lungs about sixteen to eighteen times a minute. A child breathes faster than this. So does an adult when exercising. Also, when a person's body temperature is increased, as in a case of fever, the rate of breathing becomes faster than usual.

Ordinarily, in quiet breathing, about one pint (450 ml.) of air is taken into the lungs with each breath. It is possible, of course, to inhale much more than one pint of air. When an average young adult fills his lungs to their limit and then breathes out all the air that he possibly can, he has exhaled about seven pints (3150 ml.) of air. Even then another two pints (900 ml.) of air remain within the lungs and air passages.

In the present chapter we are considering the various organs of the body concerned with the transport of the air which is breathed. These organs make up the respiratory system. The respiratory system consists of (1) the nose, (2) the pharynx (throat), (3) the larynx (voice box), (4) the trachea (windpipe), (5) the bronchi (branches of the trachea), and (6) the lungs.

The Nose

The nose is designed to prepare the air for its trip into the lungs. We might say that the nose is the air conditioning unit of the respiratory system. The nose filters the air, adds moisture to it, and warms it. Most of the filtering is done in the nostrils. Inside the nostrils are many hairs which trap the larger dust particles before they have opportunity to pass into the other respiratory organs.

The membranes lining the nose are kept constantly moistened by the watery fluid produced by tiny glands located in these same membranes. It is estimated that these glands in the membranes of the nose produce about 900 ml. (nearly a quart) of water each day. This fluid moistens the incoming air so that it will not be irritating to the tissues of the lungs.

Inside the cavities of the nose, both on the right and on the left, are three barlike structures called conchae or turbinates. They are found on the lateral (outside) wall of each nasal cavity. The conchae are shelves of bone covered with the same kind of membrane that lines the rest of the nasal cavity. Many tiny blood vessels are located within the covering membranes, and these carry large amounts of blood just beneath the surface of the membrane. The incoming air, as it is inhaled, is warmed by passing over the conchae.

Perhaps you have noticed that on a very cold day the air you breathe seems to irritate your lungs. This happens because you are breathing too rapidly for the cold air to be warmed as it passes through the nose.

The nose also contains the organs of smell. These are located high up in the nasal cavities, one on each side. When a person wishes to smell something carefully, he must sniff. Sniffing directs the incoming air into the upper parts of the nasal cavities where it comes in

contact with the organs of smell. When you have a cold, the nasal cavities become partly filled with mucus. This keeps air from reaching the organs of smell. As a result, smelling is difficult or impossible.

The Nasal Sinuses

The nasal sinuses are spaces within the bones of the head and face which connect with the nasal cavities. They are lined with the same kind of membrane that lines the inside of the nose. Two of these sinuses are located just

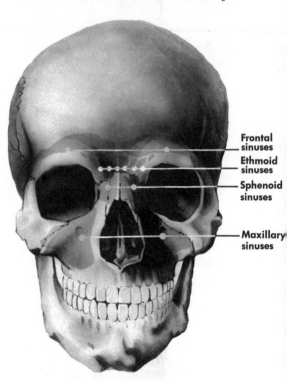

Frontal sinuses
Ethmoid sinuses
Sphenoid sinuses
Maxillary sinuses

Outline showing location of sinuses of the face.

behind the eyebrows. Another pair is located in the upper jawbone on either side of the nostrils. Other small sinuses are found above and behind the nasal cavities.

The nasal sinuses are empty spaces which improve the quality of one's voice, just as the space inside a violin gives the instrument a better tone.

Sometimes the linings of the sinuses become inflamed. An inflammation of the linings of the nasal sinuses is what constitutes sinusitis.

The Pharynx

The pharynx is the space located behind the nasal cavities and behind the mouth. The upper openings into the pharynx include the right and left nasal cavities and the mouth. Below, the pharynx connects with the larynx and with the esophagus (the passage for food). The pharynx, then, is the passageway for both air and food. The tonsils are located in the sides of the pharynx (where it opens into the mouth) and adenoid tissue is located in its posterior wall. The auditory tubes (eustachian tubes), right and left, also open into the upper and back part of the pharynx. These connect the pharynx with the middle ear cavities.

The Larynx

The larynx or voice box is located just below the pharynx and just in front of the upper part of the esophagus. Below, the larynx is directly continuous with the trachea (windpipe).

The walls of the larynx are reinforced with cartilage. This cartilage makes the walls of the larynx firm enough so that they do not collapse and at the same time permits the larynx to bend rather than to break when it is compressed from the outside. You can feel some of the cartilage in your larynx ("Adam's apple") as it moves up and down when you swallow or speak. At the very top of the larynx there is a small flap of membrane-covered cartilage called the epiglottis. This serves as sort of a trapdoor and helps to keep food and fluid from entering the larynx and trachea. When a person swallows, the entire larynx is pulled upward by muscles so that it contacts the epiglottis. This serves to close the opening into the larynx while food or fluid is being swallowed.

Inside the larynx is a pair of shelflike folds of tissue known as the vocal cords. The vocal cords can be tight-

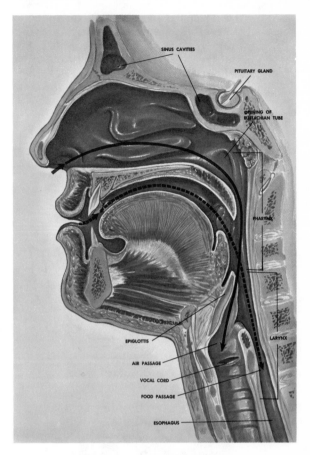

A drawing of the head, showing the route taken by air (solid line) and food (broken line).

ened or loosened by the action of small muscles in the walls of the larynx. When you speak, air coming from the lungs is forced past the vocal cords. When drawn tight, the vocal cords are caused to vibrate by the stream of air as it passes by. These vibrations produce sound. When the vocal cords are pulled very tight, the sounds are high-pitched. When the vocal cords are more relaxed, the sounds have a lower pitch. When a great deal of air passes through the larynx, the sound made by the vocal cords is loud. When there is a small volume of air passing through, the sound is not as loud. When not being used, the vocal cords fold back against the walls of the larynx so that the air can pass in and out in silence. When they are being used, however, the vocal cords almost touch each other in the midline of the larynx.

The tongue, lips, teeth, and other parts of the mouth cooperate in forming

Position of vocal cords during quiet breathing (top); during deep breathing (center); during high, shrill note (bottom).

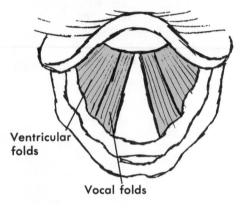

Ventricular folds

Vocal folds

Cushion of Epiglottis

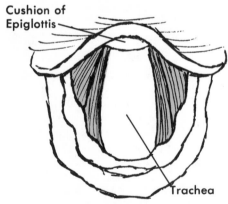

Trachea

Upper lip of epiglottis

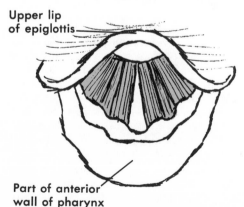

Part of anterior wall of pharynx

words from the sounds produced in the larynx.

The reason that a man's voice is deep-pitched as contrasted with a woman's voice is that a man's larynx is larger and therefore his vocal cords are longer than those of a woman. When a boy enters manhood, his larynx grows very rapidly during a few months. It is at this time that his voice is said to change as it becomes deeper-pitched. A girl's larynx does not enlarge as much when she becomes a woman. So a woman's voice is higher pitched than a man's throughout life.

The Trachea (Windpipe)

The trachea is a straight tube which carries air from the larynx above to the midportion of the chest, where the trachea branches to form the bronchi. The trachea is held open by many rings of cartilage built into its wall.

An interesting feature of the trachea, as also of the nasal cavities and bronchi, is that its lining membrane is studded with millions of tiny hairlike structures called cilia. The cilia wave quickly toward the pharynx and slowly in the opposite direction. Working in unison, they function like a built-in broom which keeps sweeping out all the tiny dust particles not trapped by the hairs in the nostrils. They also bring up mucus that may have collected in the air passages. When ciliary function becomes inadequate to move secretions and possible foreign materials into the pharynx, a forceful cough is effective in keeping the trachea open.

But for the combined actions of the cilia and the coughing mechanism, mucus and other substances which might get into the trachea and bronchi could interfere seriously with airflow and thereby impair ventilation in the lungs. Thus a person could suffocate in the secretions produced by his own tissues.

The walls of the trachea are well supplied with circulating blood. Thereby, it assists the nose and pharynx in warming and moistening air as it moves through it toward the lungs.

The Lungs

The lungs consist of two major parts—the right lung and the left lung—located near the center of the chest cavity a little more to the left side than to the right. The heart is between the lungs and in front of the trachea and bronchi. Because the heart encroaches on the space in the left side of the chest, the lung on this side is smaller than the right lung. The left lung has only two lobes, whereas the right lung has three.

As the trachea reaches the central portion of the chest, it branches suddenly to provide three bronchi for the right lung (one for each lobe) and two for the left lung. These major bronchi branch quickly into smaller tubes and these into still smaller, and so on, until the final branchings of what we call the "bronchial tree" number about one billion units. The final branchings of this system are the so-called air sacs in which the actual exchange of oxygen and carbon dioxide occurs.

The lungs have two sources of blood: the pulmonary arteries which bring blood from the right side of the heart, and the bronchial arteries which accompany the bronchi in their repeated branchings. The reason for this double blood supply is that the pulmonary arteries, coming from the right side of the heart, carry blood from which the oxygen has already been removed by the tissues through which it has passed. This blood would not be able to nourish the tissues of the lungs. Therefore the bronchi and lungs must have their own supply of fresh blood through the bronchial arteries which come from the left side of the heart by way of the aorta.

Like all arteries, the ones that carry blood from the right side of the heart to the lungs branch and keep on branching until they become capillaries. Within the lungs the air sacs and the capillaries lie side by side in such a way that only a layer of thin cells separates the air from the blood. This layer of cells is so thin that it permits oxygen to pass freely from the air to the blood and car-

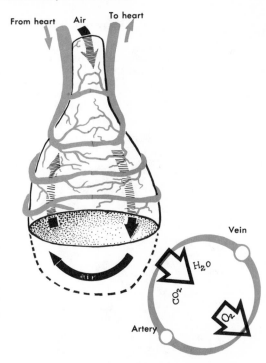

A diagram showing how an air sac in the lung allows the blood and air to come very close together.

bon dioxide to pass freely from the blood to the air.

The Mechanism of Respiration

Until now we have discussed breathing without explaining what causes the air to enter the lungs. The lungs themselves have no way of pulling air through the nose. Air is brought into the lungs by the action of certain muscles. These muscles increase the size of the chest each time a person breathes. As the chest increases in size, the lungs are expanded. Air rushes in to fill the extra space thus made available. Then when the muscles relax, the chest returns to its previous size and the air is forced out the way it came in.

The muscles which increase the size of the chest (the muscles of respiration) are the diaphragm, the muscles between the ribs (intercostal muscles), and certain muscles in the neck. These are the muscles used when air is taken into the lungs. The diaphragm is a large

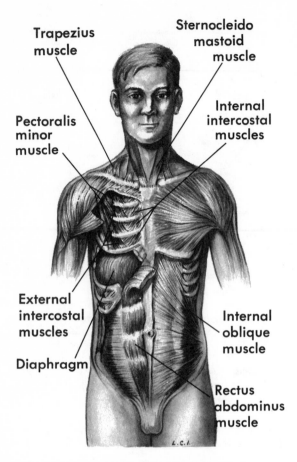

Trapezius muscle

Sternocleido mastoid muscle

Pectoralis minor muscle

Internal intercostal muscles

External intercostal muscles

Diaphragm

Internal oblique muscle

Rectus abdominus muscle

The muscles of the human body that make breathing possible.

can see this effect by holding a tape measure around your chest when you take a deep breath. The muscles between the ribs contract at the same time the diaphragm contracts and therefore help the diaphragm to expand the lungs.

The muscles in the wall of the abdomen produce an effect just opposite to that of the diaphragm and muscles between the ribs. When the muscles in the wall of the abdomen contract, they crowd the abdominal organs and diaphragm upward. This causes the air to leave the lungs quickly or else builds up a pressure within the chest. Such air pressure gives force to the voice in talking and singing.

Try holding one hand in front of your abdomen while you take a deep breath. After you have filled your lungs, hold your nose while you act as though you were trying to force the air out of your lungs. This exercise builds up air pressure inside your chest. Notice how tight the muscles in the wall of your abdomen become. It is such pressure that helps you to shout or to sing loudly.

The action of the muscles of respiration is controlled by nerves, as is the case with all of the body's muscles. As you already know, it is possible to make yourself breathe faster or deeper or to hold your breath for a while. This capability comes from your having voluntary control of the nerves and muscles concerned with breathing. Ordinarily, however, the process of breathing is controlled automatically by a nerve center in the lower part of the brain. This center sends out nerve impulses to the breathing muscles so that they contract and relax alternately. The nerve center even controls how fast and how deeply you breathe. When you exercise, the breathing center sends out its impulses in a faster rhythm than when you rest. There are even times when this breathing center makes you stop breathing temporarily. For example, when you swallow, your breathing stops until the food or water passes the opening into your larynx.

The breathing center also controls

dome-shaped muscle located at the level of the lower ribs, which separates the chest from the abdomen. The heart and lungs are in the chest cavity above the diaphragm. The liver, stomach, spleen, and the other abdominal organs are below the diaphragm. When the diaphragm contracts, it pulls downward against the organs in the abdomen. This action allows the lungs (situated above the diaphragm) to expand.

The ribs do not go around the chest on a horizontal plane, but slant downward from back to front. When the muscles between the ribs contract, they pull the front ends of the ribs upward. This movement has the effect of increasing the chest measurement. You such actions as coughing and sneezing. Whenever the lining of the air passages is irritated, the breathing center sends out nerve impulses which cause the abdominal muscles to contract quickly. This interaction forces the air out of the lungs almost all at once. In coughing, the air is forced out through the mouth; in sneezing, through the nose and mouth. The quick action of coughing or sneezing helps to carry out whatever substance was causing irritation in the air passages.

Snoring is quite a different matter. Snoring is caused by the vibration of soft tissues in the walls of the air passages as air moves in and out of the lungs. As a person sleeps, the muscles that operate during wakefulness to control the soft palate, the pharynx, and the larynx may relax to the extent that the column of moving air causes these tissues to vibrate noisily. There is no real remedy for snoring except for the sleeper to change his position so that the relaxed tissues of his air passages vibrate in a different direction.

The Covering of the Lungs

The lungs are covered by a smooth, moist membrane. At the roots of the lungs, where the blood vessels enter and leave and where the air passages enter the lungs, this smooth covering membrane doubles back on itself and forms a complete lining for that part of the chest in which each lung resides. These two layers of smooth membrane—the one that covers the lungs and the one that lines the chest cavity—are together spoken of as the pleura. Normally no space separates these two layers—they rest in contact with each other. Because their surfaces are smooth and moist, they glide past each other without friction as the lungs expand and contract.

In certain diseases, the pleura becomes irritated, rough, and painful. This condition is spoken of as pleurisy. In a case of pleurisy, each breath causes pain.

Sometimes a disease will cause fluid to accumulate between the two layers of the pleura. Because this fluid takes up a certain amount of space, the lungs are not able to expand completely. Sometimes, in treating such a case, the physician will introduce a needle between the ribs and remove the fluid which has accumulated between the two layers of the pleura.

For a fuller treatment of this subject see the following chapter.

In Summary

As we conclude our description of the organs for breathing and speaking, it seems proper to hesitate a moment to contemplate the marvels of the respiratory system. How remarkable is the way in which the air we breathe is automatically warmed and moistened as it enters the body! Even the excess tears, which have already worked one shift in keeping the eyes moist and clean, are carried through the tear ducts into he nose and there help to add moisture to the air that is breathed. Every breath of air, as it comes and goes, also does two jobs: It brings in a supply of oxygen and takes away a load of carbon dioxide. As it goes out, it can even be made to do a third job by providing the means for talking and singing.

The rate at which one breathes and the depth of each respiration is controlled automatically. One breathes oftener and more deeply whenever his body cells need more oxygen.

Breathing is not only necessary to life, but also a pleasant activity. The air we breathe brings the odors of flowers, of food, and of the countryside.

Diseases of the Respiratory Organs

The lungs rank along with the heart in having to function moment by moment in order to sustain the body's necessary activities. It follows, then, that diseases which affect the lungs or the air passages constitute a threat to life.

In the shifting patterns of disease that have occurred during the present century, the lungs have both gained and lost. Some diseases prevalent at the turn of the century have now come under partial control. Pneumonia and influenza, which topped the list of causes of death in the United States in 1900, now stand in fifth place, responsible for less than 3 percent of total deaths. This improvement stems largely from the beneficial effects of sulfa and antibiotic drugs. Most cases of tuberculosis involve the lungs. Tuberculosis was responsible for 10 percent of the total number of deaths in 1900. Though cases of tuberculosis still occur, it no longer appears among the first ten causes of death in the United States.

On the other hand, cancer of the lung, as well as the chronic obstructive pulmonary diseases, has increased at an alarming rate. This tragic increase is largely chargeable to the use of cigarettes.

Certain of the diseases of the respiratory organs are considered in volume 3. Those that pertain to the nose and pharynx are included in chapter 9. Cancer of the lung is considered in chapter 11, along with cancers which occur in other parts of the body.

A. Diseases of the Larynx

The two most common symptoms of laryngeal disease are hoarseness and obstructed breathing. Hoarseness may progress to complete loss of the voice (aphonia), and obstruction to breathing may become so severe as to cause death from asphyxia.

LARYNGITIS

Laryngitis, an inflammation of the soft tissues of the larynx, occurs most frequently as part of a viral upper respiratory infection such as the common cold. It may also occur as part of such illnesses as influenza, pneumonia, whooping cough (pertussis), and measles. Hoarseness, its most common symptom, is often accompanied by a sensation of rawness and an urge to clear the throat.

Care and Treatment

Resting the voice and the swallow-

ing of warm fluids helps to relieve the discomfort of laryngitis. The breathing of steam, with care not to inhale so vigorously as to burn the membranes of the air passages, may hasten symptomatic improvement. When laryngitis occurs as part of some other illness, the primary illness should be treated appropriately.

VOCAL CORD DAMAGE

Damage to the vocal cords or the adjacent tissues of the larynx may result from abuse of the voice, as in prolonged screaming or shouting; it may come from continued public speaking in which the voice is not used properly; or it may come from inhalation of irritating fumes or cigarette smoke. Such irritations may cause the development of small polyps on the vocal cords or the appearance of small, firm nodules on the free edge of the vocal cords. In some cases small ulcers develop in the membrane lining the larynx. Persisting hoarseness is the usual symptom in these cases.

Care and Treatment

Examination should be made by a physician to determine the exact nature of the problem. This move is especially important because of the possibility of a beginning cancer which, if treated early, can usually be treated satisfactorily. Otherwise, the treatment consists of the surgical removal of polyps or nodules, if present, a limitation on the excessive use of the voice, and lessons in voice therapy to develop proper habits of using the voice.

CANCER OF THE LARYNX

Cancer of the larynx develops most commonly among smokers. The significant symptom is hoarseness. Persistent hoarseness, particularly in the smoker, gives urgent reason for a careful examination by a physician. When cancer of the larynx is discovered early, immediate treatment offers about a 90 percent chance of recovery. Even in cases treated early, it may be necessary for

the surgeon to remove part or all of the larynx. For further facts on cancer of the larynx, see chapter 11, volume 3.

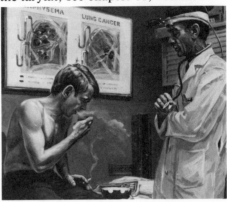

B. Cardinal Symptoms of Pulmonary Disease

Most of the diseases that affect the respiratory organs produce symptoms caused by altered functions. Some of these changes, such as fever and lack of energy, represent the body's broad response to illness. Others relate specifically to the respiratory organs. We will mention three cardinal symptoms:

COUGH

The membrane lining the air passages is very sensitive to irritation. When it is irritated the glands within the membrane produce an excess of mucus. Dust particles or noxious gases in the air cause this reaction. Very hot or very cold air also irritates the membranes. Cigarette smoke is an irritant and causes an excess of mucus to be produced.

Even a small excess of mucus may plug some of the smaller air passages. When the irritation is intense and many air passages become closed, the person coughs. A cough consists of a sudden expulsion of air from the lung, which dislodges the mucus filling the air passages. After coughing, the person is often able to resume normal breathing.

Coughing can be associated with many conditions, some serious and some not so serious. Cigarette smoking paralyzes the tiny cilia, the hairlike processes in the lining of the airways which normally sweep out the mucus. Without these fine "hairs," coughing is the primary mechanism smokers have for clearing the airways. Coughing can also be a symptom of a cold, emphysema, bronchitis, pneumonia, lung cancer, or tuberculosis of the lungs. Persistent coughing should attract the attention of the individual and his doctor to the basic cause while it is still early enough to do something about it. For a broad discussion of cough as a symptom of various problems, see chapter 6, volume 2.

Care and Treatment

Cough is a protective mechanism serving to open the air passages once they become blocked. However, some people think of cough more as a disease than as a symptom, and so they "treat" the cough by using medicines designed to suppress the cough. In many cases it is better to let the cough serve its purpose of opening up the air passages than to suppress it and thus hinder the natural process by which excess mucus and purulent material are expelled from the lungs. Fundamentally and ideally, treatment should be directed toward the basic cause of the cough rather than to suppressing it. Gentle inhaling of steam, either from an open vessel in which water is boiling or from an inhalator device, will often relieve the irritation in the air passages. When the cause of the coughing is in doubt or when a cough persists for more than a week, a physician should be consulted.

SHORTNESS OF BREATH (DYSPNEA)

Even a normal, healthy person becomes short of breath when he exercises so vigorously that the demand for oxygen throughout his body is greater than his lungs and heart can provide. And this overdraft gives a clue on the meaning of shortness of breath when it occurs in connection with a disease. It means that the body's tissues are not getting as much oxygen as they need at that time.

Other causes account for shortness of breath besides disease of the lungs. The heart may be unable to pump a sufficient volume of blood to carry the amount of oxygen needed. Or because of some form of anemia the blood is not able to carry as much oxygen as would be normal. Shortness of breath may even result from a shortage of blood, as following a severe hemorrhage. These various other causes of shortness of breath are considered in chapter 6, volume 2.

In the present chapter, we are concerned with the shortness of breath that results (1) from disease of the lungs that interferes with the transfer of oxygen from the air to the blood or (2) from conditions in which the airways leading to and from the lungs become obstructed so that the usual volume of air does not reach the lungs' air sacs.

COUGHING UP OF BLOOD (HEMOPTYSIS)

A few streaks of blood in the sputum may have no serious import, for this symptom occurs occasionally in cases of bronchitis and other forms of inflammation of the respiratory organs. But larger amounts and more frequent bleeding from the lungs may be associated with some life-threatening condition.

In any case in which blood is coughed up or expectorated it is important to discover the source of the blood. It may have come from the nasal cavities or nasal sinuses. It may have come from the stomach by way of the esophagus. But if the blood is of bright red color and comes from the lungs in quantities greater than 2 or 3 teaspoonfuls, it indicates a severe hemorrhage and requires a prompt and thorough examination by a physician to determine the cause and nature of the hemorrhage.

C. The Common Cold

The common cold is an infection of

the upper air passages (nose, sinuses, pharynx) by any one of a large group of viruses. The virus infection is easily transmitted from person to person by infected droplets of moisture or contaminated dust floating in the air. The symptoms develop from one to two days after exposure. A person who harbors the infection can transmit it to other persons a few hours before his own symptoms begin and for as long as five days after his symptoms have appeared.

Exposure to cold or to wind, extreme fatigue, loss of sleep, or other causes of reduced vitality make a person more susceptible to the common cold.

Inasmuch as the common cold may be caused by any one or more of a large number of viruses, protection by immunization is difficult. Even having an attack of the common cold makes a person immune to only the particular virus or viruses which caused his recent illness. He is still vulnerable to other viruses. Therefore, the practical means of prevention is by maintaining good general health and vigor and by avoiding excesses of fatigue and exposure.

Symptoms of the common cold usually begin with a roughness or irritation in the throat, followed by sneezing and by the discharge of watery fluid from the nose. In most cases systemic symptoms such as mild chilliness, general aching, and a feeling of indisposition also appear.

As the tissues of the upper air passages become irritated because of the virus infection, they then become vulnerable to invasion by common bacteria, always present in the air passages. It is such a secondary infection by common bacteria that is responsible for the complications that may develop, such as infection of the middle ear (otitis media), infection of the nasal sinuses, bronchitis, and even pneumonia.

Care and Treatment

The person with a common cold should avoid becoming fatigued and should be protected against exposure to wind and unfavorable temperatures.

As a courtesy to other people, one suffering from a common cold should cover his face with a handkerchief when he sneezes or coughs and should avoid being near other people while his symptoms last. Such precautions help to protect the spread of the virus infection.

Antibiotic medications are not effective in combating virus infections. They are therefore not useful in treating the common cold unless complications develop because of the invasion of common bacteria.

The use of large doses of vitamin C has been recommended by some authorities for the prevention or treatment of the common cold. Controlled experiments indicate that vitamin C does not uniformly prevent the occurrence of common colds, even though it may have a slight favorable effect on the severity and duration of symptoms.

The use of nose drops and of steam inhalations may help to relieve the discomfort of the common cold.

Heating compresses to the throat or to the chest, particularly during the night, will help to relieve the symptoms and hasten recovery from the common cold. See chapter 25, in volume 3.

D. Chronic Obstructive Pulmonary Disease (Chronic Bronchitis and Emphysema)

Beginning about 1970 there developed an alarming increase in the number of cases of chronic obstructive pulmonary disease, until within the succeeding ten years it accounted for over 50,000 deaths per year in the United States. An estimated 200,000 persons in the United States are confined to bed because of chronic obstructive pulmonary disease. An additional half million must limit their regular activities because of it. The disability and death caused by this disease

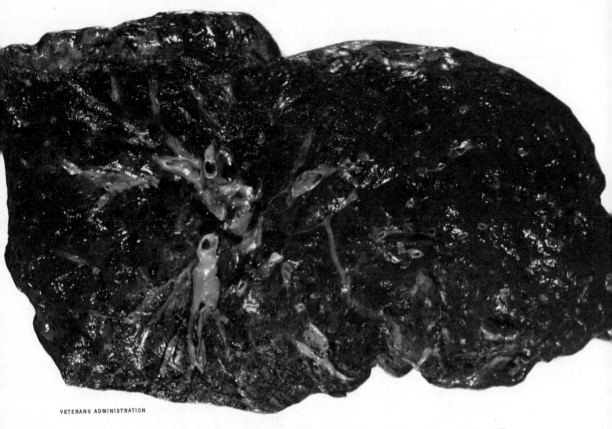

VETERANS ADMINISTRATION

Emphysema diffused throughout the lung. The enlarged alveoli, characteristic of the disease, may be observed on the surface.

is exceeded only by heart disease. It affects an estimated 15 percent of older men. About eight times more cases occur among men than among women. However, the incidence among women is increasing.

The term chronic obstructive pulmonary disease includes the two ailments of chronic bronchitis and emphysema. These used to be described as separate diseases, but because they result from the same causes and because they both interfere with the flow of air to and from the lungs, these two illnesses are now being described as part of the same disease process. In some cases the damage to the tissues of the air passages (chronic bronchitis) is more pronounced than the damage to the delicate tissues in the air sacs of the lungs

(emphysema). But in every case, both the air passages and the lungs suffer damage. Thus it is proper to consider chronic bronchitis and emphysema as part of the same manifestation of disease.

When chronic bronchitis is the principal manifestation, there has developed an inflammation and swelling of the tissues forming the walls of the air passages. The glands which produce mucus become enlarged and are more active than normal. The principal symptoms are cough and the raising of much mucus.

When the emphysema predominates, large-scale destruction of the walls of the air sacs located at the ends of the smallest air passages takes place. The lung loses some of its elasticity which normally enables it to expand with each breath. Cavities form as a result of the breakdown of the walls of the air sacs, and these cavities contain an accumulation of contaminated mucus. The efficiency of the lungs is greatly reduced, and the patient suffers much because of coughing and shortness of breath.

Because the lung cannot repair itself, chronic obstructive pulmonary disease is a serious form of illness. Once established, the only benefit of treatment is to make life a little more comfortable for the months, or perhaps a few years, during which the disease progresses. In mild cases, the patient experiences progressive invalidism for a period of ten or more years. In more severe cases, death may occur as soon as two years after the diagnosis of the disease.

Because chronic obstructive pulmonary disease is not curable, once established, we focus our attention on prevention, which brings us to the consideration of its causes. Cigarette smoking is the major factor. It is recognized that certain irritants such as cotton fibers, asbestos fibers, and coal dust, carried by the air into the lungs, may play a part in causing or aggravating this disease. But the influence of these other irritants is minor as compared with the damaging effect of cigarette smoke. Smoking interacts with air pollution to produce higher rates of this disease than would be caused by either factor by itself.

Early Detection

We have said that no cure exists for chronic obstructive pulmonary disease once it becomes established—only palliative treatment which makes the patient a little more comfortable. But let us tarry a moment on the expression "once established." During a very early phase of this disease it may be possible to prevent its further development, provided the aggravating factor or factors are removed. Practically, this observation means that when evidence indicates the beginning of chronic obstructive pulmonary disease, prompt discontinuance of smoking, in addition to the avoidance of irritants in the air, may prevent the further development of this tragic illness.

This suggestion of hope brings us to the question, How can a person recognize chronic obstructive pulmonary disease in its very early stages?

The usual first evidence is the development of a persistent, productive cough. By this description we mean that the usual "smoker's cough" gradually changes to a cough in which mucus is raised from the air passages during a coughing episode. If the mucus contains pus, this symptom is even more significant.

An additional evidence that helps a person to know whether his air passages and lungs are becoming involved with chronic obstructive pulmonary disease is the rate at which he can empty the air which has been drawn into his lungs. The patient can perform a simple home test to measure this rate. It requires that the person inhale all the air he possibly can. Then, with his lungs filled to their limit with air, he measures the time in seconds required to completely expel all the air his lungs contained. This requires the use of a stopwatch. The person with normal lungs and air passages can expel this air in a period of three seconds. If the emptying time in a given case exceeds five seconds, good evidence exists that chronic obstructive pulmonary disease is already present.

Care and Treatment

We must emphasize that prevention is the only satisfactory way of avoiding chronic obstructive pulmonary disease. As mentioned in the previous paragraphs, if this disease can be detected in its very early stages, it may be possible to arrest its progress or even to partially reverse the damage already done, by discontinuing smoking and avoiding aggravating irritants in the air. These irritants include cotton dust, certain plastic vapors, the fumes of welding operations, and the high levels of nitrous and sulfur dioxides contained in

smog. By all means the most important factor is to abstain from smoking cigarettes.

The person with chronic obstructive pulmonary disease must be protected as far as possible from the infections that affect lungs and air passages. He should receive flu shots every year as a means of preventing, as far as possible, the flu that would aggravate his condition. When he develops infections, these should be treated vigorously, under a doctor's direction. As the word *obstructive* implies, he has difficulty in keeping his air passages open. The sticky mucus which tends to close off certain of the air passages must be coughed up in order to allow sufficient air to reach his lungs and thus to provide his need for oxygen. As the obstruction to his breathing becomes more serious, he will need to be taught the methods of postural drainage by which he can rid the air passages of the accumulations of mucus. He will also receive benefit from breathing oxygen or an oxygen-rich mixture with air.

E. Other Involvements of the Bronchi

BRONCHIAL ASTHMA

Asthma is a chronic disease characterized by attacks of coughing, wheezing, and difficult breathing in which the patient feels that once he has drawn air into his lungs it is almost impossible to expel it. An attack of asthma may last for a few minutes or many hours. Between attacks, the patient is relatively free from symptoms, even though the basic problems in the tissues persist.

Three changes in the air passages account for the symptoms of asthma: (1) A contraction in the smooth muscle cells in the walls of the air passages causes their lumen to become smaller. (2) A swelling of the tissues lining the air passages still further encroaches on the space through which air passes to and from the lungs. (3) The glands in the lining of the air passages become overactive and produce excess amounts of mucus.

An estimated 2.5 percent of the population suffers from asthma in one degree or another. Sixty-five percent of all asthma patients develop their symptoms before the age of five years. Thus we see that more than half the cases of asthma begin during childhood. It is said to be the most common chronic disease of childhood. Boys and men are afflicted with asthma more than girls and women in a ratio of about 2 to 1. The asthma that begins early in childhood often declines in severity as a child becomes older, so that about half of those who have had asthma in their early childhood have become symptom-free by the time they reach adulthood.

Asthma can be controlled quite satisfactorily by the use of appropriate medications, so that most persons who have asthma can, by following a proper treatment program, live relatively normal lives. Even so, about 5000 deaths per year in the United States can be attributed to asthma, the victims being mostly persons who have neglected to arrange for a treatment program adapted to their particular cases.

The attack of asthma may begin gradually or suddenly. It is characterized by a feeling of tightness in the chest, accompanied by coughing and wheezing. These symptoms become more severe until the patient actually struggles to force the air out of his lungs. In doing so, he typically leans forward as he rests his face against his crossed arms. His lips and even his skin take on a dark blue coloration due to the decrease in the oxygen which his blood receives as it passes through the lungs. The patient actually experiences a certain panic because of his difficult breathing and may become agitated and somewhat mentally confused. He labors actively to breathe, bringing into use all the muscles of respiration. Thus his heartbeat becomes rapid. As he coughs, he expels thick, tenacious mucus.

Many factors have their influence in

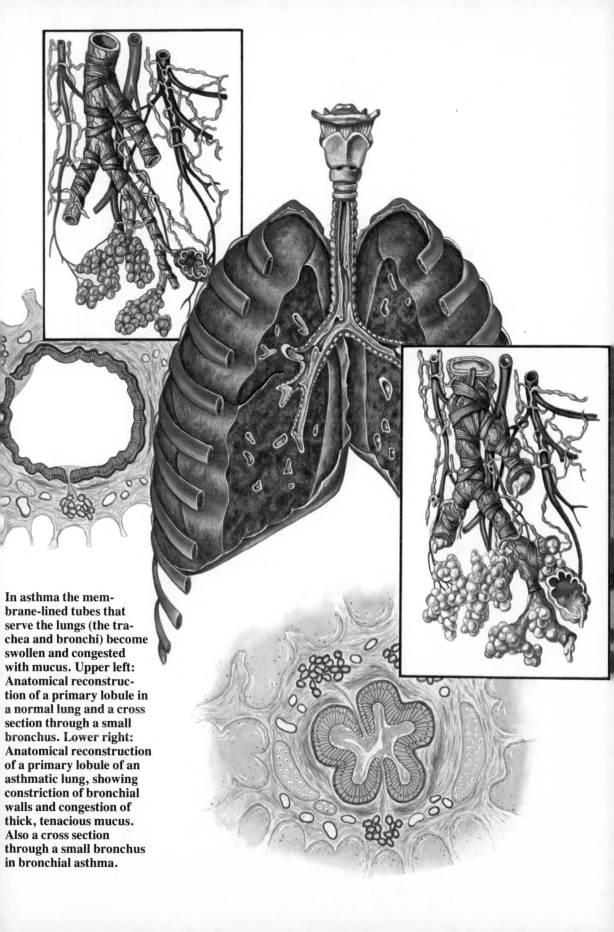

In asthma the membrane-lined tubes that serve the lungs (the trachea and bronchi) become swollen and congested with mucus. Upper left: Anatomical reconstruction of a primary lobule in a normal lung and a cross section through a small bronchus. Lower right: Anatomical reconstruction of a primary lobule of an asthmatic lung, showing constriction of bronchial walls and congestion of thick, tenacious mucus. Also a cross section through a small bronchus in bronchial asthma.

causing asthma. Basically, the problem stems from an inherited predisposition manifested by the unusual sensitivity of the air passages to certain irritants or allergens. We may say, then, that in most cases of asthma the important element of allergy plays a part. Certain irritants may trigger an attack of asthma, some persons being sensitive to particular irritants and other persons being sensitive to different ones. The list of irritants includes house dust, pollens, animal dander, tobacco smoke, and grain dust. In some cases a food sensitivity such as the eating of eggs, shellfish, or chocolate may provoke an attack of asthma. Some people are sensitive to certain pollutants in the air, such as sulfur dioxide. Infections of the organs of breathing, especially viral infections, may trigger an attack. Vigorous exercise itself may precipitate an asthmatic attack in certain people.

Certain circumstances may lower a person's resistance to the extent that, if he has a predisposition to asthma, he will, under those circumstances, have an attack. These include exposure to cold air, exertion and fatigue, emotional stress, and excitement. In many cases it is not possible to identify the exact circumstance that triggers the attack of asthma. It is common for the attack to occur during the night.

Care and Treatment

For Immediate Relief. When an attack of asthma is not too severe, a warm drink or the inhalation of vapor from a vaporizer or pan of boiling water may be helpful. A cone made of newspaper is useful in directing the vapor to the face of the patient. Care must be taken, however, to prevent the hot vapor from burning the face or the membranes of the air passages.

In more severe attacks, it is preferable for the patient to be admitted to a hospital so that he can be under the immediate care of a physician. Certain medications have the effect of relaxing the spasm of the muscle cells in the walls of the air passages so that air can move more freely into and out of the lungs. Also, the corticosteroid medications, properly selected and administered, have a very beneficial effect. Care must be given to the patient's water balance so as to prevent his becoming dehydrated. In some cases allowing the patient to breathe oxygen is a help at the time of an acute attack.

Long-range Treatment. It is important to discover the particular circumstances that trigger an attack of asthma. The various irritants and conditions that set the stage for an attack should be carefully avoided. In some cases the patient's sensitivity may be reduced by a series of desensitizing injections arranged by the physician. The use of flu shots each year may help to reduce the infections of the organs of breathing which often set the stage for asthmatic attacks. Physical exercise should be limited to the individual's ready tolerance. Extremes of cold and of humidity should be avoided. Many patients who have asthma derive benefit from the use of aerosol-administered medications such as may be selected by the physician in charge. Several of the effective medications are taken by mouth at specified times throughout the twenty-four hour period.

BRONCHIECTASIS

In this condition the medium-sized and smaller bronchi, usually in the lower part of one or both lungs, dilate and become pockets in which chronic infection persists, with the formation of large amounts of pussy mucus.

Bronchiectasis is characterized by fits of coughing and the raising of much mucus, especially in the first hour or two after rising in the morning and immediately upon lying down at night. Another important symptom is coughing up of blood (hemoptysis), which usually occurs at times of recurrent infection.

Bronchiectasis usually develops as an aftermath of pneumonia, especially the pneumonia that occurs as a complication of whooping cough or measles.

The outcome of a case of bronchiectasis depends upon whether it is possible to control repeated and persistent infections of the lung tissues. When such infections can be controlled, either by the use of antibiotic medications or by the surgical removal of a portion of the lung, life expectancy is approximately normal. In cases where the infection cannot be controlled, the patient's life will be correspondingly shortened.

Care and Treatment

Two forms of treatment may be used in caring for the patient with bronchiectasis: medical and/or surgical. The choice between these two depends upon observations made during the thorough examination of the lungs, which includes not only X-ray studies but the use of the bronchoscope (an instrument by which the physician observes the interior of the air passages).

The medical form of treatment consists of controlling infections of the lung by the use of antibiotic medications, along with helping the patient to obtain relief by postural drainage. Postural drainage involves positioning the patient so that the accumulated mucus can be raised and expectorated. In the usual procedure, the patient lies across a bed with his face and chest hanging downward. His elbows rest on a pillow on the floor and his body is turned so that the most seriously affected side of his chest is uppermost. This position places the head and neck at a lower level than the lungs. The patient should assume this position three or four times a day, especially in the morning when rising, and hold the position for at least ten minutes each time. Coughing will probably be spontaneous, but this is desirable because it promotes drainage of the mucus that has accumulated. If the patient is a smoker, his smoking must be discontinued.

Surgical removal of a portion of a lung is beneficial when the disease is largely limited to one part of one lung. By the surgical removal of this part, the coughing, the production of excess quantities of mucus, and the tendency to hemorrhage will thereby be eliminated.

CYSTIC FIBROSIS

Cystic fibrosis is a serious disease of hereditary origin which begins in infancy and continues through childhood as long as the patient survives—an average of 15 to 20 years—though this statistic is now improving with better patient care. This disease affects the glands which produce secretions in the air passages of the lungs, the pancreas, and the skin. The involvement of the lungs is characterized by chronic cough, wheezing, the excessive production of thick mucus, and recurring infections of the air passages. For a further discussion of this disease together with suggestions for care and treatment, see chapter 17, volume 1.

F. The Pneumonias

Several forms of pneumonia prevail which, though differing in causes and manifestations, consist of an acute infection of the delicate tissues of the lungs. Several kinds of bacteria, viruses, and fungi may cause such infection. When the infection involves principally a certain lobe of a lung, the disease may be called lobar pneumonia. When the infection is scattered throughout the lungs and involves the delicate tissue closely related to the bronchi, it may be called bronchopneumonia.

Pneumonia is a serious disease for two reasons: (1) The toxemia is relatively great. (2) One's very life depends on the continuous functioning of the lungs. In diseases of the digestive organs a person may go without food for a while, thus giving the affected organs a rest from their usual function during the process of healing. But the lungs must function continuously, day and night, whether involved with disease or not. If their involvement with disease

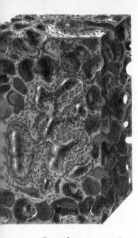

Bronchopneumonia

Purulent exudation in the terminal bronchiole is spreading into the attached alveoli, with a surrounding cuff of serous exudation and hyperemia.

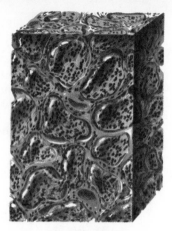

Lobar Pneumonia

Lobar pneumonia, showing alveoli filled with fibrinous exudate containing polynuclear leukocytes; the exudate traverses the alveoli and is of uniform composition throughout the section.

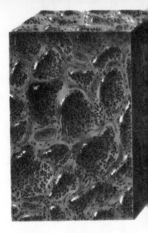

Friedländer's Pneumonia

The alveoli are packed with polynu clear leukocites and necrotic mucoi material; note necrosis of part of th alveolar walls, with early formation microabscesses.

Lobar Pneumonia

Lobar pneumonia of the right middle lobe, gray hepatization, with acute fibrinous pleuritis.

Friedländer's Pneumonia

Lobar pneumonia of right upper lobe; Friedländer's bacillus; the pleura shows fibrinous exudate and the cut surface has a thick nucopurulent surface over a diffusely purplish-gray consolidation.

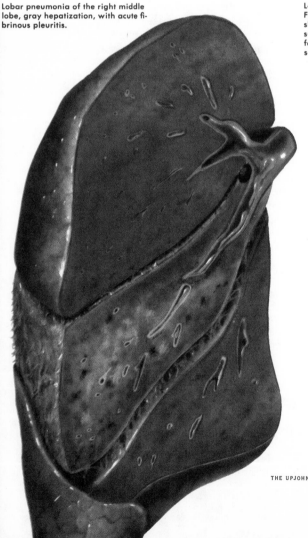

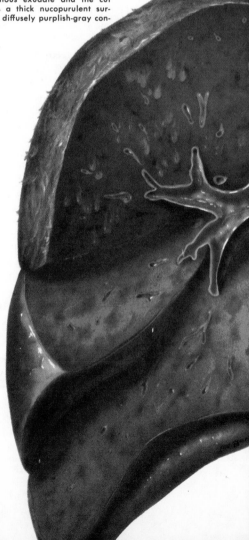

curtails their function too much, death results.

Prior to the advent of antibiotic drugs, pneumonia in its various forms was one of the major killers. Infection of the lungs, once established, had to run its course as the body endeavored to build up resistance to the particular germ causing the pneumonia. If resistance was developed soon enough, the patient got well, but if the infection overwhelmed the body's defenses, the patient died.

Now the picture is different. Pneumonia, untreated, is still a serious, even fatal, disease. But with the early and proper use of antibiotic drugs, most of the organisms that cause pneumonia can be rendered harmless even while the resistance to the organisms is being developed. As for the care of the pneumonia patient, it is well to use general measures to build up his vitality while the antibiotic drugs are taking effect. The germs and viruses which cause the various forms of pneumonia are widely prevalent, and almost every individual is exposed to them repeatedly. The reason that more cases of pneumonia do not spring up is that when the body's defenses are functioning well, the organisms are disposed of before they become established in the lung tissues. Under conditions of lowered vitality and consequent lowered resistance to infection, a person becomes ill with pneumonia.

Understandably, pneumonia often follows the common cold. It occurs in alcoholism or in cases of malnutrition or general debility. It may result from exposure to extremes of temperature or may follow injury to the tissues of the lungs.

PNEUMONIA CAUSED BY THE PNEUMOCOCCUS

Pneumonia that is caused by the pneumococcus bacterium is characterized by a sudden onset of symptoms: a violent chill accompanied by a rapidly mounting fever (up to 105° F. or 40.6° C.), chest pain on breathing (in which the pain may also involve the abdomen or the shoulder), cough, and the spitting of rust-colored (blood tinged) sputum. The breathing becomes rapid, with respirations up to 40 per minute.

When untreated, pneumococcal pneumonia runs its course in about two weeks, ending in death in more than 30 percent of cases and in prompt improvement (by "crisis") in the remaining 70 percent. Common complications are pleurisy, empyema, lung abscess, infection of the heart (pericarditis or endocarditis), and meningitis.

In cases treated early and adequately with antibiotic drugs or sulfonamides the mortality rate is less than 5 percent.

Care and Treatment

The patient with pneumococcal pneumonia is in urgent need of care by a physician, preferably in a hospital. The first procedure will be to take samples of the patient's blood and sputum so that it can be determined in the laboratory just what germ is responsible for the patient's illness. On the basis of the laboratory findings, the doctor will select the antibiotic medication or the sulfonamide most suitable for the particular case. In cases in which the pneumococcus is the proven cause of the illness, penicillin G is the preferred drug to be used. Other antibiotics and sulfonamides may be used to advantage in selected cases.

Patients with this type of pneumonia respond favorably to the proper medication within a matter of hours or at least three or four days. The medications must be continued, however, until the patient has been without fever for about 40 hours.

Complete bed rest, the administration of sufficient fluids to avoid dehydration, and the use of oxygen for the patient to breathe are important during the period of illness. Hydrotherapy treatments are helpful in building up the patient's resistance to the infection. These can be given two or three times a day during the acute phase of the illness. The treatment room should be sufficiently warm when such treatments are given. A hot footbath in bed, in addition to four or five hot fomentations to the chest, followed by a brisk, cold mitten friction, constitute a suitable adjunct to antibiotic treatment. For further details on the use of hydrotherapy in such a case, see chapter 25, volume 3. Also, see chapter 2, volume 2, for mention of polyvalent vaccine which provides protection from pneumococcal pneumonia.

PNEUMONIA CAUSED BY OTHER BACTERIA

During recent years an increasing proportion of pneumonias are caused by organisms other than the pneumococcus. These infecting germs include streptococcus, staphylococcus, and Friedländer's bacillus (Klebsiella pneumoniae). Usually these cause bronchopneumonia. The illness in these cases may have either a sudden or a gradual onset. It usually develops secondary to some other illness, such as a virus infection, viral pneumonia, influenza, measles, or some debilitating disease. Common complications of these cases include pleurisy, empyema, and lung abscess.

Care and Treatment

The plan for care and treatment is essentially the same as that for pneumonia caused by the pneumococcus as described above. Here again it is important that laboratory tests be made as early in the disease as possible to determine what germ is causing the infection. This information is an important guide to the physician in determining what antimicrobial medication to use.

MYCOPLASMAL PNEUMONIA

Mycoplasmal pneumonia, formerly called primary atypical pneumonia, is caused by infection of the lung tissues by a tiny organism, the *Mycoplasma pneumoniae* (formerly called the Eaton agent), which is smaller than some viruses and larger than others. This type of pneumonia accounts for approximately 7 percent of all forms of pneumonia.

Mycoplasmal pneumonia is most common in the 10- to 30-year-old age group. The time from exposure until the beginning of symptoms is about two to three weeks. The onset of the illness is gradual, with symptoms of headache, fever, and cough. The disease sometimes reaches epidemic proportions, especially in schools and military camps where young people associate closely together. Recovery is usually spontaneous in about ten days. The illness is usually transmitted from one person to another by droplets produced by sneezing or coughing by someone who is ill with this disease.

Care and Treatment

Mycoplasmal pneumonia does not respond well to the penicillins but is benefited by erythromycins and tetracyclines which, at least, serve to shorten the course of the illness. Other than this therapy, general supportive care, which includes bed rest, adequate fluid, mild diet, and hydrotherapy as outlined under PNEUMOCOCCAL PNEUMONIA, is beneficial.

VIRAL PNEUMONIA

Viral pneumonia is an illness in which the delicate tissues of the lungs are affected by one of several kinds of viruses. Inasmuch as viruses are responsible for the common cold and inasmuch as some cases of viral pneumonia are mild and are caused by extension of the infection of a common cold, the involvement of the lungs is not always recognized as a form of pneumonia and may even pass for a severe cold. There are many cases of this mild form of viral pneumonia—so many that viral pneumonia, in one degree or another, accounts for about 75 percent of the acute pulmonary infections.

We must not assume that viral pneumonia is always a mild disease. Severe

but they also permit a sidewise motion by which the chin can be moved from side to side. Inasmuch as the teeth are anchored in the upper and lower jaws, the provision for a sidewise movement of the lower jaw aids in the grinding of food as it is crushed between the upper and lower teeth. The movements of the lower jaw are produced by muscles which reside in the deeper portions of the face and neck.

The Salivary Glands

The entire internal mouth is lined by a membrane designed to resist the friction with food and at the same time permit the free movement of this food as it is manipulated by the tongue and crushed by the teeth. This membrane is kept moist at all times by the saliva

Showing the position of the salivary glands.

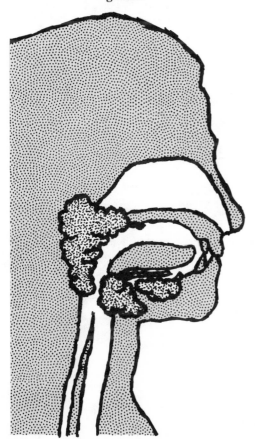

produced by three pairs of salivary glands. The parotid glands, right and left, are located in the deep tissues of the face, just in front of the ears. Each gland produces a watery secretion of saliva which is conveyed by a tiny duct within the upper part of the cheek, which opens into the vestibule opposite the upper second molar tooth. The sublingual salivary glands lie in the floor of the mouth on either side of the base of the tongue. The secretion which they produce is delivered through a row of several small ducts which open beneath the sides of the tongue. The submandibular salivary glands lie in the floor of the mouth toward the front and near the midline. The duct from each of these glands opens beneath the tip of the tongue, one on the right and one on the left.

The Tongue

The tongue is a marvelous organ designed for active and precise movements which aid in the manipulation of food as it is being chewed and which assists in the proper shaping of the mouth for the enunciation of spoken words. The bulk of the tongue's substance is composed of interlacing muscle fibers so placed as to permit movement of the tongue in many directions. The tongue is covered on its sides and undersurface by the same type of membrane that lines the remainder of the mouth. On its upper surface, however, the covering of the tongue is modified by the presence of many tiny papillae which make the surface rough enough to move the food from place to place as it is being chewed. The tongue is abundantly supplied with nerves, some of which control the muscle fibers that permit its various movements and many of which make the tongue sensitive to sensations of temperature, touch, pressure, and pain. Also there are embedded in the surface of the tongue many tiny taste buds capable of responding to the fundamental tastes of sweet, sour, bitter, and salt as may be contained in the food taken into the mouth.

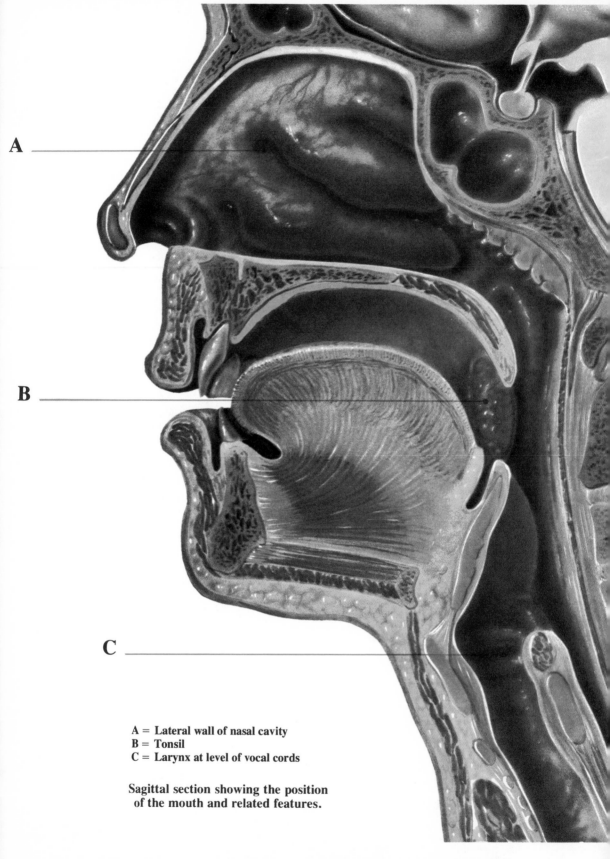

A = Lateral wall of nasal cavity
B = Tonsil
C = Larynx at level of vocal cords

Sagittal section showing the position
of the mouth and related features.

B. The Teeth

Development of the Teeth

During his lifetime a person has two sets of teeth. The first set consists of 20 teeth, called the primary, deciduous, or baby teeth. A later set of 32 teeth are called secondary teeth or permanent teeth. As indicated in the accompanying diagram on page 228, the individual teeth of these two sets make their appearance in the mouth according to a schedule which begins in infancy at about $7^1/_2$ months of age and continues through childhood and on to about 21 years of age.

The ages given in the diagram are those at which the teeth erupt through the soft tissues of the gums and thus become available for chewing. But before that, the teeth are in process of formation for many months—several years in some cases.

The development of the primary teeth begins about seven weeks after conception. These 20 primary teeth, already well formed within the tissues of the jaws at the time of birth, make their appearance by pushing through the soft tissues of the gums as indicated on the diagram. Permanent teeth begin their development at about the middle of the period of intrauterine life (5 months after conception). Thus the preschool child has two sets of teeth present in his mouth—the primary teeth, already in place and available for chewing, and the permanent teeth, still hidden within the deeper tissues of the jaws awaiting their respective dates for erupting.

The reason for having two successive sets of teeth is that the teeth of the primary set are smaller and thus adapted to the smaller size of the young child's jaws. As the jaws become large enough to accommodate large-sized teeth, the primary teeth are replaced by the permanent teeth.

The permanent set of teeth consists of 32 teeth—12 more than compose the primary set. This means that three molar teeth of the permanent set eventually emerge in each side of each jaw behind the position of the last tooth of the primary set. The first molars of the permanent set come into the mouth at about the same time that the central incisors of the primary set are being replaced by the central incisors of the permanent set. The replacing of the incisors attracts attention, for the child notices that his front teeth become loose and are soon ready to be pulled. Then there grows into the available spaces other, slightly larger teeth—the central incisors of the permanent set.

The erupting of the first molar tooth of the permanent set is not spectacular. It comes into the mouth silently and is often unnoticed. When it is noticed, it sometimes is mistakenly assumed that it belongs to the primary set. This is unfortunate, for this first permanent molar tooth is destined to remain throughout life or until destroyed by disease. Very often the child and his parents neglect to take proper care of this first permanent molar tooth, and so it becomes the most susceptible of all the teeth to damage by dental caries.

Even when the permanent teeth begin to make their appearance in the mouth, the jaws are still growing. For this reason the third permanent molars (the "wisdom teeth") do not erupt until after the seventeenth year—there is not room enough for the entire set of 32 teeth until this age is reached.

Occasionally a person's jaws do not grow enough to provide room for this third molar even by the time he reaches adulthood. That is, some jaws never become large enough to accommodate the complete set of 32 permanent teeth. In such cases, the third molar teeth move into abnormal positions, sometimes being directed against the second molar teeth in a manner that keeps them from erupting. Such teeth are said to be impacted. It is usually advisable to have them removed by dental surgery.

The teeth seem to compete to some extent for space in the mouth. In a case where the jaw is not large enough to permit all 32 teeth of the permanent set

JAWS OF CHILD ABOUT 6 YEARS OLD

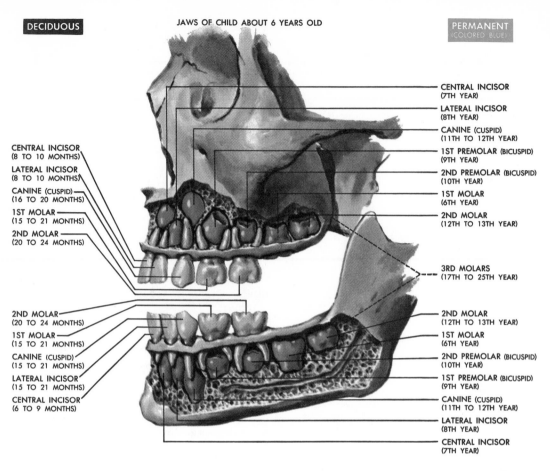

CENTRAL INCISOR
(7TH YEAR)

LATERAL INCISOR
(8TH YEAR)

CANINE (CUSPID)
(11TH TO 12TH YEAR)

1ST PREMOLAR (BICUSPID)
(9TH YEAR)

2ND PREMOLAR (BICUSPID)
(10TH YEAR)

1ST MOLAR
(6TH YEAR)

2ND MOLAR
(12TH TO 13TH YEAR)

3RD MOLARS
(17TH TO 25TH YEAR)

2ND MOLAR
(12TH TO 13TH YEAR)

1ST MOLAR
(6TH YEAR)

2ND PREMOLAR (BICUSPID)
(10TH YEAR)

1ST PREMOLAR (BICUSPID)
(9TH YEAR)

CANINE (CUSPID)
(11TH TO 12TH YEAR)

LATERAL INCISOR
(8TH YEAR)

CENTRAL INCISOR
(7TH YEAR)

CENTRAL INCISOR
(8 TO 10 MONTHS)

LATERAL INCISOR
(8 TO 10 MONTHS)

CANINE (CUSPID)
(16 TO 20 MONTHS)

1ST MOLAR
(15 TO 21 MONTHS)

2ND MOLAR
(20 TO 24 MONTHS)

2ND MOLAR
(20 TO 24 MONTHS)

1ST MOLAR
(15 TO 21 MONTHS)

CANINE (CUSPID)
(15 TO 21 MONTHS)

LATERAL INCISOR
(15 TO 21 MONTHS)

CENTRAL INCISOR
(6 TO 9 MONTHS)

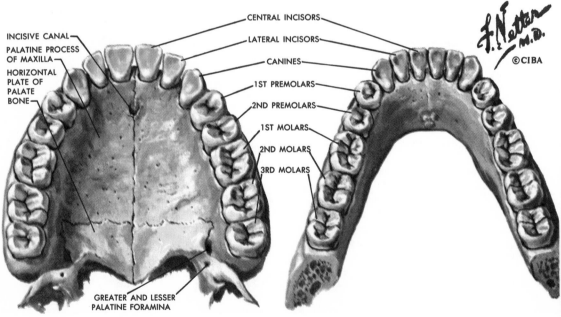

INCISIVE CANAL

PALATINE PROCESS
OF MAXILLA

HORIZONTAL
PLATE OF
PALATE
BONE

CENTRAL INCISORS

LATERAL INCISORS

CANINES

1ST PREMOLARS

2ND PREMOLARS

1ST MOLARS

2ND MOLARS

3RD MOLARS

GREATER AND LESSER
PALATINE FORAMINA

UPPER PERMANENT TEETH

LOWER PERMANENT TEETH

F. Netter
M.D.

©CIBA

to be accommodated in normal fashion, the crowding may cause some teeth to be misplaced, and we then say this person has crooked teeth. A child with this condition should receive care from an orthodontist—a dentist especially trained in the treatment of misplaced teeth. It sometimes becomes necessary for one or more of a child's teeth to be removed in order to make room for other teeth. In some cases the orthodontist guides the misplaced teeth into more favorable positions by exerting gentle pressure through temporary mechanical devices which he fastens to the teeth.

Because the primary teeth serve as space retainers for permanent teeth, it is unfortunate when a primary tooth is lost too soon. After the loss of a primary tooth, the adjacent teeth tend to crowd into the space thus made available, without leaving room for the permanent tooth due to come into this same space at a later time. For this reason a child's primary teeth should receive adequate care—to preserve them in a healthy state so they may contribute to the proper alignment of the permanent teeth. For this reason, also, primary teeth should be treated by a dentist if caries develop.

A young child should be taught to give care to his primary teeth by brushing them after meals, just as he will care for his permanent teeth later on. If it becomes necessary to have a primary tooth removed before its time, it is often advisable to have it replaced by a false tooth or by a dental retainer such as the dentist may recommend, in order to maintain the space into which its permanent successor may grow.

Certain faulty habits may interfere with the favorable positioning of a child's teeth. Thumb-sucking, nail-biting, lip-biting, tongue-thrusting, and pencil-biting are practices which may exert pressure against a child's teeth when the tissues of his jaws are still pliable. In helping such a child to break these habits, the parent must not only be firm but understanding and discerning. Perhaps the child who takes recourse to such habits needs more evidence of his being welcome in the family and more manifestations of affection.

Structure of the Teeth

Although the shape of teeth varies all the way from chisel-shaped incisors to the heavy-faceted molars, all teeth have certain essential parts in common. The surface layer of the exposed portion of a tooth (crown) is composed of enamel, the hardest substance in the body. Enamel consists largely of the salts of calcium and phosphorus. Once formed, enamel becomes inert and incapable of self-repair. This unique characteristic places it in contrast to most of the tissues of the body, which do have provision for healing. Because enamel cannot be repaired or replaced naturally, any cavity occurring in a tooth tends to become larger and deeper unless treated by a dentist. The conventional method of treatment is to drill out the damaged walls of the cavity and then fill the space with some inert material such as gold or amalgam.

A tooth is composed mostly of dentin, a substance softer than enamel though slightly harder than bone. Once the enamel covering has been penetrated, the dentin underneath is very sensitive to stimuli—a fact which explains why some individuals receive painful sensations from teeth involved with dental caries. At the root portion of a tooth, the dentin is covered by a bonelike substance called cementum. No enamel covers the root of a tooth—just cementum.

The very central portion of a tooth contains soft tissue called dental pulp, which contains tiny blood vessels and nerve filaments.

The root of a tooth is embedded in the bone of the jaw. Fortunately, a cushion of firm tissue lies between the root and its bony socket. This intervening tissue, called the periodontal ligament, is very strong, but it does permit the tooth to move just enough to prevent possible fracture in case one should bite something very hard.

229

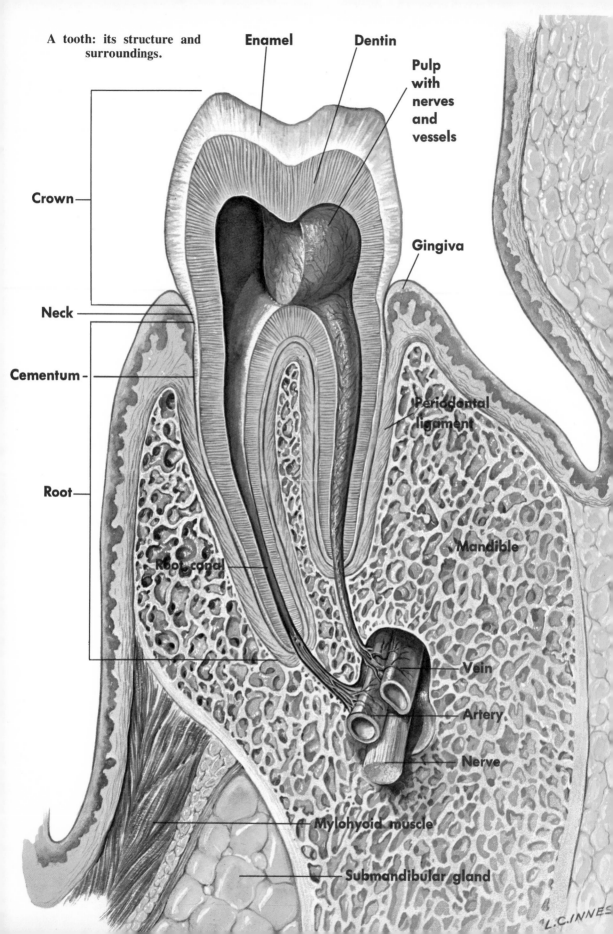

A tooth: its structure and surroundings.

Enamel

Dentin

Pulp with nerves and vessels

Crown

Gingiva

Neck

Cementum

Periodontal ligament

Root

Mandible

Root canal

Vein

Artery

Nerve

Mylohyoid muscle

Submandibular gland

L.C.INNES

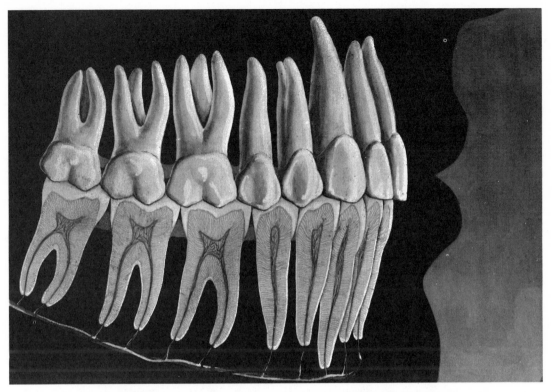

Adult dentition, showing right side of jaw. Note how each tooth depends on the one next to it for support and how when all the teeth are straight they match properly with their opposites—an ideal situation not only for mastication but also for appearance.

The various teeth are adapted for different purposes. Incisor teeth, shaped like chisels, are adapted to shearing off portions of food to be eaten, such as when one bites a piece out of an apple. The cuspid teeth are spade-shaped and are capable of tearing or shredding food. The premolar teeth are built to tear and crush food. They are best for handling tough and stringy food such as celery. The molar teeth are designed to complete the process of chewing food by grinding it to small bits. They have broad surfaces, able to withstand great pressure as food is ground between the upper and lower molars.

Home Care of the Teeth

When a person neglects to care for his teeth they become susceptible to dental decay. This impairment consists of the erosion of a portion of the enamel of a tooth and the possibility that this erosion may even penetrate into the dentin. The dentist speaks of this destructive process as caries. The site of destruction is often called a cavity. Cavities in the teeth resulting from caries are actually holes, sometimes with ragged margins. When neglected, dental caries will result in toothache and eventual loss of the tooth.

Dental caries result from a combination of three factors: (1) the presence of germs in the mouth, (2) an untidy condition of the teeth caused by particles of food left in contact with the teeth, and (3) an inherited susceptibility to caries. No one of the three factors will, by itself, cause cavities to develop in a tooth. It takes a combination of all three.

Germs are constantly present in the mouth. A person can doubtless reduce the number of germs by keeping his teeth clean, but he can never render his mouth germ-free regardless of how much highly advertised toothpaste or antiseptic mouthwash he may use.

Food particles remain in the mouth after a person eats. Fragments of food cling to the surfaces of the teeth, especially in the fissures of the grinding surfaces and in the spaces between the teeth and between the teeth and the gums. When a person neglects to clean his teeth after eating, the food particles become part of a gelatinous film which envelops the teeth and tends to remain.

With continued neglect, additional layers are added to the film day after day. There is then a tendency for calcification to develop in the thickened film. Then we say that tartar has formed on the surface of the teeth. This deposit irritates the soft tissues of the gum, favoring the development of periodontal disease (pyorrhea) as described in the chapter that follows. Periodontal disease is a major cause for the loss of teeth.

Germs thrive in food residue left clinging to the teeth. They bring about certain chemical changes and thereby produce an acid. It is this acid that damages tooth enamel and causes caries to develop.

With respect to the third factor in tooth decay—the factor of susceptibility—it must be admitted that some persons have tissues more resistant than the same tissues in other persons. A few fortunate individuals have teeth so resistant that caries do not develop despite the presence of germs and food particles. But these persons are rare. It is possible that their resistance to dental caries depends as much upon an active flow of saliva, which tends to wash away the acids which develop next to their teeth, as upon the inherent resistance of their teeth to decay.

Of the three factors just listed as causes of dental caries, there is only one (the second) over which you have personal control. It is the middle link of the caries-producing chain that must be broken in order to prevent the development of cavities in the teeth. In other words, a person can prevent the development of dental caries if he follows a program of keeping his teeth free from food particles. This requires simply that he clean his teeth thoroughly after each meal and, if he eats between meals, after each snack.

Cleaning the teeth should be done promptly after eating, for the damage done to the teeth by the combination of germs and food particles is done quickly. When a person waits even half an hour after eating before cleaning his teeth, the damage has probably already been done.

In the matter of finding a means of adequate home care for one's teeth, the dentist is in a position to help. He can suggest acceptable methods that will suit particular circumstances. Here we suggest methods that will be satisfactory in most cases:

When a toothbrush is not available, thorough rinsing of the mouth with plain water will remove most of the food particles that have remained following a meal. Such rinsing can well be supplemented by the use of dental floss or dental tape. The use of dental floss or dental tape will actually enable one to clean portions of the teeth that cannot be reached by a toothbrush. Care must be used not to snap the floss or tape into position between the teeth, for this practice injures the delicate tissues of the gums. By rinsing the mouth thoroughly with plain water before and after the use of dental floss or dental tape, practically all food particles can be removed. A convenient container for dental floss or dental tape is available at most drugstores and can be carried easily in one's pocket, or purse.

In selecting a toothbrush, many people make the mistake of choosing one too large. The ideal toothbrush is of medium size, with small head and straight handle. The brushing surface should be flat and the bristles resilient and firm, but not so brittle as to injure the gums. Obviously, toothbrushes for children should be smaller than those for adults. Following use, the toothbrush should be placed where it can dry quickly. A toothbrush should be replaced when its bristles become loose or soft.

The choice of a toothpaste or tooth powder is not so important as the method of using the toothbrush and the timing of cleaning the teeth. No essential difference exists between paste and powder in their effectiveness for cleaning the mouth and the teeth. Fluoride-containing dentifrices have been shown to have some value in preventing dental caries. The individual who has special needs should consult his dentist for a choice of a dentifrice.

Advertising claims for the control of bad breath by the use of some particular toothpaste are unfounded. Bad breath stems from factors beyond control by simple cleansing of the teeth. It can be caused by diseased soft tissues of the mouth, by poor digestion, by conditions of nervous tension, and by general conditions of ill health.

In using a toothbrush, a person does well to imagine that he is using a broom to sweep a cracked wooden floor. In sweeping such a floor he moves the broom in the same direction as the cracks in the floor. Teeth should be brushed in a similar fashion, moving the toothbrush in small strokes up and down so as to clean the spaces between the teeth. The bristles of the toothbrush should be pressed into the tiny spaces between the teeth.

There is danger in using a vigorous motion with the toothbrush so as to scour the teeth. Dental scouring is justified on the grinding surfaces of the molar teeth but not on the sides of the teeth. The bristles of the toothbrush will have the effect, in the long run, of actually grinding away the enamel of the teeth when a scouring motion is used.

The accompanying illustrations show the accepted method of using a toothbrush. The bristles of the toothbrush should be placed against the gum and then the toothbrush rotated in such a

Brush the biting and chewing surfaces of the teeth.

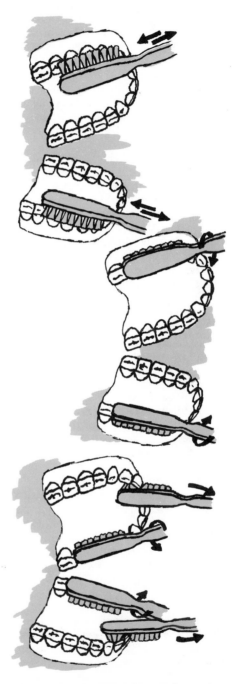

Brush the outside of teeth from the gums to chewing edge. Brush the inside similarly.

manner that these bristles come into the spaces between the teeth. It is wise to ask a dentist, each time you have your teeth checked, whether you have been using the best method of brushing your teeth.

Dentists recommend that the toothbrush also be used to massage the gums. This should be done gently with the tips of the bristles placed against the gum at the junction between gum and teeth while the toothbrush is caused to "vibrate."

It is a mistaken idea that chewing gum after meals will take the place of cleaning the teeth by toothbrushing and dental tape. The use of chewing gum is actually harmful because of the sugar in the gum. Any sugar, even that contained in the gum, serves as a medium for the growth of germs and therefore favors the production of acid which damages the teeth. The same principle applies to sweet drinks taken between meals.

The consideration of diet and its relation to health centers around two important questions: When? and What?

A controlled study on the incidence of dental caries indicated that eating snacks between meals is more directly related to the occurrence of caries than other factors. Logically, then, if persons who eat between meals would take time to clean their teeth thoroughly after each snack, the damage to their teeth would be reduced.

The excessive use of sugar in candies, sweetened drinks, and pastries has the effect of depriving a person of the amount of wholesome food which he would otherwise eat. Candy, pastries, et cetera, lack the vitamins and minerals necessary for building healthy tissues and maintaining tissue resistance to disease.

With respect to calcium, so important to the building of teeth and bones, the child will obtain a sufficient amount of this element by simply drinking the usually recommended quart of milk a day. His diet must, of course, also include an adequate amount of vitamin D so that the calcium in his diet becomes available for building bones and teeth.

Fluorine

Fluorine is a trace element of outstanding importance in the development and health of the teeth. Scientific studies indicate that children reared in areas where the drinking water lacks traces of fluorine have a higher incidence of dental caries than do children reared in areas where traces of fluorine are available. This finding is the basis on which authorities now recommend that communities add fluorine to the drinking water, up to 0.7 parts of fluorine per million parts of water, when this element is otherwise lacking. It has already been established that the addition of this small amount of fluorine in the drinking water will have the effect of reducing the cases of dental caries by 60 percent.

Care by the Dentist

Taking good care of teeth starts with taking good care of a child's primary teeth. Even a child needs to have periodic appointments with the dentist, and these should begin when the child is about three years of age.

One of the most critical periods of life with respect to the care of one's teeth occurs at about six years of age. As mentioned previously, the appearance of the first permanent molar teeth often does not attract attention. They erupt just behind the last molars of the primary set and therefore do not cause any of the primary teeth to be shed. But these first molars of the permanent group need even more careful attention than do other permanent teeth.

These newly formed teeth contain certain fissures on their grinding surfaces in which food can easily become lodged. The fissures are relatively narrow and deep and the enamel at the bottom of them may not be fully fused. Thus the inherent shape of these first molar teeth, plus the usual carefree attitude of a child, forms a combination of circumstances that makes the first permanent molars more susceptible to caries than any of the other teeth.

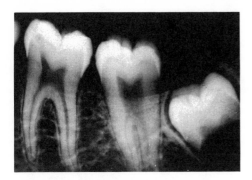

X ray showing position of a third molar before it emerges.

Dentists are trained to watch for unwholesome changes in first molar teeth. When such changes are detected early the dentist can repair the teeth with small fillings and thus preserve their usefulness for the usual lifespan.

A dentist can tell a great deal by simply making a survey of each tooth. But as we have noticed from the previous description of the structure of the teeth, only a portion of each tooth is available for direct observation. In order to get the full story of the condition of one's mouth and teeth, the dentist must have the advantage of a radiographic examination (X-ray study). He will recommend this from time to time.

Radiographic studies of a child's mouth will indicate whether the development of his teeth is following the normal schedule. It will show whether any teeth are developing in abnormal positions. Such studies of the teeth in either a child or an adult will show the presence of caries still too small to be detected by direct examination.

This early detection of caries is especially important when caries develop in the hidden areas where one tooth is in contact with another. A radiographic study will show beginning caries beneath old fillings. It will indicate early stages of disease in the supporting tissues surrounding the teeth. It will indicate destruction of bone about the roots of the teeth, such as occurs in long-standing disease of these tissues.

The question is often asked, Is there danger in having one's teeth examined by X ray?

In recent years scientists have issued warnings about the dangers of exposure to X rays and to other forms of radiation. Now that we have come into the atomic age, these warnings are timely. It is therefore proper to find the answer.

Carefully controlled experiments have been made to determine the tolerance of the tissues of the human body for radiation produced by radiographic (X-ray) equipment. It is now understood that the effects of radiation are cumulative—that a person's exposures to radiation at various times must be added together to determine the cumulative effects on his tissues. Passing X rays through one portion of a person's body produces no appreciable effect on the tissues of other portions of his body. Thus the occasional radiographic examinations made of a person's mouth do not reduce his tolerance for X-ray studies that may be made later of his chest.

In summary, it may be stated that human tolerance for radiation permits as many as 70 complete radiographic studies of the mouth and teeth within a span of 30 years. In other words, it is safe for a person to have a complete radiographic study of his mouth and teeth as often as every year or even every six months should the dentist feel such frequency advisable.

C. Functions of the Mouth

The mouth is one of the organs of speech. The tongue, the teeth, the cheeks, and the lips play important parts in articulating words and in molding and modifying the sounds that originate in the larynx.

The mouth is concerned with the expressing of emotion. Although a smile requires the use of muscles of the entire face, it especially brings into play the muscles around the mouth. In laughing, it is primarily the mouth that provides

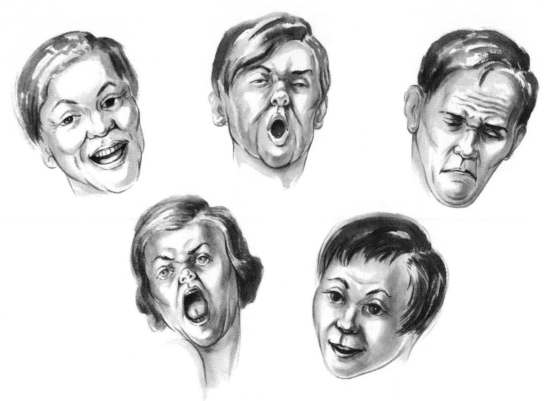

The external mouth registers emotions and mood.

the appropriate facial expression and which also makes possible the joyous sounds that are part of this emotionl experience. The mouth and its several parts contribute materially to a person's general appearance. The form of the lips, the jaws, and the teeth probably do more to make a person attractive or otherwise than even such features as the eyes and the nose.

Even with respect to the functions of digestion, the mouth does much more than merely serve as a funnel through which the food passes on its way to the stomach. The teeth grind the food into small particles, thus aiding in digestion. The tongue moves actively and cleverly in keeping the food in contact with the teeth while it is being chewed. The cheeks aid in this same function. The salivary glands pour their secretions of saliva into the mouth so that it is mixed

with the food while it is being chewed. The saliva contains a chemical substance called ptyalin, which reacts with the starch contained in the food to convert it to a simple sugar, thus initiating the process of digestion. Also, the saliva, as it mixes with the food, moistens it, making it easier to swallow and preparing it to be readily acted upon by other digestive agents.

The mouth is involved in still another function related to food—the registering of taste. The taste buds are capable of being stimulated by the various kinds of molecules in one's food. They register the fundamental tastes and relay to the brain nervous impulses, which are interpreted as either pleasant or unpleasant and which thus influence a person's attitude toward food and even modify the functions of his digestive organs.

236

Problems of the Mouth and Teeth

The present chapter deals with a part of the body that not only has several functions but is composed of an interesting array of tissues, including bone, skin, moist membrane, muscle, glands, and teeth. The discussions therefore cover a variety of problems, including inherited defects, orthopedic considerations, dental problems, various infections, gland involvements, and cancer.

Harelip (Cleft Lip) and Cleft Palate

Harelip is a congenital defect involving the upper lip, sometimes on the right, sometimes on the left, and sometimes on both sides. It results from a faulty fusion of certain of the components which in early embryonic life join one another to form the facial features. A child with harelip should be taken to a plastic surgeon soon after birth. The results of a carefully planned surgery are usually excellent, as indicated in the accompanying photographs on page 238. When harelip is neglected, however, the child may form unfortunate speech patterns and become sensitive about his disfigurement.

Cleft palate results from a failure of fusion of certain embryonic structures which normally join in the midline to form the roof of the mouth. There are various degrees of cleft palate, some involving only the soft palate and some involving also the hard palate and upper jaw. Cleft palate is often associated with harelip. It may interfere with the infant's ability to nurse. Also an untreated cleft palate interferes with the ability to pronounce words. A plastic surgeon should be consulted while the child with cleft palate is in early infancy.

Temporomandibular Joint Problems

The temporomandibular joints, right and left, are the structures which make it possible for the lower jaw to move and, thus, to open and close the mouth. These joints are located just in front of the ears. By using the tips of your fingers you can feel motion in these areas as you move the lower jaw up and down and from side to side.

The movements of the lower jaw are produced by muscles located deep in the sides of the face. Muscle action is required both to open and to close the mouth. These muscles are active much of the time, for the lower jaw moves not only with chewing but also with speaking. Also, motions of the lower jaw are involved in a person's expressions of emotion. Many persons reflexly clench their jaw when under tension or when concentrating to solve a problem. Some have habits of grinding their teeth while sleeping (bruxism).

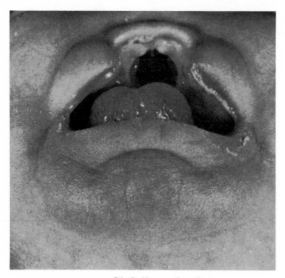

Cleft lip and palate.

With all this activity it is not surprising that many persons develop symptoms of difficulty in the region of the temporomandibular joint. These may consist of limited motion of the lower jaw, noise or clicking sounds when the jaw is moved, or pain in the face which seems to originate in the ear and may be transmitted to the temple, the neck, or the angle of the jaw. In a few cases the muscles which move the jaw upward go into spasm, thus "locking" the jaw for the time being.

Most of the symptoms relating to the temporomandibular joint result either from habits produced by nervous tension (such as grinding or clenching the teeth) or by malocclusion of the teeth (the teeth failing to meet properly when the jaw is closed). Malocclusion can re-

Harelip can usually be corrected by surgery. Upper (both cases), before surgery; lower, after surgery.

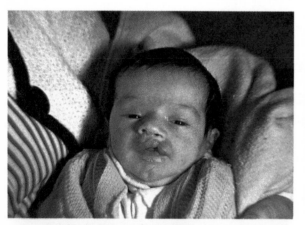

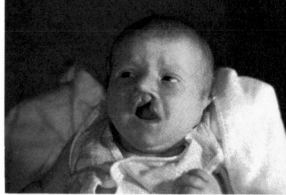

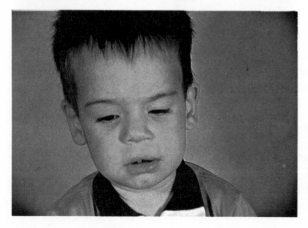

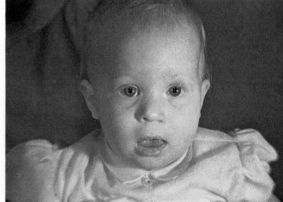

sult from a slight shifting of the teeth when one or more teeth have been removed or even by a dental filling or crown positioned "too high" so that it strikes the opposing tooth too soon.

The remedy for symptoms relating to the temporomandibular joint centers around two considerations: (1) attention to emotional or psychological problems that cause the patient to resort to clenching his jaw or grinding his teeth and (2) correction by the dentist of problems of malocclusion.

In occasional cases the lower jaw becomes dislocated as the result of an accident or by sudden muscle action when the individual yawns widely. The dislocation consists of a forward movement of the articulating portion of the lower jaw within the temporomandibular joint, and the person cannot close his mouth. The emergency treatment for this condition is described in chapter 23, volume 3.

Dental Problems

DENTAL CARIES (TOOTH DECAY)
Ninety-five percent of all Americans

suffer some tooth decay at one time or another. One half of all children three years of age have one or more teeth already affected by caries. The average child in the grades has three or more teeth in which dental cavities have occurred. The average sixteen-year-old has seven teeth which have either been affected by dental caries or have been filled or are missing. Nine out of ten high school students have suffered from some degree of dental caries.

Three factors combine to cause the development of caries. These are listed and discussed in the preceding chapter.

The essentials for preventing dental caries are (1) prompt cleaning of the teeth after each meal, (2) an adequate diet consisting largely of natural foods, and (3) a limitation on pastries and confections because of the large amount of sugar they contain. Even under ideal circumstances the possibility of developing caries still exists.

Prevention and Treatment

A neglected cavity in a tooth will grow in size and eventually penetrate the deeper layers of the tooth, eventu-

Dental caries begin first by a tiny opening in the enamel. If left untreated, the cavity grows deeper and larger, eventually reaching the pulp and causing toothache and finally total loss of tooth.

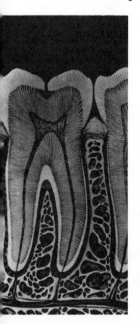 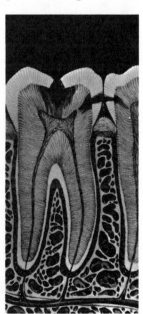 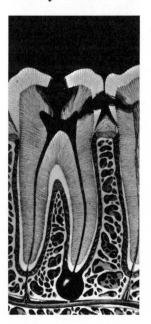 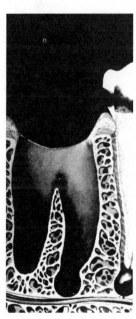

ally causing the tooth to be lost. Even though a person has no knowledge of caries in his teeth, he should visit his dentist at least once a year (some recommend every six months) so that his teeth may be inspected and treated as indicated.

Teeth should be cleaned promptly after each meal, preferably using dental floss or dental tape between the teeth, followed by gentle brushing with a toothbrush and thorough rinsing.

Food and sweetened drinks should not be taken between meals. Candies, pastries, and highly refined foods should be kept to the minimum in one's diet by giving preference to whole grains, nuts, vegetables, and fruits.

PULPITIS

Pulpitis is the major cause of toothache. As the term implies, pulpitis consists of an inflammation of the pulp (the most central tissue of a tooth). Typically and usually pulpitis occurs as the result of neglecting the treatment of a carious cavity. Dental pulp is a sensitive tissue because it contains many nerve filaments. In pulpitis, therefore, sharp pain develops, which may be throbbing, shooting, and intermittent. Strangely, it may be difficult for the person affected to know exactly which tooth is causing the trouble, for the pain may be referred to other teeth.

Care and Treatment

For the first-aid treatment of the toothache caused by pulpitis, the cavity should be located and cleansed by rinsing. Clove oil when instilled into the cleansed cavity may provide some relief of pain. Mixing clove oil with zinc oxide powder to form a paste which is then packed into the cavity of the tooth provides relief which may endure for a few hours. The permanent treatment of pulpitis by the dentist involves his removing the infected pulp tissue, closing the tooth's root canal and then filling the cavity that has been produced by the caries. Oth-

erwise, the affected tooth may have to be removed.

PERIAPICAL ABSCESS

The apex of a tooth is that portion most deeply situated in the bony socket. At the apex there is an opening through which tiny blood vessels and nerve filaments find their way into the tooth's pulp. By definition, a periapical abscess is an area of infection that develops around the apex of a tooth. The usual route by which an infection reaches the apical area is by the extension of an infection of the pulp through the root canal to this deepest part of the bony socket. That is, in most cases a periapical abscess is the first result of the neglect of caries. Occasional cases of periapical abscess are caused by mechanical damage to the tooth.

Periapical abscess causes a continuous type of pain which is aggravated when the tooth is brought into firm contact. Pain is increased by hot or cold foods or drinks.

Care and Treatment

For the immediate relief of pain, the application of either heat or cold (whichever the patient tolerates best) is usually helpful. This treatment is best administered by the patient holding a mouthful of hot or cold liquid in his mouth for about a minute. If hot solution is used, it should be about the temperature of the usual hot breakfast drink. The corrective treatment for periapical abscess as administered by the dentist consists of the use of antibiotic medication to combat the infection plus root canal therapy if the tooth is to be retained in place.

PERIODONTAL DISEASE (PYORRHEA)

Periodontal disease consists of an infection caused by bacteria which affects the tissue surrounding a tooth. The infection begins as an inflammation of the gum (gingivitis). The infection may persist in the tissues of the gum for months or even years, but usually it progresses to affect the support-

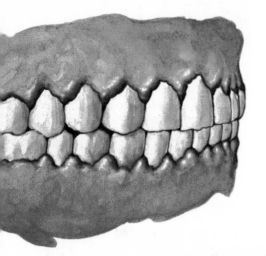

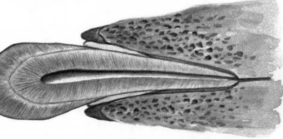

Diagram showing how pyorrhea in periodontal tissue initiates destruction in surrounding bone.

ing tissue which anchors the tooth to its bony socket. Deep pockets develop between the gum and the root of the tooth. These pockets harbor bacteria, and as the process continues, some of the fibers which normally anchor the tooth to the bony socket are destroyed and the tooth then becomes loose. Periodontal disease is the principal cause of the loss of teeth after the age of 30 years.

The early signs of periodontal disease consists of tenderness and redness of the gums, with the tendency for them to bleed.

The circumstances that lead to the development of periodontal disease are simply neglect in brushing and flossing the teeth after each meal. The purpose of such brushing and flossing is to remove the food remnants that tend to persist on the surfaces of the teeth.

When such remnants remain, there develops a gelatinous film on the surface of the teeth, particularly at the gum margins. When not removed, it becomes firm by the deposit of calcium and is called tartar or dental calculus. Sometimes the deposits of tartar or calculus are spoken of as plaque. The hazard of such deposits is that germs are thus harbored and cause inflammation of the gums (gingivitis), which progresses to periodontal disease.

Even with consistent brushing and flossing of the teeth after meals, the film of calculus may build up slowly. And this possibility constitutes one of the reasons why a person should consult his dentist at intervals of six months to one year. The dentist or his dental hygienist assistant will then use appropriate instruments to remove the film of calculus so that the surface of the tooth is freed from the germ-laden layer of foreign material.

Care and Treatment

In treating periodontal disease the dentist's first effort is to remove the layer of tartar or calculus that may still be present on the surface of the teeth. If deep pockets have already formed next to the roots of an affected tooth, he will explore these pockets and remove the tartar or calculus from the surface of the tooth's root, reaching as deeply as the gum has been separated. This latter process is called deep scaling.

The patient will be instructed to maintain a consistent program of brushing and flossing his teeth after each meal. In cases where periodontal disease persists even after deep scaling has been performed, it may be necessary for the dentist to perform a minor surgical procedure in which the diseased tissue at the depth of the deep pockets is removed, thus allowing the remaining healthy tissue to reattach to the surface of the tooth.

ACCIDENT INVOLVING A TOOTH

A tooth which has been fractured may need a protective covering which the dentist can supply until permanent repair can be made at a later time. Even teeth moved out of position by accident may gradually move back into their normal position, especially when this involves primary teeth (deciduous or baby teeth).

Surprising as it may seem, a tooth knocked out by accident may possibly be successfully reimplanted. For this reason a tooth which has been accidentally removed should be preserved in warm salt solution (half a teaspoonful of salt to the glass of water) until the dentist has an opportunity to decide whether an attempt to reimplant it is feasible. Such a situation, of course, requires prompt action.

GLOSSITIS (INFLAMMATION OF THE TONGUE)

The tongue may become inflamed either by local damage or on account of some systemic disease. The local involvements usually occur in connection with an injury such as biting or burning or repeated exposure to irritants such as alcohol, tobacco, or hot foods or drinks. Following such injury, germs already present in the mouth invade the injured area and cause the tongue to become inflamed. The systemic diseases that may involve the tongue include some of the anemias, some generalized skin diseases, and some cases of vitamin deficiency, particularly those involving the B vitamins.

The symptoms and manifestations of glossitis vary, depending upon the cause of the difficulty. Usually, the tongue becomes swollen, ulcerated, and sore. In a severe form of infection, the lymph nodes in the neck are swollen and tender. Frequently the flow of saliva is so excessive as to be troublesome. There may be fever and other symptoms commonly caused by infection.

Care and Treatment

Each case of glossitis deserves individual study. Once the cause is identified, the treatment is planned accord-ingly. Jagged teeth or ill-fitting dentures should be corrected by a dentist. Irritants such as tobacco, alcohol, and hot foods should be avoided. A bland diet should be arranged, and the temperature of the food taken should be moderate. The mouth may be rinsed several times a day with alkaline aromatic solution, a standard preparation available at most drugstores. Antibiotic medications and other specific remedies may be arranged by the physician when an infection persists.

Problems Within the Mouth

VINCENT'S INFECTION (TRENCH MOUTH)

Vincent's infection is a severe infection characterized by painful bleeding gums, excessive production of saliva, a fetid breath, and small ulcers on the gums, particularly between the teeth. It is caused by a combination of two kinds of germs, a bacillus and a spirochete. The infection appears not to be transmitted from one person to another. It occurs under circumstances in which a person has allowed his general resistance to decline or in which some systemic illness has caused him to lose vigor or in which the tissues of the mouth have been neglected or insulted, as by excess smoking. In addition to the local evidences of the infection, swallowing and talking are painful.

Care and Treatment

A hot mouth wash every 30 to 60 minutes throughout the day is beneficial. A suitable preparation is half-strength hydrogen peroxide (prepared by mixing equal parts of water and hydrogen peroxide as it comes from the drugstore). The affected areas may be painted between mouth washes with a paste prepared from sodium perborate powder to which a few drops of water have been added. The patient should rest a great deal, and his diet should consist of bland, soft food. Smoking should be eliminated. Antibiotic medications prescribed by a physician or a dentist may hasten recovery, but usually local treatment is sufficient. After the acute phase of the illness subsides, a dentist should make an examination and instruct the patient on methods of care for his mouth, gums, and teeth.

THRUSH (ORAL CANDIDIASIS)

Thrush usually, but not always, affects babies rather than older persons. It is caused by a species of fungus *(Candida albicans)* which produces a white velvetlike growth on the tongue, the roof of the mouth, and inside the cheeks and lips. The grayish-white patches on the membranes resemble damp blotting paper. In appearance, the lesions may be confused with milk curd, except that the lesions of thrush are difficult to remove. The symptoms include fever and poor appetite which, in the case of an infant, may involve a refusal to nurse. The patient becomes restless and may have diarrhea. In an infant, thrush is a serious disease, for if not treated it may threaten the infant's life by spreading throughout the digestive and respiratory organs.

Care and Treatment

The antibiotic drug nystatin is the specific remedy for thrush. For an infant, a preparation containing 100,000 units of nystatin per ml. is used. One ml. (¼ teaspoonful) of this preparation is dripped into the infant's mouth every six hours. For an adult, tablets each containing 500,000 units of nystatin are available. One tablet should be taken every 12 hours, and the tablet should be allowed to dissolve in the mouth. The patient's general resistance to illness should be improved by good hygienic measures and an adequate diet. If the patient is a breast-fed child, its mother's breasts and nipples should be washed with a saturated solution of boric acid and then rinsed with cooled boiled water, both before and after nursing. If the patient is a bottle-fed infant, its nursing bottles and nipples should be washed and boiled after each using.

Only bottles and nipples that have been thus sterilized should be given the child, either for its formula or for its drinking water.

MOUTH INVOLVEMENT ACCOMPANYING SYSTEMIC DISEASE

Involvements of the membrane lining the mouth may occur in such systemic diseases as measles, certain skin diseases, pellagra (a vitamin deficiency disease), and syphilis. In each of such cases, the treatment should be directed toward the particular systemic disease.

CANKER SORES

Canker sores usually begin as small red swellings or tiny blisters on the membrane which lines the mouth or on the under surface of the tongue. They

Canker sores in the mouth.

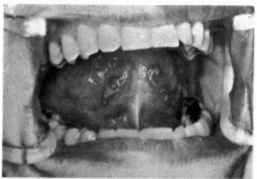

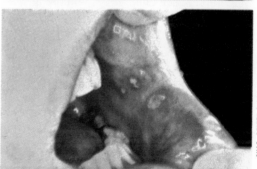

become painful as soon as an ulcer forms at the summit of the swelling. The lesions are one eighth to one fourth of an inch (3-6 mm.) in diameter.

There appears to be no single cause for canker sores. Girls and women are affected more than boys and men. Canker sores occur when one's general resistance is low. They also tend to occur when the membranes of the mouth are irritated by jagged teeth or by poor mouth hygiene. The disease is usually self-limited, occurs only once or twice a year, and causes little inconvenience except for the soreness in the mouth.

Care and Treatment

The application of anesthetic ointments may serve to relieve the discomfort of canker sores. Suitable preparations are dibucaine ointment (1%) and lidocaine ointment (5%).

COLD SORES (ORAL HERPES SIMPLEX)

Herpes simplex is a systemic disease caused by a virus. The virus may enter a person's body during infancy (see chapter 17, volume 1,) or at most any time later in life. The first attack is more severe than later attacks and is called primary herpes simplex. The virus remains in a person's body throughout life once he has had the attack of primary herpes simplex. Periodically throughout the remainder of life he experiences manifestations of this virus infection, typically the development of cold sores, usually appearing on the margin of the lips. For a more complete discussion of herpes simplex, see chapter 25, volume 2.

Leukoplakia

Leukoplakia is a curious involvement of the membranes of the lips, cheeks, tongue, floor of the mouth, and palate. The disease is characterized by the appearance of yellowish-white areas with a leathery consistency. The size of the areas varies. Cracks, fissures, and even ulcers may develop. Leukoplakia occurs most commonly in men over the age of 40 years.

Leukoplakia is considered to be the result of prolonged irritation of the membranes of the mouth and related structures. Tobacco smoking or chewing is given a large share of the blame for this. Repeated and prolonged irritations by jagged teeth or dental restorations may cause it. Poor oral hygiene may be a factor, as may also the use of highly seasoned foods and the habitual drinking of hot beverages. Leukoplakia is considered to be a step toward the development of cancer; therefore, patients suffering with this ailment are urgently advised to see a physician and to report to him periodically even after successful treatment. Usually the condition responds favorably to the avoidance of all irritating agents.

Salivary Gland Involvement

PTYALISM

Ptyalism is a symptom, not a disease. It consists of an increased flow of saliva from the salivary glands. The function of the salivary glands is regulated by nerves which operate in a reflex manner to stimulate the glands when there is food in the mouth and even when there are thoughts of eating. This same reflex operates automatically when a condition in or around the mouth exists that produces pain or when there is some interference with swallowing. Ptyalism also occurs in cases of poisoning by mercury or by one of the iodides.

XEROSTOMIA

In xerostomia the mouth is dry. This disorder may occur when there is disease of the salivary glands or when a major duct of a salivary gland has become obstructed by a stone. Xerostomia occurs reflexly when a person is anxious or under emotional tension, as in the case of the public speaker. Xerostomia may also occur when a person is dehydrated.

INFLAMMATION OF THE SALIVARY GLANDS

The most common cause of inflammation of the salivary glands is mumps, which is a virus disease involving one or both of the parotid glands. For a more detailed description of mumps see chapter 16, volume 3.

The parotid gland is sometimes involved by an infection unrelated to mumps and caused by germs which have worked their way from the mouth through the duct of the parotid gland into the gland tissue proper. Such an infection causes a painful swelling of the gland. The treatment is that of any other similar infection and consists essentially of the use of an antibiotic medication.

A submandibular salivary gland may become inflamed because of an obstruction to its duct which prevents its secretion from reaching the mouth. Such obstruction occurs more commonly in this gland than in the other salivary glands, probably because of the uphill course of its duct. This condition causes a swelling in the floor of the mouth at one side of the tongue. The swelling becomes most noticeable at mealtime when the gland would otherwise be active in producing a large volume of saliva. The obstruction is caused by a stone in the duct and the treatment consists of the minor surgical procedure of removing this stone.

TUMORS OF THE SALIVARY GLANDS

It is the parotid gland which is affected in 80 percent of the cases of salivary gland tumors. A tumor of the parotid gland usually develops slowly and produces a firm, round, painless swelling just above the angle of the jaw. It is important to have such a tumor examined by a physician at the earliest possible opportunity, because a certain percentage of these are truly malignant. The physician will want to arrange for a sample of the tumor to be examined microscopically. Thus it can be determined whether the tumor is of the malignant type. If so, it should be removed promptly by surgery. In some cases it is advisable for the surgery to be followed by radiation therapy.

Cancer of the Mouth

Cancer in the region of the mouth accounts for about 2 percent of all cancers. Any ulcer of the lining of the mouth that does not heal within two weeks should be investigated by a physician. In the early stages, cancer of the mouth often does not produce symptoms. Therefore a lesion which does not heal should be investigated even before pain or other symptoms develop. Cancer of the lower lip is the most common form of cancer in the vicinity of the mouth; but cancer may develop in the gums, in the palate, in the tongue, in the cheek, or in the floor of the mouth. The most reliable method of determining whether or not a lesion is cancerous is by biopsy examination of a sample of removed tissue.

The factors which predispose to cancer of the mouth include longtime exposure to the sun, as in sailors and farmers, the use of chewing tobacco and snuff, chronic drinking of alcoholic beverages, and the smoking of tobacco.

Further details on cancer are provided in chapter 10, volume 3, and material relating to cancer of the mouth is contained in chapter 11, volume 3.

245

The Stomach and Intestines

The organs concerned with the digestion of food constitute the digestive system. The mouth and the pharynx through which food passes first serve not only in the handling of food, but in the handling of air as well. But beginning at the lower boundary of the pharynx food passes into the esophagus and air passes through the larynx and trachea. The digestive system includes the esophagus, the stomach, the small intestine, and the large intestine.

The Esophagus

The esophagus, or gullet, is a simple tube about 10 inches (25 cm.) long which conveys food from the pharynx above to the stomach below. As it passes through the upper part of the chest, the esophagus lies behind the trachea (windpipe). As it approaches the stomach, the esophagus passes through an opening in the diaphragm (the muscular partition that separates the organs of the chest, above, from those of the abdomen, below). The esophagus is lined by a membrane which is kept moist and lubricated by the secretion of tiny glands. The wall of the esophagus contains muscle fibers which, as they contract, propel the food on its way toward the stomach.

Swallowing

Food does not merely fall from the mouth into the stomach. It is possible for a person to swallow even while standing on his head. Swallowing consists of a progressive action of the muscles in the walls of the mouth, pharynx, and esophagus. As they contract they push the food on its way.

Swallowing must be accomplished quickly, for the pharynx serves as a passageway not only for food and drink, but also for air moving to and from the lungs. The flow of air must not be interrupted for long.

At the beginning of swallowing the tongue presses upward and backward against the roof of the mouth, thus pushing the food into the pharynx. The soft palate is forced upward so as to close off the nasal cavities. The larynx (voice box) is drawn upward to contact the epiglottis so that, for the moment, the opening into the lower air passages is closed. Thus the bolus of food has no other way to move but into the esophagus. The muscles in the pharynx and esophagus work together in producing a ring of contraction which moves

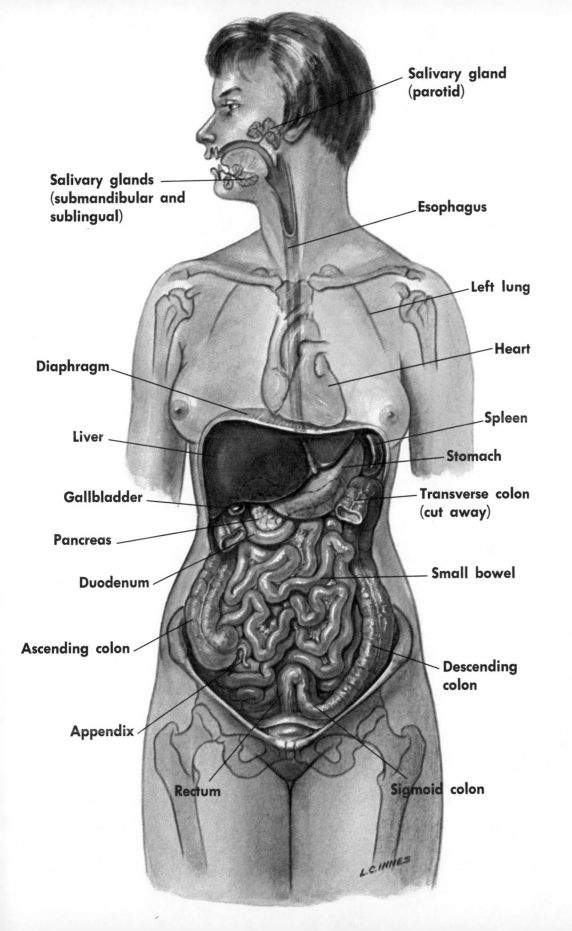

Salivary gland
(parotid)

Salivary glands
(submandibular and
sublingual)

Esophagus

Left lung

Heart

Diaphragm

Spleen

Liver

Stomach

Gallbladder

Transverse colon
(cut away)

Pancreas

Duodenum

Small bowel

Ascending colon

Descending
colon

Appendix

Rectum

Sigmoid colon

L.C. INNES

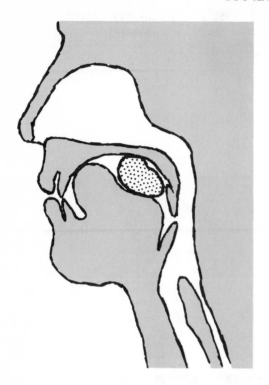 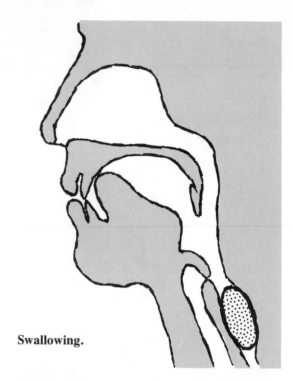

Swallowing.

downward, forcing the food ahead of it.

The Stomach

The stomach is located below the diaphragm. It is not a very large organ when empty, but its walls can stretch enormously. The stronger part of the stomach wall is composed of smooth muscle. When the stomach contains food, the muscle contracts in a way that churns the food as it mixes it with the digestive enzymes. After a person eats a meal, the stomach may hold the food for as long as three or four hours, churning it all the while.

The delicate lining of the stomach contains many tiny glands which produce digestive enzymes and hydrochloric acid. These enzymes and the hydrochloric acid, together with the water in which they are dissolved, make up the gastric juice. Two or three quarts (2 or 3 liters) of gastric juice are produced each 24 hours. The hydrochloric acid of the gastric juice helps the enzymes to do their work and also softens the food and kills most of the

germs which may have been swallowed with the food. Pepsin, one of the important enzymes of the gastric juice, acts on the protein molecules of the food and begins the process by which they are broken down into smaller molecules.

Notice that the function of the gastric juice is to digest protein. Protein is an important constituent of food. Also, however, protein is a constituent of the body's tissues, including those that compose the stomach. And this raises the question that medical scientists have wrestled with for many years: Why is it that normally the gastric juice does not digest the wall of the stomach? What protects the lining of the stomach from being eroded?

Erosion of the lining of the stomach does occur in cases of stomach ulcer, as mentioned in the following chapter. It must be that in a case of stomach ulcer something has gone wrong with the normal means by which the lining of the stomach is protected. We know further that the taking of certain sub-

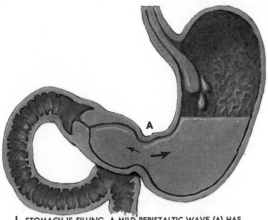

1. STOMACH IS FILLING. A MILD PERISTALTIC WAVE (A) HAS STARTED IN ANTRUM AND IS PASSING TOWARD PYLORUS. GASTRIC CONTENTS ARE CHURNED AND LARGELY PUSHED BACK INTO BODY OF STOMACH

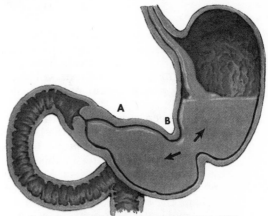

2. WAVE (A) FADING OUT AS PYLORUS FAILS TO OPEN. A STRONGER WAVE (B) IS ORIGINATING AT INCISURE AND IS AGAIN SQUEEZING GASTRIC CONTENTS IN BOTH DIRECTIONS

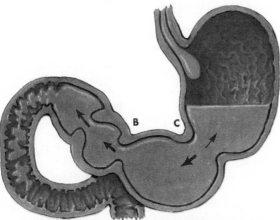

3. PYLORUS OPENS AS WAVE (B) APPROACHES IT. DUODENAL BULB IS FILLED AND SOME CONTENTS PASS INTO SECOND PORTION OF DUODENUM. WAVE (C) STARTING JUST ABOVE INCISURE

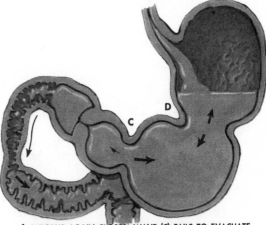

4. PYLORUS AGAIN CLOSED. WAVE (C) FAILS TO EVACUATE CONTENTS. WAVE (D) STARTING HIGHER ON BODY OF STOMACH. DUODENAL BULB MAY CONTRACT OR MAY REMAIN FILLED, AS PERISTALTIC WAVE ORIGINATING JUST BEYOND IT EMPTIES SECOND PORTION

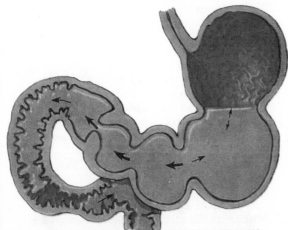

5. PERISTALTIC WAVES ARE NOW ORIGINATING HIGHER ON BODY OF STOMACH. GASTRIC CONTENTS ARE EVACUATED INTERMITTENTLY. CONTENTS OF DUODENAL BULB AREA PUSHED PASSIVELY INTO SECOND PORTION AS MORE GASTRIC CONTENTS EMERGE

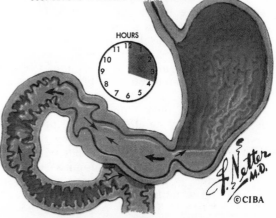

6. 3 TO 4 HOURS LATER STOMACH ALMOST EMPTY. SMALL PERISTALTIC WAVE EMPTYING DUODENAL BULB WITH SOME REFLUX INTO STOMACH. REVERSE AND ANTEGRADE PERISTALSIS PRESENT IN DUODENUM

stances, such as aspirin and alcohol, is often associated with erosions of the stomach. But we do not yet understand fully the means by which nervous tension and psychological pressures can predispose to ulcer of the stomach.

It has been assumed that the stomach's lining is protected by the layer of mucus produced by certain mucus-producing cells. In addition to this, however, there normally exists a barrier to prevent the penetration of gastric juice. Perhaps the barrier consists of a layer of fat molecules. At any rate, the normal stomach does not digest itself!

After the gastric juice and food have been churned in the stomach for three or four hours, the muscle surrounding the stomach's outlet relaxes and allows the stomach contents to pass into the duodenum, the first portion of the small intestine.

Vomiting

Vomiting is sort of an emergency function by which the contents of the stomach are expelled upward through the esophagus and mouth to the outside. It occurs as a symptom of certain illnesses. It is prompted by irritation or stretching of the tissues of the digestive organs (stomach or intestines). It also occurs under conditions of excessive nervous excitability, as in emotional shock. Its causes and significance are considered in chapter 6, this volume.

There is a so-called vomiting center located in the lower part of the brain which, when stimulated, activates the various muscles concerned with expelling the stomach contents. Vomiting occurs automatically without the person's being able to willfully control the sequence of events.

First, the person takes a deep breath. This has the effect of lowering the diaphragm and thus increasing the pressure within the abdominal cavity. Then the muscles of the abdominal wall contract, producing more pressure among the abdominal organs, including the stomach. The soft palate is raised and the opening into the larynx closes so that the vomitus, as it is expelled, can-

not enter either the nasal cavities or the lower air passages. Lastly, the muscle tissue at the junction of the esophagus and the stomach relaxes so that the stomach contents can escape upward. Actually, the stomach plays only a passive role in the process as it is squeezed by the increased pressure within the abdominal cavity.

Small Intestine

As the food which has been churned within the stomach for three or four hours leaves this organ, it enters the duodenal portion of the small intestine. The small intestine is a narrow tubular structure which opens terminally into the large intestine. It is described as having three divisions: (1) the duodenum, about 10 inches (25 cm.) in length, (2) the jejunum, about 9 feet (2.5 meters) long, and (3) the ileum, the terminal portion, about 13 feet (4 meters) in length. The latter opens into the large intestine; and together these three divisions total nearly 23 feet (7 meters).

The many coils of the small intestine are located centrally in the abdomen, where they are held in place by a ribbonlike reflection of the peritoneal lining of the abdominal cavity called the mesentery. The small intestine performs two functions: (1) to continue and complete the process of digesting food and (2) to provide for the absorption of the simple molecules of food substance made available by the chemical processes of digestion.

The duodenum receives (1) stomach contents (a mixture of food and gastric juice), (2) bile (which has been produced by the liver and is delivered through the common bile duct), and (3) pancreatic juice (which contains digestive enzymes produced in the pancreas and delivered through the pancreatic duct). Thus, within the duodenum the processes of digestion are continued at a rapid rate.

The jejunum and the ileum are concerned with completing digestion and absorbing the small food molecules that digestion produces. Certain of the cells in the lining of the jejunum and ileum

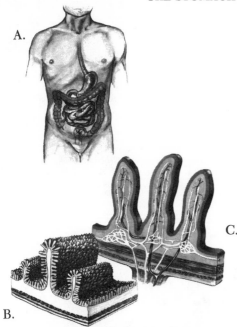

The wall of the small intestine contains smooth muscle very much like that found in the stomach. Muscle contractions churn the food, mixing it with the digestive enzymes. The rings of muscle contractions (peristaltic waves) progress slowly toward the large intestine, thus moving the intestinal contents in this direction.

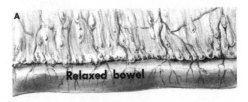

A. The coils of the small intestine. B. A small section of the wall of the small intestine enlarged to show the fingerlike villi. C. A magnification of three villi showing capillaries and lymph vessels.

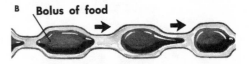

Diagram of segmental contractions.

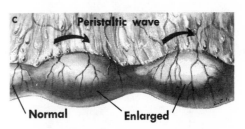

A typical portion of the small intestine, showing how muscle contractions move the food along.

contain enzymes that finish the dismantling of the large molecules of carbohydrate, protein, and fat so that the small molecules can now pass through the lining membrane and enter the blood or the lymph and be transported to their proper locations within the body.

The lining of the small intestine is not a simple, smooth lining. Observation through the microscope reveals millions of tiny, fingerline projections called villi (singular, villus). These serve to greatly increase the surface area of the lining membrane and thus to facilitate the process of absorbing the food materials. Each villus contains a network of blood capillaries and a small lymph vessel. The blood carries away the small molecules that have been formed by the digestion of the carbohydrates and proteins, as well as some of the simpler products of fat digestion. The remaining portions of digested fat are transported by the lymph.

The Large Intestine

The large intestine is the terminal part of the digestive tube. It extends for about four and a half feet (1.5 meters) from its junction with the ileum in the lower right side of the abdominal cavity, in a large circular sweep upward, across the midline to the left, and downward to the rectum and anal canal. The contents of the large intestine consist of the food residue not absorbed in the small intestine, plus the inert bulk, such as cellulose,

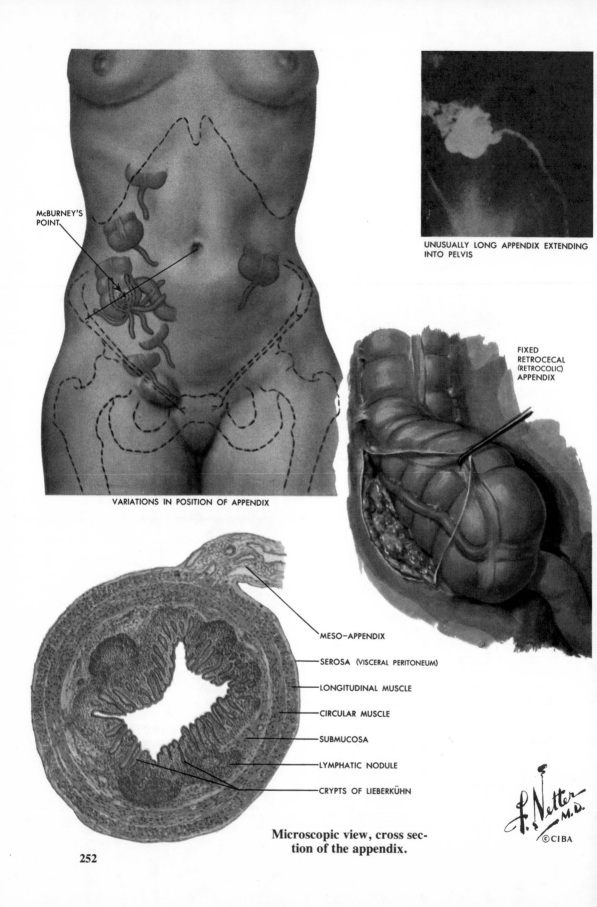

McBURNEY'S POINT

VARIATIONS IN POSITION OF APPENDIX

UNUSUALLY LONG APPENDIX EXTENDING INTO PELVIS

FIXED RETROCECAL (RETROCOLIC) APPENDIX

MESO–APPENDIX

SEROSA (VISCERAL PERITONEUM)

LONGITUDINAL MUSCLE

CIRCULAR MUSCLE

SUBMUCOSA

LYMPHATIC NODULE

CRYPTS OF LIEBERKÜHN

Microscopic view, cross section of the appendix.

compositionally not susceptible to being broken down by digestive enzymes.

The function of the large intestine is to absorb the excess water from the intestinal contents and thus compact what is left for convenient elimination as feces. No digestive enzymes are produced here. The glands located in the wall of the large intestine produce large quantities of mucus that serve as lubricant and also as a bonding agent for the feces.

The large intestine is classically divided into seven subdivisions: (1) the cecum and appendix, which normally lie in the lower, right portion of the abdominal cavity; (2) the ascending colon, which extends upward on the right side from the point of junction with the ileum to a site just below the liver; (3) the transverse colon, which extends from the right to left in front of the other abdominal organs to a point just below the spleen; (4) the descending colon, which continues downward into the lower left quadrant of the abdominal cavity; (5) the sigmoid colon, which curves as it descends into the pelvic portion of the abdominal cavity; (6) the rectum, which is about five inches (12 cm.) long and extends downward to the (7) anal canal, a little more than one inch (2.5 cm.) in length, which opens to the outside at the anus.

The internal structure of the large intestine differs from that of the small intestine in that no villi are attached to the membrane which lines it.

The appendix, a pencil-shaped, narrow extension of the cecum, measures less than half an inch (less than 13 mm.) in diameter and approximately three inches (8 cm.) in length. A great deal of lymphoid tissue is present in the wall of the appendix. This organ therefore is topically described among the lymphoid structures in chapter 11 of this volume.

The above description of the location of the various parts of the large intestine is based on the usual, classic position of these structures. It should be explained, however, that the cecum and appendix are not always located in the lower right portion of the abdominal cavity. They may be located at various positions along the right side and, in the rare cases of transposition of the organs, they may even be located on the left side of the body.

Defecation

The descending colon and the sigmoid colon serve as a reservoir for retaining the fecal material until such time as defecation (bowel movement) occurs. There is a mild reinforcement of the muscle in the wall of the intestinal tube at the junction between the sigmoid colon and the rectum, and this allows the rectum to remain empty most of the time. But once the mass of fecal material builds up sufficiently to force its way into the rectum, delicate nerve endings in the wall of the rectum initiate a desire for defecation. The process of defecation is not entirely automatic, however. In the wall of the anal canal two masses of circular muscle called sphincters serve as valves to restrain the oncoming feces. These are designated as the internal and external anal sphincters. A person has voluntary control of the external sphincter and is thus able to inhibit and postpone defecation if circumstances are not convenient at the time the impulse first develops. With undue delay, however, the accumulation of fecal material may cause the reflex desire for defecation to become compelling.

A person may form the habit of ignoring the desire for defecation, and this tendency may contribute to a problem of constipation. The desire for defecation may be strongest following a meal when peristaltic activity of the entire digestive tube is at its height. Forming the habit of responding to the desire for defecation at a certain time each day may help to prevent constipation.

Diseases of the Digestive Organs

We include in this chapter the health problems that affect the esophagus, the stomach, and the small and large intestines. Technically, when we use the term *digestive organs,* we must include also the liver, gallbladder, and pancreas. For the sake of organization, however, these latter organs are considered in the two chapters which follow.

Diseases of the entire group of digestive organs, including the liver, gallbladder, and pancreas, affect about 18,000,000 Americans. These diseases are the leading cause of hospitalization in the United States. They are the second major cause of days lost from work. They are second only to the cardiovascular diseases as reasons for visits to physicians.

A. Ailments of the Esophagus

GASTROESOPHAGEAL REFLUX AND ESOPHAGITIS

The term *gastroesophageal reflux* denotes a condition in which the stomach contents move upward into the lower part of the esophagus. Being strongly acid, the stomach contents irritate the esophagus, causing an inflammation for which we use the term *reflux esophagitis.*

The muscle in the wall of the lower part of the esophagus is reinforced somewhat at the junction of the esophagus with the stomach. This heavier muscle ring functions like a sphincter, which normally prevents the stomach contents from moving upward into the esophagus. This sphincter relaxes, of course, during the process of swallowing to allow the food that passes through the esophagus to enter the stomach. One of the causes, then, of gastroesophageal reflux is an inefficiency of this sphincter. Other contributing factors include obesity, overeating so that the stomach is filled beyond its usual capacity, and increased pressure within the abdomen as when the individual strains or bends over while wearing a tight belt.

Heartburn is the typical symptom of esophagitis. It consists of a burning type of pain that seems to originate behind the lower part of the sternum (breastbone). The discomfort can usually be relieved by standing up, by drinking fluid to wash the contents back into the stomach, or by the swallowing of an antacid preparation.

Care and Treatment

The first consideration in treating gastroesophageal reflux is to avoid

overloading the stomach. This discipline requires taking less food at each meal and refraining from eating during the last two or three hours before retiring at night. Excess fat in the diet and the use of cigarettes reduce the efficiency of the lower esophageal sphincter. Therefore these should be avoided. Tight belts and garments which constrict the abdomen should be discarded. For a person with reflux esophagitis it is helpful to elevate the legs of the head of the bed in which he sleeps by the use of blocks four to six inches high. The use of pillows or elevation of just the mattress produce an angle in the mattress making it difficult to roll over.

The consistent use of an antacid preparation partially neutralizes the acid contents of the stomach and thus relieves the irritation of the esophagus when stomach contents are refluxed. The preferable antacid preparations are liquid ones and those which do not contain calcium. Two to three tablespoonfuls should be taken about 30 minutes after each meal and at bedtime. The antacid preparation should be taken straight and not followed by food or drink.

NARROWING OF THE ESOPHAGUS

A narrowing of the esophagus can be produced by tumors growing within the organ or pressing on it from surrounding areas. Severe narrowing (stenosis or stricture) can result from the shrinking of scars caused by the accidental drinking of some caustic substance such as acid or alkali (lye) or by longstanding esophagitis. A temporary narrowing is more likely to be caused by a spasm of the muscles in the walls of the organ—a condition commonly called achalasia or cardiospasm.

Permanent narrowing of the esophagus usually causes a sense of fullness under the breastbone when the patient attempts to swallow (dysphagia). He is compelled to eat slowly; and, as the condition gets worse, there is a return of food to the mouth because it cannot enter the stomach. Seldom does the patient experience nausea, and regurgitated food has no sour taste as it would have if it came from the stomach. Pain may be troublesome, and a danger of lung infection threatens should some of the regurgitated food enter the air passages.

Care and Treatment

When the narrowing is the result of a contracting scar, the esophagus may be kept open by stretching it with special equipment which the physician is prepared to use. Repeated stretching from time to time may be necessary. For narrowing from other causes, appropriate forms of surgery may be required.

HIATUS HERNIA

In hiatus hernia a part of the stomach is pushed or pulled upward through the opening (hiatus) in the diaphragm through which the esophagus normally passes. The hernia consists of a pouch in which portions of both stomach and esophagus are present and which may contain partly digested stomach contents. Inflammation or an actual ulcer may develop in this displaced tissue, though many people with hiatal hernias have no symptoms at all. When symptoms do develop, they are usually from an esophagitis and are aggravated by the same things that aggravate reflux esophagitis.

Care and Treatment

Inasmuch as the symptoms of hiatus hernia are caused by the presence of acid stomach contents in the hernial pouch, the immediate treatment is similar to that recommended above for reflux esophagitis. For cases in which these simple measures do not bring relief, it may rarely be necessary to arrange for surgery to return the displaced tissues to their normal position.

B. Diseases of the Stomach

INDIGESTION (DYSPEPSIA)

Indigestion as usually understood

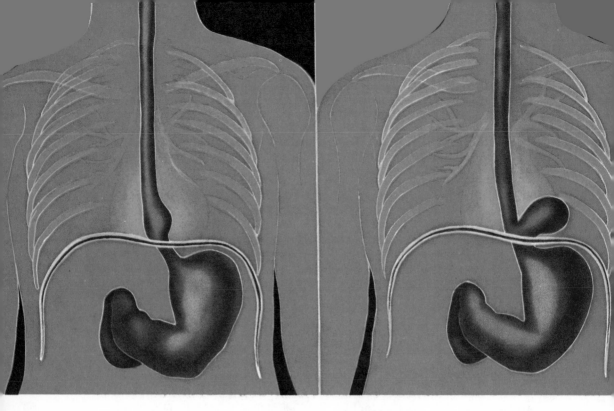

Hiatus hernia, whether the sliding type (left) or the rolling type (right), results in an abnormal pouch at the lower end of the esophagus just above the diaphragm.

consists of distress after eating. Many people suffer from delayed digestion. In such cases, food fermentation occurs, accompanied by gas formation. Belching of gas gives relief from the distress for a time. Gas may gurgle and rumble in the intestines causing bloating and abdominal distress. Intestinal irritation and gas formation may cause diarrhea. There may be headache and a sensation of mental dullness.

It is now recognized that an important cause in many cases is a congenital deficiency of lactase—an enzyme concerned with the assimilation of lactose, one of the carbohydrates contained in milk. In such a case milk taken into the digestive organs ferments instead of being digested and assimilated. The use of milk, even when used in cooking, will continue to cause symptoms.

Care and Treatment

During an attack of indigestion, it is best to let the stomach and intestines rest by not eating solid food for 24 hours. Liquid intake should consist only of water, or clear liquids such as fruit juice or clear broth.

If the indigestion recurs when eating is resumed, try abstaining from milk in all forms—this because of the possibility that the indigestion may be caused by a deficiency of lactase as mentioned above. If the attacks continue, consult a physician.

ACUTE GASTRITIS

Gastritis is an inflammation of the membrane which lines the stomach. Acute gastritis typically causes an uncomfortable feeling in the stomach, distention of the abdomen, headache, nausea, a coated tongue, and a bad taste in the mouth. In severe cases there may be upper abdominal pain, tenderness, vomiting, fever, and sometimes bleeding from the stomach. The latter may appear either as bright red blood in the vomitus or "coffee grounds" material in the stool.

Probably the most common cause of

acute gastritis is a viral infection. This often affects the intestines as well, when it is called gastroenteritis. It may cause nausea with or without vomiting, or intestinal cramps and diarrhea. This is usually a self-limiting disease and is often called the "flu," though the term is best reserved for respiratory infections.

Another cause of acute gastritis is the misuse of aspirin, such as taking large doses on an empty stomach. This damage can be prevented either by taking aspirin at mealtime or by using aspirin preparations that contain antacid.

Gastritis also occurs in acute alcoholism, in which the lining of the stomach becomes inflamed because of direct contact with alcohol.

A form of acute gastritis known as stress ulceration often develops in cases of severe burns, multiple injuries, or major surgical operations. The exact means by which stressful situations produce erosions in the lining of the stomach is not known. It is assumed, however, that an interference with the usual blood supply takes place which allows the delicate cells in the stomach's lining to deteriorate. In the usual case of stress ulceration, healing takes place promptly once the stressful situation is corrected.

The most dangerous cases of acute gastritis are those caused by the swallowing of corrosive acids or alkalies, or irritating poisons.

Care and Treatment

For the usual cases of acute gastritis, the patient should abstain from all food for a day or two. Repeated doses of a nonabsorbable, liquid antacid (available in the drugstore) may be helpful in some types of gastritis. Applying heat locally over the abdomen by fomentations or by a heating pad serves to relieve the discomfort. As the patient's condition improves, he may be allowed small amounts of bland food, with a gradual return to normal diet. If the symptoms persist, a physician should be consulted to determine whether there may be a serious underlying condition such as cancer.

In cases in which a corrosive poison has been swallowed, treatment of the poisoning should receive first attention. (See chapter 22, volume 3.)

In cases of stress ulceration following severe burns or multiple injuries, the essential consideration is the restoration of blood volume, as in the treatment of systemic shock. Once the underlying cause has been properly treated, the gastritis usually heals promptly.

CHRONIC GASTRITIS

The symptoms of chronic gastritis are similar to those of acute gastritis, with the possible addition of discomfort in the upper abdomen after meals, tenderness over the stomach, and a general feeling of semi-invalidism. Chronic gastritis may be caused by long indulgence in improper food, eating an excess of fat or greasy food, hasty eating, drinking large amounts of fluid at mealtime, drinking iced beverages, eating at irregular times, excessive use of spices and condiments, the use of tobacco and liquor, or eating when worried or extremely tired. Chronic gastritis may develop after repeated attacks of acute gastritis.

When the errors that cause chronic gastritis have been practiced for a long time, the glands in the lining of the stomach which produce the gastric juice begin to deteriorate, and in such cases a complete cure is not to be expected.

Care and Treatment

The person with chronic gastritis should review his habits of eating with a determination to correct unhealthful ones. He should masticate his food thoroughly, eat at regular times, avoid drinking excess fluid at mealtime, avoid the use of very hot or very cold drinks, totally abstain from tobacco and alcoholic drinks, and eat sparingly at each meal. There should be a study of personal circumstances with an effort to avoid factors that cause worry, anger, and other emotional upsets. If certain foods aggravate the condition, these should be eliminated from the diet.

PEPTIC ULCER

The term *peptic ulcer* includes (1) gastric ulcers that occur in the stomach and (2) duodenal ulcers that occur in the first part of the duodenum just beyond the stomach's outlet.

The term *ulcer*, as used for lesions in any part of the body, implies a raw area in which the normal covering of the underlying tissue is no longer present. So a peptic ulcer consists of a relatively small area in the inner wall of the stomach or the duodenum no longer covered by the soft tissue normally present. On examining the site of a peptic ulcer it appears that the lining tissue has been punched out at this site.

The gastric juice, the digestive agent produced by glands in the stomach's lining, contains an enzyme, pepsin, which, together with hydrochloric acid, has the ability to disintegrate protein substances. Because the soft tissues of the stomach contain protein, they may be affected. Hence it is a marvel that the lining of the stomach and the duodenum is not all destroyed. Normally the cells that compose the lining of the stomach and duodenum possess a protective mechanism, as yet not fully understood, which keeps them from being digested by gastric juice. It must be, then, that at the site of a peptic ulcer this protective mechanism has failed. Beyond this, we do not know the precise cause. We do know, however, several factors that predispose to peptic ulcers.

We often hear people say, "I was so distraught that I almost got an ulcer over the situation." It is true that persons under stress and persons who drive themselves beyond their reasonable limitations stand in greater danger of developing peptic ulcer than those who live calmly and peaceably.

Presumably, even an hereditary element figures in the predisposition to peptic ulcer. It would be hard to separate this factor, however, from the factor of psychic stress mentioned above. It may be that what the individual actually inherits is a tendency to work under pressure.

Circumstances and customs prevail in the environment that predispose to peptic ulcer. The taking of aspirin into the stomach has a corrosive effect on the stomach's lining. Coffee, tea, and cola drinks increase the stomach's production of acid and thus favor the development of peptic ulcer. Persons who drink liquor are more subject to peptic ulcer than those who abstain. The use of cigarettes has a detrimental effect on the lining of the stomach and duodenum. One scientific study has indicated that peptic ulcers show up a little more than twice as frequently among men who smoke as compared with those who don't smoke. For women, the incidence of peptic ulcer is 1.6 times greater among smokers.

The incidence of gastric ulcer (ulcer in the stomach) is about the same for men and for women. Strangely, duodenal ulcer is ten times more frequent in men than in women.

The principal symptom of peptic ulcer is pain. Besides this, there may be a sensitive spot, especially noticeable on deep pressure, just below the lower end of the sternum (breastbone). Other symptoms of ulcer include heartburn, belching of acid, nausea, loss of appetite, and loss of weight. The pain of duodenal ulcer typically appears two or three hours after a meal. This pain may be quickly relieved by taking more food or by using an antacid preparation, preferably in liquid form. Taking an antacid does not cure the ulcer, but only neutralizes the acid irritating the raw bed of the ulcer.

Ulcers that occur in the stomach (gastric ulcers) may represent the early phase of cancer of the stomach. Duodenal ulcers, by contrast seldom become malignant. It is because of this probability of cancer that every gastric ulcer should be evaluated by a physician or by the members of a diagnostic clinic. It is now possible for the interior of the

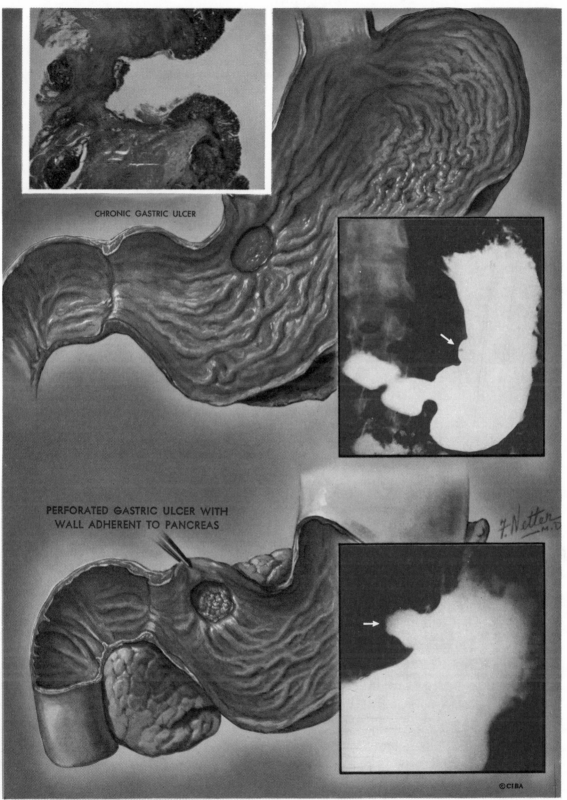

CHRONIC GASTRIC ULCER

PERFORATED GASTRIC ULCER WITH
WALL ADHERENT TO PANCREAS

F. Netter
M.D.

©CIBA

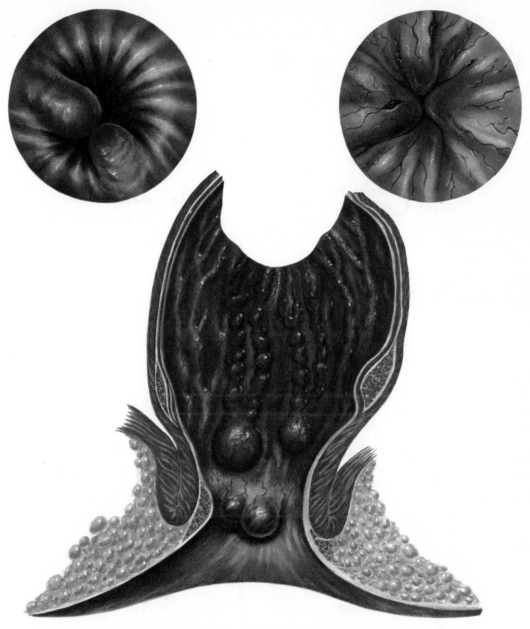

Hemorrhoids are swellings containing dilated veins situated in the mucous membrane of the anal canal.

level teaspoonful of salt to the pint [500 ml.] of water) and then gently pressed into place while the patient is lying down with his head lower than his hips.

A daily hot sitz bath with the patient sitting for 30 minutes in hot water may help to relieve the discomfort which hemorrhoids produce. When bleeding from the hemorrhoids persists, a physician should be consulted. Hemorrhoids of long standing are best treated by surgical removal.

ANAL FISSURE

An anal fissure consists of a small tear in the membrane which lines the anal canal. This problem usually occurs in a person troubled with constipation when a firm or sharp mass of fecal ma-

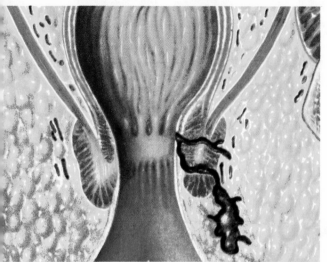

THE UPJOHN COMPANY

A common cause of anal fistula is a perianal abscess. Note fistulous tract leading from the abscess to the anal canal.

terial breaks through the lining membrane while the feces are being expelled. The outstanding symptom is severe pain at the time of defecation. Healing of the fissure may be delayed if constipation is not remedied. The hazard of an anal fissure is that infection developing in the denuded area may penetrate into the deeper tissues, causing an abscess.

Care and Treatment

The usual treatment of anal fissure is to relieve the condition of constipation as far as possible and to insert an anesthetic ointment within the anal canal before each defecation.

PERIANAL ABSCESS

When an infection penetrates the deeper tissues in the vicinity of the anus, there may be a breakdown of the cells in the area of infection, with the formation of an abscess. An abscess in this area causes extreme discomfort, with deep pain radiating into the buttock.

Care and Treatment

Treatment consists of a surgical incision into the cavity of the abscess to allow the pus to escape. It is often advisable to pack the incision with sterile gauze so as to keep the drainage route open while healing proceeds from the depth of the incision.

ANAL FISTULA

When untreated, a perianal abscess tends to burrow its way to the nearest surface—either to the membrane lining the anal canal or to the skin surrounding the anal opening. Such a channel provides a route for the escape of the pus contained in the abscess. But the process of healing when such a development occurs is slow and tedious. In some cases there is an opening both to the interior of the anal canal and to the skin surrounding the anus. Such fistulous canals tend to remain infected. The persisting inflammation causes extreme discomfort.

Care and Treatment

The only satisfactory treatment for an anal fistula consists of the surgical removal of all of the infected tissue.

274

The Liver, Gallbladder, and Pancreas

A. The Liver

The liver is the body's largest gland. It weighs about 4 pounds (1.8 kg.) in the adult and performs more than a hundred important functions necessary to health. The lowest five or six ribs protect this soft, fleshy organ located just below the diaphragm, more on the right than on the left.

The liver functions as a multipurpose manufacturing plant, producing blood cells in early fetal life, storing and releasing certain substances the body urgently needs, producing bile (an important aid to the body's assimilation of fat), producing important protein substances for the blood plasma, bringing about chemical transformations in many substances which the body requires for energy or tissue building, preparing leftover or expended substances for elimination, and rendering certain toxins less noxious.

All of the liver's functioning cells lie close to flowing blood. In fact, blood bathes practically every liver cell on at least one of its surfaces. This interrelationship is important, because the liver performs its chemical magic on substances brought in and carried away by the blood. It is no surprise, then, that the liver has a double blood supply—one consisting of fresh blood coming quite directly from the lungs and heart, and the other of blood which comes to the liver after it has been through the tissues of the small intestine. The blood from this second source carries the food substances which it absorbed while flowing through the small intestine.

The liver's ability to perform many tasks becomes the more remarkable when we notice its nearly homogenous structure. No special regions in the liver perform its sundry functions. All gland cells in the liver look alike. It seems that the cells switch jobs as the occasion requires.

Despite the liver's many activities, it also serves as a storehouse. Although the blood passing through the liver always keeps moving, the amount of blood contained within the organ varies from time to time. When the liver distends with blood, it serves, to this extent, as a reservoir.

The liver amasses within its cells supplies of the fundamental food elements and liberates them into the blood as needed to meet the body's moment-by-moment requirements. For example, the liver reserves a sufficient amount of carbohydrate (the body's prime energy food) to provide up to 500

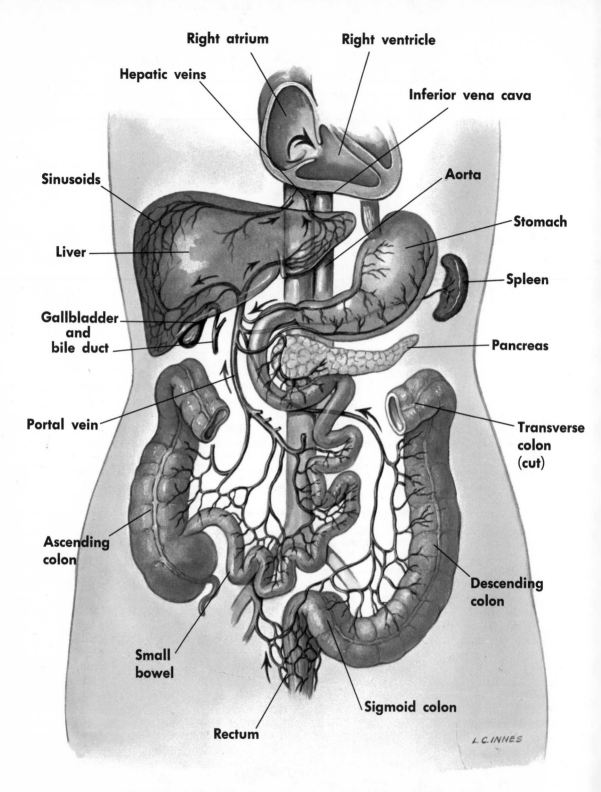

Right atrium   Right ventricle

Hepatic veins

Inferior vena cava

Sinusoids

Aorta

Stomach

Liver

Spleen

Gallbladder
and
bile duct

Pancreas

Portal vein

Transverse
colon
(cut)

Ascending
colon

Descending
colon

Small
bowel

Sigmoid colon

Rectum

L. C. INNES

The liver not only receives its own supply of pure blood, but also
receives through the portal vein the blood that comes from the intestines (shown in blue) laden with newly absorbed food. The liver
also secretes the bile, a fluid which is drained away by the common
bile duct (green) and poured into the duodenum.

calories of food energy. This is only about one fifth of the average daily energy requirement; but it serves as a working capital always available on short notice to fill the need while the body mobilizes other, less accessible stores of energy food.

In a similar manner the liver stocks modest amounts of amino acids—the building blocks for the various proteins—so that it can assemble quickly just the particular kind of protein that may be momentarily in short supply. The liver stores a small amount of fat, even though most of the body's fat is located elsewhere.

The liver contains deposits of vitamins A, B, and D, holding these ready for utilization by other tissues. The liver conserves the body's precious store of iron.

The liver produces bile, and by this function it comes closest to qualifying as a typical gland, for it includes a system of tiny canals which carry away the bile secreted by the gland cells. These canals unite to form ducts, which in turn unite to form a single tube which carries the bile toward the duodenum, with a detour for storage purposes in the gallbladder. The liver produces almost a quart (1 liter) of bile each day.

The bile contains chemical substances (bile salts) which help to emulsify the fat contained in the food entering the small intestine, and it facilitates the digestion of fat prior to its being absorbed. Thus bile aids in the digestion of fats and makes possible the absorption from the intestine of the fat-soluble vitamins—vitamins A, D, E, and K.

The bile contains pigments, which are some of the end products in the destruction of hemoglobin. When the flow of bile is blocked, these pigments cause the yellow color of the skin and eyes characteristic of jaundice.

The liver takes the material brought to it by the blood and custom-builds some of the particular chemical substances required by the body. Take protein as one example. The chemical composition of human protein differs from the protein of plants and other animals. When we eat protein, the digestive system first disassembles the protein molecule to its individual amino acids. These are carried to the liver, where some of them are reorganized into certain types of human protein.

The liver disposes of discarded protein. Protein is unique among the basic food substances because it contains nitrogen and because its molecules are so large that the kidneys cannot eliminate them. The liver breaks down the large protein molecules and salvages the parts it can transform for other uses. It converts the residue to urea, a nitrogen-containing substance consisting of molecules small enough to be eliminated by the kidneys.

Finally, in our consideration of the liver we come to its ability to handle toxic substances. The chemical mechanisms available in the liver either disrupt the molecules of noxious substances or they bring about chemical combinations which are harmless, or at least less harmful.

Considering the many things the liver does to further the welfare of the body, it is understandable that diseases of the liver, when they occur, pose a serious threat to health and even to life itself.

B. The Gallbladder

The gallbladder is a small, hollow, pear-shaped organ, which serves as a storage reservoir for the bile produced by the liver. The liver produces bile continuously, but bile is needed only periodically to aid in the digestion of food within the intestine. So the bile is stored, between times, in the gallbladder. The gallbladder is so small that it is surprising that it can function thus as a reservoir. It can hold only about one twentieth the volume of bile produced within a 24-hour period. The explanation is that the lining of the gallbladder absorbs water and thus concentrates the bile about fivefold.

In response to the presence of food in the duodenum, the delicate muscle located in the wall of the gallbladder contracts, forcing the concentrated bile

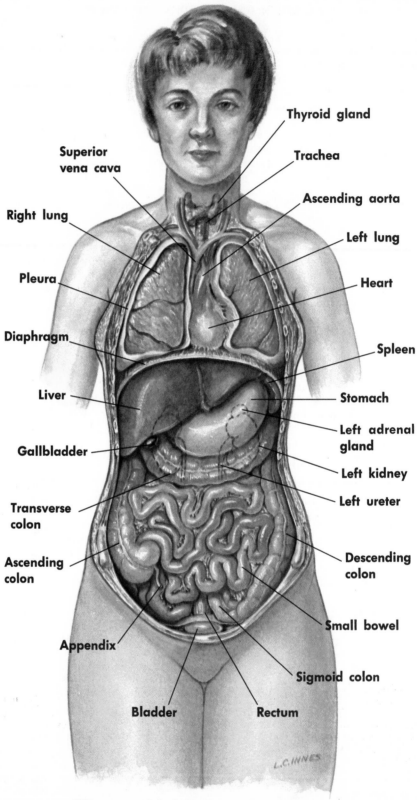

Thyroid gland

Trachea

Ascending aorta

Left lung

Heart

Spleen

Stomach

Left adrenal gland

Left kidney

Left ureter

Descending colon

Small bowel

Sigmoid colon

Rectum

Superior vena cava

Right lung

Pleura

Diaphragm

Liver

Gallbladder

Transverse colon

Ascending colon

Appendix

Bladder

L.C.INNES

The organs of the body as seen from in front.

out of the gallbladder and into the duodenum, where it aids in the digestion process.

C. The Pancreas

The pancreas, like the liver, is classed as an accessory digestive organ. It is a long, soft, lumpy organ, which stretches across the deeper wall of the abdominal cavity from the duodenum on the right to the vicinity of the spleen on the left.

The pancreas is really two glands in one—an exocrine gland and an endocrine gland. It is an exocrine gland because it produces pancreatic juice, which contains digestive enzymes that are emptied through the pancreatic duct into the duodenum at the site at which bile is discharged into the duodenum. It is an endocrine gland because scattered throughout its substance are many tiny islands of tissue (islets of Langerhans) which discharge hormones into the bloodstream. The exocrine tissue which produces the pancreatic juice constitutes about 99 percent of the bulk of the pancreas, while the islets of Langerhans account for only about 1 percent.

Pancreatic juice contains enzymes which aid in the digestion of all three of the major types of food: proteins, carbohydrates, and fats. It also contains bicarbonate ions, which counteract the acidity of the stomach contents as delivered to the duodenum.

The islets of Langerhans have no connection with the system of ducts which carries the pancreatic juice to the duodenum. They contain two kinds of functioning cells. One kind produces insulin; the other, glucagon. Insulin has an important influence on the rate at which glucose (blood sugar) is used as energy fuel throughout the body. This hormone will be considered in greater detail in chapter 1, volume 3. Glucagon, the other hormone produced by the islets of Langerhans, acts in emergency situations to release the body's stores of glucose.

Diseases of the Liver, Gallbladder, and Pancreas

A. Diseases of the Liver

As indicated in the previous chapter, the liver performs many important functions, many of them extremely important to the well-being of the individual. Therefore, any form of liver disease becomes at once a serious problem. Fortunately, the liver has a remarkable capacity for self-healing. Nevertheless, certain liver ailments continue to pose a threat in the practice of medicine.

Common Symptoms Produced by Liver Disorders

A multitude of different symptoms may appear in liver disease. This abundance is understandable because of the many functions which the liver normally performs. We mention three common symptoms here:

JAUNDICE (ICTERUS)

Jaundice consists of a yellow coloration of the skin and, particularly, of the whites of the eyes. This symptom is caused by any one of several conditions which interferes with the liver's

dismantling of the hemoglobin (red pigment) released by worn-out red blood cells. In the normal process, the molecules of hemoglobin are broken down into smaller molecules, which become components of the bile and are eliminated through the intestinal tract. One product of the breakdown of hemoglobin is yellow in color and another is green. When elimination of these is interfered with, they accumulate in the blood, and the color of these so-called bile pigments shows up in the skin and in the whites of the eyes.

ENLARGEMENT OF THE LIVER (HEPATOMEGALY)

Enlargement of the liver occurs when the liver is inflamed, as in hepatitis, when the bile duct is obstructed so that the bile cannot leave the liver, when cirrhosis develops (except in the late stage of this disease), when cysts or abscesses occur in the liver, or when a tumor develops in the liver. Normally, the lower margin of the liver can be felt at or just slightly below the lowest rib on the right side. When the liver becomes enlarged, its lower border can be felt through the abdominal wall at a lower position than normal.

FLUID IN THE ABDOMEN (ASCITES)

Several possible causes exist for the accumulation of free fluid in the abdominal (peritoneal) cavity, and several of these are not related to the liver. Conditions of the liver which may cause ascites include cirrhosis of the liver, chronic active hepatitis, and obstruction of the vein which carries blood away from the liver.

Acute Hepatitis

Hepatitis is an inflammatory involvement of the liver which causes damage to its functioning cells. Several possible causes might account for the problem, including viruses, toxins, drugs, and poisonings. However, the usual cause of acute hepatitis is a viral infection.

VIRAL HEPATITIS

The term *viral hepatitis* includes several similar diseases caused by separate types of virus and typically transmitted by different means. These are designated as hepatitis type A, hepatitis type B, and non-A, non-B hepatitis.

1. *Hepatitis Type A* (previously called *infectious hepatitis*). This type of hepatitis is most common among children. The virus is usually transmitted by person-to-person contact, especially among those living under crowded conditions. The virus can be transmitted by contaminated food or water. The symptoms of the illness begin two to six weeks after the virus was transmitted to the individual. The onset of symptoms is usually abrupt, and the duration of the illness is six to eight weeks—shorter than the duration for hepatitis type B. Hepatitis type A is seldom associated with serious complications, there being a mortality rate of only about 0.1 percent. Hepatitis type A can be prevented or at least modified by the administration of an immune serum globulin, even after contacts have been made with persons ill with the dis-

ease. The protection afforded by the use of immune serum globulin lasts up to six months.

2. *Hepatitis Type B* (previously called *serum hepatitis*). Hepatitis type B typically affects adolescents and adults. The virus is usually transmitted by accidental injection by means of some contaminated instrument, such as a hypodermic needle (as used in drug abuse), a tattooing needle, or the in-

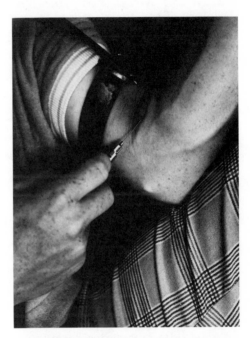

Hepatitis is often spread by hypodermic needles used in drug abuse.

strument for piercing earlobes; or, occasionally, by way of blood transfusion. Presumably it can also be acquired by sexual contact. The incubation period (time lapse between transmission of the virus and the onset of symptoms) is four to twenty weeks. The onset of symptoms is usually gradual. The duration of illness is three to four months. Serious liver damage occurs in 5 to 10 percent of cases. The mortality rate is between 1 and 10 percent.

The illness with hepatitis type B can

be made less severe by the administration of a special serum globulin.

A vaccine effective in 90 percent of persons for protection from hepatitis type B was approved in 1981 for use in the United States. It is known as Heptavax-B and is administered intramuscularly in three doses over a period of six months. It is recommended for all persons possibly at risk of contracting hepatitis type B.

3. *Non-A, Non-B Viral Hepatitis.* This type of hepatitis is caused by one or more viruses other than type A or type B. The acute hepatitis that sometimes develops following a blood transfusion in which contaminated blood was instilled, is most frequently of this type. At the time of writing the exact identity of the viruses causing this type of hepatitis is still being studied.

The course of the illness in viral hepatitis may be described in three phases: a prodromal phase, an icteric phase, and a recovery phase. (1) In the prodromal phase the patient has symptoms similar to those of influenza—malaise, loss of appetite, nausea, and fatigue. (2) In the icteric phase the functions of the liver are altered, causing jaundice (icterus, a yellow coloring of the skin and whites of the eyes), dark-colored urine, and light-colored stools. The jaundice reaches its maximum in 7 to 14 days, and thereafter subsides progressively. (3) In the recovery phase the symptoms and jaundice gradually disappear. The patient is usually quite comfortable during this phase, but is still weak and should not overexert himself.

Care and Treatment

Viral hepatitis should be taken seriously and the patient should be under the care of a physician. The physician will arrange for repeated tests of the liver's function. The information thus provided will enable the physician to judge the seriousness of this particular case so that he can modify the treatment accordingly.

Rest throughout the period of ill-

ness is very important, and the patient's strength and vitality should be carefully conserved. In spite of poor appetite it is important for the patient to have adequate nourishment throughout the illness. In some cases, it may be necessary to supplement the diet by intravenous feeding.

Surgical procedures during the period of illness should be avoided if at all possible. The effects of an anesthetic can be damaging to the liver during this time when the liver's functions are already diminished.

The condition of jaundice usually causes the skin to itch. This discomfort may be somewhat relieved by the application to the skin of calamine lotion.

It is important that the patient recovering from viral hepatitis be restrained from resuming his normal activities too soon.

OTHER TYPES OF ACUTE HEPATITIS

Some cases of acute hepatitis are caused by sensitivity to drugs. When administered to a sensitive person, many drugs can cause this type of illness. The treatment in such cases is, of course, discontinuance and further avoidance of the drug.

Another cause of acute hepatitis is poisoning by the eating of wild mushrooms. Even small amounts can cause serious damage to the liver, and in these cases the mortality rate is high.

Another form of acute hepatitis is that which occurs as part of Reye's syndrome, a childhood disease described in chapter 17, volume 1.

CHRONIC HEPATITIS

Chronic hepatitis is a persisting illness involving the liver for which in many cases no cause is known. In some cases it is a continuation of an episode of acute hepatitis. There are two types, but in the early course of the illness it may be necessary to use laboratory tests and make a microscopic examination of a small sample of liver tissue to know which type is present.

CHRONIC ACTIVE HEPATITIS

This is a serious disease, often related to hepatitis B, which tends to progress toward cirrhosis of the liver and, without treatment, tends to end fatally within a few years. The symptoms include fatigue, abdominal pain, loss of appetite, jaundice, ascites (fluid in the abdomen), and enlargement of the liver. Many of these cases respond favorably to corticosteroid medication. This type of treatment must be carefully regulated by a physician, but, even so, it is hazardous because of the possibility of serious side effects.

CHRONIC PERSISTENT HEPATITIS

The symptoms of chronic persistent hepatitis are mild and may consist only of fatigue. The illness persists for years, does not respond to any known form of treatment, but does not endanger the patient's life.

LAENNEC'S CIRRHOSIS (ALCOHOLIC CIRRHOSIS)

Cirrhosis is a condition in which the functioning cells of the liver are damaged to the extent that many of them are finally displaced by fibrous tissue. In the meantime, there are scattered areas throughout the liver in which islands of regeneration appear, but the general architecture of the liver becomes so distorted that liver function cannot return to normal. Several possible causes for cirrhosis can be cited, but in the United States and Western Europe the most common cause is the prolonged intake of alcoholic drinks. The alcohol acts as a toxic agent, causing direct damage to the functioning liver cells.

The development of Laennec's cirrhosis is progressive over a period of years. In its early stages, the disease may be arrested by the permanent discontinuance of alcoholic drinks. But once a sufficient amount of liver tissue has been damaged, the disease progresses to a fatal outcome, even though the patient then abstains from alcohol.

In the early stages the liver becomes enlarged and is more firm than normal.

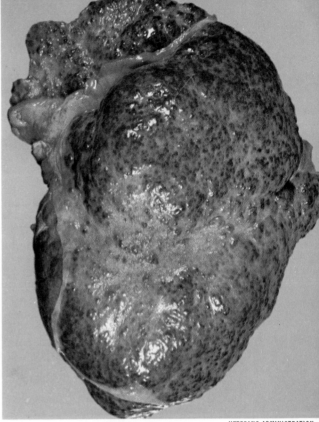

Cirrhosis of the liver.

In the advanced stage the organ becomes shrunken and rock-hard. With this development, a decline takes place in the usual functions of the liver, along with a resistance to the passage of blood, so that blood carried by the portal vein, which would normally pass through the liver, meets resistance and follows alternate courses on its return to the heart.

The symptoms include a general loss of vitality, loss of weight, loss of appetite, jaundice, and the accumulation of fluid in the abdomen (ascites). One of the alternate routes now taken by the blood is by way of veins in the wall of the esophagus. These dilated veins are called varices and are prone to rupture.

Care and Treatment

The first consideration in the treatment of cirrhosis resulting from the chronic use of alcohol is to persuade the patient to completely abstain from alcohol in the future. At best, the patient's prospect of a five-year survival is listed at about 70 percent. Without abstaining from alcohol, the prospect is reduced to 40 percent. Other than abstaining from alcohol the care consists of providing an adequate diet with vitamin supplements.

BILIARY CIRRHOSIS

This is a chronic disease of unknown cause which typically affects women between the ages of 35 and 55. The early changes in the liver are different from those of Laennec's cirrrhosis, but in the end the inability of the liver to perform its functions is comparable to what occurs in Laennec's cirrhosis. The primary change in the liver is one in which the tiny ductules which normally carry bile toward the hepatic duct becomes obliterated so that bile produced by the functioning cells has no route of escape.

This disease is slowly progressive over a period of 10 to 20 years, and the serious symptoms develop so slowly that the patient may live a relatively normal life for several years after the onset of itching, which is the usual first symptom. Often the skin becomes brown-pigmented. Eventually enlargement of the liver and jaundice develop.

One of the effects of the liver damage in this case is a failure to activate vitamin D, a failure that causes the bones to lose part of their normal content of calcium. Thus there may be pain in the bones and even multiple fractures.

Care and Treatment

There is no satisfactory treatment for biliary cirrhosis. The care of the patient consists of relieving the symptoms as far as possible and maintaining the patient's courage and comfort during the several years of the downhill course of the disease.

Liver Abscesses

An abscess is a fluid-filled cavity which occurs in an area of tissue destruction caused by the invasion of bacteria or parasites. A great volume of blood flows through the liver slowly; and if it happens to carry bacteria or parasites, these may lodge in the liver, causing one or more local infections. The white blood cells crowd into any such area of infection; and in the resulting conflict between white blood cells and germs, some of the liver cells are destroyed. Thus one or more abscesses develop right in the substance of the liver.

PYOGENIC LIVER ABSCESS

The germs which cause the ordinary type of liver abscess may come from an infection in the common bile duct, as may occur when a gallstone lodges in this duct. Another possible source of such germs is some infection in the intestines. In other cases, the germs may originate in an area of peritonitis, such as results from a rupture of the appendix or a perforation of a duodenal ulcer.

The symptoms of a liver abscess are those typical of a severe infection, plus those relating to involvement of the liver. There is fever, sweats, weight loss, and vomiting. The liver is usually enlarged and tender, and there is pain in the right side of the abdomen and in the region of the right shoulder.

Care and Treatment

The patient with liver abscess is in serious condition. The mortality rate, even with treatment, is quite high. The treatment consists of surgical drainage of the abscess, in addition to the aggressive use of antibiotic medications to combat the infection.

AMEBIC LIVER ABSCESS

Amebic liver abscess is a complication of an infection of the large intestine by the amoeba *Entamoeba histolytica*. This infection is rare in the United States but relatively common in some tropical countries. The liver abscess in such a case is usually single and results from the arrival in the liver of a parasite which has traveled by the bloodstream from the infected large intestine.

The symptoms of amebic liver abscess are similar to those caused by

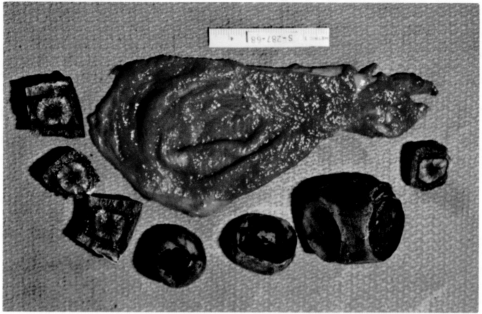

An operation to remove gallstones usually includes removal of the patient's gallbladder also.

pyogenic liver abscess, except that in this case the illness develops more gradually. The treatment is directed to the control of the parasitic infection in the intestine. See chapter 20, volume 3, for the details of this treatment.

Cancer of the Liver

There are many cases in which cancer involves the liver, but in most of these the cancer has originated in some other part of the body with the transplant of cancer cells to the liver by way of the blood. Cancer of the liver is always serious. For further information on this, see chapter 11, volume 3.

B. Diseases of the Gallbladder and Bile Ducts

GALLSTONES (CHOLELITHIASIS)

Gallstone disease affects about 10 percent of the total population and about 30 percent of persons over 65 years of age. Stonelike concretions form within the gallbladder. These tend to move down the cystic duct and into the common bile duct. Gallstones begin as tiny granules and gradually enlarge until, in an occasional case, one stone will virtually fill the gallbladder.

The hazard of gallstones is that they are often associated with inflammation in the gallbladder or in the bile ducts, they may obstruct the common bile duct and thus cause a stoppage of the flow of bile, and they increase the risk of cancer of the gallbladder.

Gallstones occur twice as commonly among women as among men. Obesity seems to predispose to the formation of gallstones, as does also infection of the gallbladder or the bile ducts. Gallstones are composed of some of the substances which normally occur in the bile. Just why these substances precipitate out of solution to become concretions is not clear. It is known, however, that an excess of cholesterol in the bile, as well as the presence of estrogen and a high rate of destruction of red blood cells, favors the formation of gallstones.

The symptoms vary all the way from no symptoms at all (in about half the

cases) to extreme symptoms of excru-
ciating pain, chills, and fever. Jaundice
is a prominent symptom when a
gallstone in the common bile duct prevents the flow of bile into the duodenum.

The diagnosis of gallstone disease is
sometimes difficult to make. Symptoms, when present, may be similar to
those caused by other conditions. X-
ray studies are often helpful, but some
types of gallstones do not cast shadows
on the X-ray film. Once the diagnosis is
confirmed, however, treatment should
be arranged. Otherwise serious complications may develop.

Care and Treatment

**The traditional treatment for
gallstones is surgical removal, usually
accomplished by removing the gallbladder. A person whose gallbladder
has been removed carries no handicap on this account. In some cases
treatment with bile acid medications
may bring about the partial dissolving
of the gallstones, especially of those
composed largely of cholesterol.**

INFLAMMATION IN THE
GALLBLADDER (CHOLECYSTITIS)

Inflammation of the gallbladder in its
acute form is usually caused by the
lodging of a gallstone in the cystic duct
(the duct that leads to and from the
gallbladder). This sudden obstruction
of the cystic duct interferes with the
blood supply to the gallbladder and
thus sets the stage for inflammation. In
about three fourths of the cases, the
symptoms subside in three or four
days, with the patient feeling normal
again. In many of such cases, however,
repeated attacks occur later in what is
called chronic inflammation of the
gallbladder (chronic cholecystitis).

In the one fourth of cases in which
the symptoms persist or become more
severe, the gallbladder must be surgically removed to avoid the possible
complication of perforation of the
gallbladder.

The symptoms of acute inflammation
of the gallbladder include pain in the
right upper part of the abdomen, vomiting, fever, and possibly jaundice.

Care and Treatment

**The only definitive treatment for
inflammation of the gallbladder is the
surgical removal of the organ. The
decision on whether to operate immediately or wait for a possible remission of symptoms must be made by
the physician in charge.**

Obstructive Jaundice

Obstructive jaundice is not a disease
in itself, but an indication of a blockage
in the outflow of bile. The obstruction
may be a gallstone lodged in a bile
duct, especially the common bile duct.
A tumor of the pancreas, a cancer, or
an inflammation of the bile ducts or
structures around them may cause obstruction. Obstructive jaundice needs
to be distinguished from jaundice
caused by an inflammation within the
liver or that caused by excessive disin-
tegration of red blood cells.

Because of the various possible
causes of jaundice and the seriousness
of some of them, the appearance of yellow coloring of the skin and of the
whites of the eyes is a signal for a thorough examination with laboratory tests
to determine the condition of the liver
and its associated structures.

C. Diseases of the Pancreas

Pancreatitis

Pancreatitis is a condition in which
the tissues of the pancreas are inflamed. Whether in acute or chronic
form, pancreatitis is serious. Normal
pancreatic tissue is fragile; and when
an inflammation progresses to the stage
of tissue injury, the liberation of the digestive enzymes which the pancreas
produces causes destruction of the tissues of the pancreas and damages adjacent structures.

ACUTE PANCREATITIS

The acute form of pancreatitis is
typically a complication of gallstones

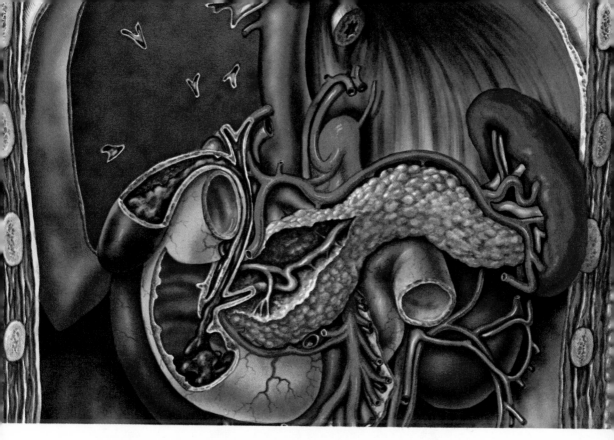

Cutaway view of the abdomen, showing pancreas (yellow) and gall-bladder (green). Note bile duct through which bile flows into the duodenum. Gallstones sometimes pass through the bile duct, causing severe pain.

or other disease in the bile passages. Other causes include mechanical injury (trauma), a perforating peptic ulcer, or an infection by the virus that causes mumps.

In the milder cases the mortality rate is less than 10 percent, but in those complicated by extensive destruction of pancreatic tissue, the mortality rate may excede 50 percent.

The outstanding symptom is severe steady pain in the upper abdomen and back. Nausea and vomiting commonly occur, and the patient may lapse into shock. In those cases in which the bile ducts are involved, there may be jaundice.

Care and Treatment

The two essentials in the treatment of acute pancreatitis are (1) sustaining the patient's vitality by the relief of pain and by the use of intravenous therapy to combat the patient's shock, and (2) reducing the activity of the pancreas. The latter is best accomplished by the continuous removal of gastric juice from the stomach, using a suction tube inserted through the nose. By removing the gastric juice, the usual stimulation of the pancreas is prevented. Complications such as kidney failure must be treated if and when they develop. In a small number of cases an abscess develops within the pancreas, and this adverse circumstance requires surgical intervention to drain the abscess.

CHRONIC PANCREATITIS

Chronic pancreatitis is commonly associated with chronic alcoholism. It may also result from obstruction of the pancreatic duct caused by cancer.

287

Care and Treatment

The long-range care of a patient with chronic pancreatitis requires complete abstinence from alcohol. In many such cases the pancreatic tissue cannot be restored to its normal condition, even though the patient abstains from alcohol. In selected cases, surgical removal of the damaged portion or portions of the pancreas has met with reasonable success. In a few cases on record total removal of the pancreas has resulted in long-range benefit. In such cases, however, the enzymes and hormones normally produced by the pancreas must be supplied by medication.

Cancer of the Pancreas

This is a serious form of cancer which is discussed in chapter 11, volume 3.

Diabetes Mellitus

This is a condition in which a reduction takes place in the amount of insulin produced by the beta cells of the isles of Langerhans of the pancreas. This condition is discussed in detail in chapter 13, volume 3.

Cystic Fibrosis

This is a childhood disease in which the pancreas is usually involved. It is discussed in chapter 17, volume 1.

Section **VI**

The Skeletal System

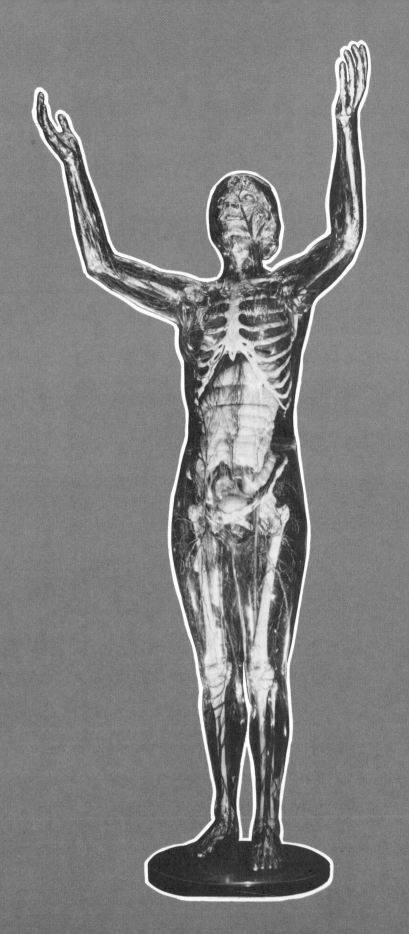

The Body's Framework

"You say that bones produce blood?" a student in physiology class asked her teacher.

"Essentially, that's what I said," the teacher replied. "But the way you state your question is not quite correct. It is the marrow inside the bones, not the bones themselves, that produces certain of the blood cells."

"Well, I thought bones were to the body something like the steel framework is to a building," the coed persisted. "I had supposed that the bones provide the body's support, and that's all."

"The bones do support the body just as you had supposed. But the human body is designed very efficiently. Many of its tissues have more than one function to perform. Bones, you know, consist of living tissue. The cells contained in bone are very much alive, just as are the cells of muscle and nerve."

Many people, like this student, think of the body's framework as consisting only of bones. It is true that bones compose the skeleton, that inner structure of the body which provides for its main support and protection and determines its general shape and posture. But just as the framework of a building consists not only of steel girders but also of studding joists, and rafters, so the body's framework includes not only bones but other related tissues which help to hold the organs of the body in place and thus make their functions possible.

Four kinds of tissue make up the body's framework: (1) connective tissue, (2) ligaments and tendons, (3) cartilage, and (4) bone. These framework tissues are designed not only to provide mechanical support for the body but to permit flexibility and movement in certain parts.

Connective Tissue

Connective tissue, a strong, pliable "packing material," is found throughout the body. It surrounds and supports the body's various organs and binds the more active tissues to the skeleton. It provides an envelope around each muscle. It forms the deeper part of the skin and is strong enough to hold the skin in place and yet elastic enough to allow the skin to move freely over the underlying structures.

Connective tissue consists of cells and fibers. One of the important functions of the cells in connective tissue is to produce the fibers which form strands and feltworks. The fibers give connective tissue its strength. The arrangement of the fibers, as they run this way and that way, makes connective tissue pliable and elastic. Some of the fibers of connective tissue can stretch and return again to their former length.

291

commonly occurs in kidney disease. Pain in the back may be an early symptom of a generalized infection. It may result from an injury.

For a further consideration of back pain and backache, see chapter 7, volume 3.

HERNIATED DISK INVOLVEMENT (SLIPPED DISK; HERNIATED DISK; RUPTURED DISK)

The vertebral column (spinal column) is the mainstay of the skeleton. It is subject to tremendous mechanical forces, as in lifting, jumping, twisting, and carrying heavy weights. Between each vertebra and its neighbor there is interposed a cushionlike disk of fibrocartilage (an intervertebral disk). It is these disks, by way of their resiliency, that permit the bending and twisting movements of which the vertebral column is capable. Each intervertebral disk is composed of an elastic central part, called the nucleus pulposus, and a surrounding ring of dense tissue, designated as the annulus fibrosus.

Between the bony processes of each vertebra and its neighbor there emerges a pair of spinal nerves—nerves leading from the spinal cord to some particular part of the body or the extremities.

Injuries to the intervertebral disks constitute the most common type of vertebral column injury. Such injury may be caused by heavy lifting, by a fall, by an automobile accident, by striking the head while diving, or, very commonly, by elusive, recurring forces of pressure that cause the disks to deteriorate. Immediately following an injury that damages an intervertebral disk, the patient will usually suffer pain for a few days, experiencing a "catch in the back" or a "crick in the neck." This discomfort is caused by torn ligaments or strained muscles. It may be some time later, possibly after several incidents of discomfort, that the nucleus pulposus at the center of the intervertebral disk actually squeezes through a damaged or weak part of the annulus fibrosus and brings pressure against an adjacent nerve root. This pressure causes severe pain and possible weakness of the muscles supplied

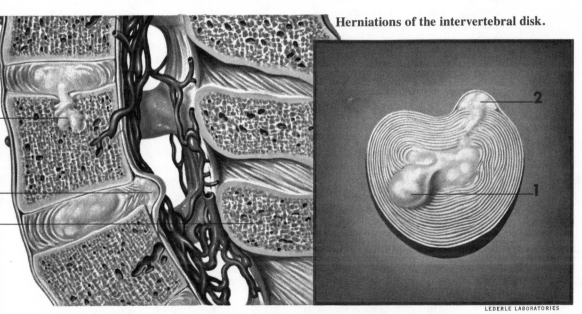

Herniations of the intervertebral disk.

LEDERLE LABORATORIES

(1) Herniation of nucleus pulposus (fibrocartilage) into the spongiosa of the vertebra. (2) Herniation of nucleus pulposus beneath the posterior longitudinal ligament. (3) Spinous process.

by the affected nerve. The terms *slipped disk* and *herniated disk* are often applied to this development.

For a description of the symptoms of pain and weakness of muscles that occur in cases of intervertebral disk involvement, see chapter 4, volume 3, where the neurological aspects of this problem are considered.

Care and Treatment

Treatment for cases of herniated intervertebral disk falls into two categories: conservative and radical. Conservative treatment consists of bedrest for several days or a few weeks in order to eliminate the mechanical pressure that has caused the intervertebral disk to collapse and bulge. In cases where the damaged disk is in the lower back, the patient's bed should be very firm so as to keep the structures of the vertebral column in the most favorable position. A relatively unyielding mattress should be used, and this should be laid on plywood or other firm foundation.

For cases in which the injury is in the neck, it is often advisable to provide traction. This is arranged by attaching a weight by a cord that runs over a pulley at the head of the bed so as to exert a continuous pull on a closely fitted head harness. As the patient improves, he may be allowed out of bed during the daytime, provided he wears a supporting collar. The traction is usually resumed at night for a longer time.

Radical treatment consists of either one of two procedures: (1) Anesthetizing the patient and injecting a chemical substance (chymopapain) into the disk to dissolve the nucleus pulposus or (2) making a surgical approach and actually removing the nucleus pulposus.

PAINFUL HEEL (CALCANEAL SPUR)

Undue weight-bearing may cause the development of a bony spur beneath the heel bone. This causes pain when weight is borne on the heel.

Care and Treatment

Attach a ring-shaped pad of felt to the skin of the weight-bearing area of the heel, with the central area of the ring over the tender spot. If the afflicted person is overweight, he should bring his weight within the normal range. Hot foot baths followed by massage, once or twice a day, will increase the circulation of blood and help to relieve the discomfort. Surgical removal of the spur is rarely necessary. Local injection can be helpful in some resistant cases.

OSTEITIS DEFORMANS (PAGET'S DISEASE)

This is a slowly progressive disease of unknown cause which usually appears only after age 30 and is said to affect about 3 percent of the population in the United States above 50 years of age. It consists essentially of a depletion of calcium in the bones, with consequent alterations in their structure. Any bone or group of bones may be affected—commonly the vertebrae, the pelvis, the skull, and the bones of the legs. The bones become thickened, misshapen, and weakened. Extreme bowing of the legs is an unusual manifestation. Spontaneous fracture may occur. Pain in the bones is a common symptom. The remodeling of the bones sometimes compresses certain nerves, causing symptoms referable to these nerves.

Care and Treatment

Several medications are proving to be somewhat beneficial in the treatment of osteitis deformans. Perhaps the outstanding of these is calcitonin, a hormone produced by the thyroid gland. It is administered by intramuscular injection, three or more times a week. It inhibits the loss of calcium from the bones.

OSTEOPOROSIS

This is a condition in which bone substance throughout the body is decreased. It may occur in cases of malnutrition, of hyperthyroidism, diabetes, vitamin C deficiency, or when there is an excess of adrenal cortical hormones. It may occur in a woman following her menopause, occurring more commonly in such cases among those who smoke. A certain degree of osteoporosis occurs almost constantly in old age in both sexes. The possible complications include pain in the bones, fracture of a bone that has become weak, kyphosis, and general debility.

Care and Treatment

Because of the several possible causes of osteoporosis, each case should be carefully studied and the program of treatment designed accordingly. For the usual case, the following procedures are useful: (1) Provide a high intake of calcium, either by the use of at least one quart of milk per day or by the intake of certain salts of calcium such as are contained in the pharmaceutical products Neo-Calglucon or Os-Cal Forte tablets. (2) Provide intensive physical therapy to keep the major muscles in good condition and thus exert a stimulating influence on the bones of the body. (3)

Arrange a program of physical exercise, consistent with the individual's degree of vitality. (4) In the case of an elderly woman with osteoporosis, abstain from smoking and consider with her physician the possible use of estrogen hormone.

TUMORS OF BONE

Among the tumors that affect the bones, some are benign (relatively harmless), some are malignant (cancerous) and originate in the bony structure, and some are malignant and have migrated from cancerous growths in other parts of the body. For a further discussion of malignant tumors (cancers) of bone, see chapter 11, volume 3.

B. Involvements of Tendons and Ligaments

TENOSYNOVITIS AND TENDONITIS

Tenosynovitis and tendonitis tend to occur together and consist of inflammation of the delicate sheath that surrounds a tendon (tenosynovitis) associated with inflammation of the tendon itself (tendonitis). Pain occurs when the involved tendon is stretched. The tendons commonly affected are in the

X-ray view of a bone tumor below the knee.

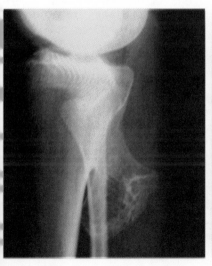

X-ray view of a bone tumor involving a finger.

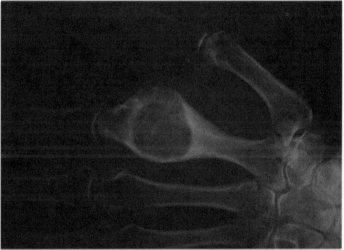

307

shoulder, wrist, palm of the hand, thumb, hip, back of the knee, and back of the ankle. Such pain may be noticed by a woman who has been accustomed to wearing high-heeled shoes when she transfers to low-heeled shoes, thus stretching the tendon at the back of the ankle.

A related condition is "tennis elbow," in which pain develops in that part of the elbow farthest from the body. This problem occurs not only in tennis players, but also among housewives who carry heavy shopping bags. The pain is aggravated by twisting motions of the wrist, such as in using a screwdriver, gripping a doorknob, or merely in shaking hands.

Care and Treatment

For the usual case of tenosynovitis and tendonitis, the affected part should be kept at rest for a few days until the pain disappears. The application of heat and/or ice to the affected area often gives comfort. For severe cases, the application of a plaster cast or splint for two or three weeks prevents the motions which stretch the inflamed tendon, thus allowing healing to take place. Antiinflammatory medication and the injection of a corticosteroid preparation into the inflamed sheath will help to relieve persistent symptoms.

BURSITIS

Bursas are membranous sacs or pockets situated chiefly near joints, especially those of the shoulder, elbow, and knee, where tendons slide over bony prominences or come in close contact with other tendons. The walls of these sacs are similar in structure to thin ligaments, and their linings secrete a lubricating fluid. The purpose of a bursa is to reduce friction.

When the lining of a bursa becomes inflamed, the condition is called bursitis. There is pain on movement, tenderness on pressure, usually some swelling, and sometimes there develops a deposit of calcium salts in the bursa or in its walls.

An example of bursitis is the so-called "housemaid's knee" in which the bursa just below the kneecap becomes inflamed and painful.

Care and Treatment

The affected part should be given as much rest as possible. Fomentations or hot and cold compresses applied to the painful area twice each day often give comfort and hasten healing. See chapter 25, volume 3, for details regarding such treatments.

When the shoulder is affected, bending the body forward and making pendulum motions with the arms as they move backward and forward and from side to side may help to restore the normal range of joint movement. Such motions should be made without undue force. Seesaw overhead pulley exercises may also be helpful.

Physicians sometimes inject an anesthetic solution mixed with a corticosteroid preparation into the affected bursa. In cases where X-ray examination reveals a deposit of calcium in a bursa, the deposit or the entire bursa may need to be removed by surgery.

SPRAINS

A sprain is an injury to a joint in which one or more of the ligaments that support the joint or the joint capsule are stretched or torn. The injury is usually caused by a sudden twist, with the weight of the body thrown onto the joint while it is in an unfavorable position. A sprain may be difficult to distinguish from a fracture; therefore an X-ray study of the joint should be made as soon after the accident as possible.

A sprain causes severe pain, swelling, tenderness to touch, black-and-blue discoloration, and difficulty in using the joint because of the pain. The joints most commonly sprained are the ankle, the knee, and the wrist.

Care and Treatment

Once it has been determined that the injury is a sprain and not a fracture, attention is given to reducing the patient's discomfort and promoting the process of healing. The application of cold by the use of an ice bag during the first one to three days after the injury serves to reduce the pain and minimize the swelling. Two or three thicknesses of cloth should be placed between the skin and the ice bag. Once the tendency to swelling has ceased, the application of cold should be replaced by hot and cold. This increases the circulation of blood to the injured tissues and hastens the healing process.

The affected joint should be kept as motionless as possible during the time of healing. This objective is accomplished by the use of a bandage and a sling (for the elbow) or crutches (for sprains of the knee or ankle). When a person with a sprained ankle or knee is able to walk by the use of crutches, his leg should be placed in a horizontal position for at least 15 minutes out of each hour, this to prevent stagnation of blood in the leg.

NECK SPRAIN (WHIPLASH)

This rather common injury is typically sustained by a person riding in a car hit by another car from the rear. The impact of the collision causes the person's head to snap backward and then rebound forward.

The symptoms of neck sprain may begin at the time of the injury or within the next few hours. They consist of pain in the neck and back, muscle spasm, localized tenderness, swelling, guarding of the injured area, headache, and, possibly, sleeplessness. The fundamental cause is an overstretching of the ligaments and muscles that support and move the head.

Care and Treatment

A physician should examine the patient after a whiplash injury to determine whether there has been actual damage to the bony structures or nerves. If so, these should be treated accordingly. Otherwise, the aim of treatment is to relieve the patient's discomfort and to promote healing.

The bed used by the patient should be reinforced with a piece of plywood between the mattress and the springs so that the mattress does not sag when the bed is occupied. The patient should wear an orthopedic type of collar suport for about an hour, three or four times each day or whenever the muscles of the neck are under stress, as when riding in a car or walking over rough ground. This support serves to rest the neck muscles. The collar should not be worn for long periods, for to do so would allow the muscles to become weak.

Dry heat to the neck area tends to relieve pain and increase the circulation of blood through the involved tissues. Heat is easily provided by suspending a 100-watt light bulb at a distance of about two feet from the patient. The skin should become warm, not hot.

The neck muscles should be gently exercised two or three times a day by deliberately moving the head in various directions. The range of motion and the extent of the exercise should be increased slightly each day. This movement serves to strengthen the neck muscles.

FLATFOOT AND ARCH STRAIN (FALLEN ARCHES)

The foot has two arches. One is a side-to-side arch, formed by the bones and ligaments in the ball of the foot. The other is a front-to-back arch, extending from the ball of the foot to the heel. The front-to-back arch consists of two parts: The inner side, which forms the true arch, is for resilience in walking, running, et cetera; the outer side, which is almost flat, is for weight-bearing. The arches are supported by muscles, ligaments, and a strong layer of fascia, which covers the sole of the foot.

Flatfoot with arch strain is caused by anything that weakens or unduly strains the muscles that support the arches, by whatever rapidly increases the load that the arches must support,

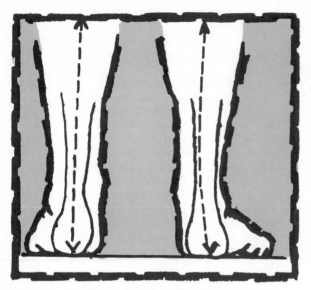

One manifestation of flatfoot is an outward deviation, shown on right, as compared with a normal foot, shown on left.

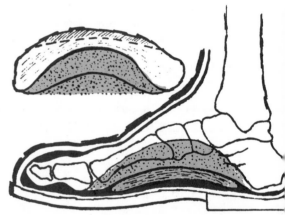

Normal distribution of body weight on the foot, the points bearing the major portion reflected in mirror.

Footprints on wet floor: A, of a normal foot; B, C, and D, of increasing degrees of flatfoot.

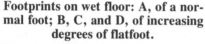

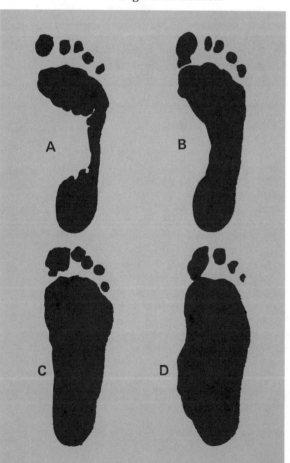

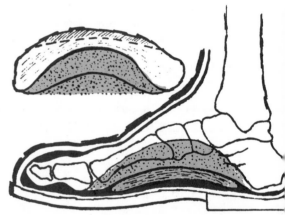

Diagram showing how arch support in a shoe helps a patient suffering from flatfoot.

or by long-continued strain on the ligaments. If a person whose leg and foot muscles are weak from too little use suddenly begins to exercise vigorously, the muscles cannot support the arches of his feet. This failure throws an added burden on the ligaments, which then stretch, causing the pain. The same result may come from a rapid increase in body weight. It may be caused by an occupation that involves the carrying of heavy weights or by standing for long periods without sufficient walking. Flatfoot may also be congenital.

In flatfoot there is a sensation of weakness and strain in the underside of the foot and ankle. After a long period of standing, a dull ache in the calf of the leg or a pain in the knee, the hip, or the back will be felt. Often, after overexertion, a sharp pain is noticed, radiating from the point of weakness. The victim finds it hard to buy comfortable shoes. Increasing discomfort from corns, bunions, enlarged great toe joints, and other deformities of the toes may develop. Coldness, numbness, and increased perspiration of the feet, caused by a poor circulation of blood, are common.

Care and Treatment

Proper treatment for flatfoot gives good prospect for a cure, except in elderly people with arteriosclerosis. The wearing of comfortable, well-fitting shoes which allow adequate room for the toes is important. When walking, the person with flat feet should direct his toes forward rather than to the outside. At the take-off for each step he should distribute his weight on all five toes rather than on just the great toe. Standing in one position for a long time should be avoided. When sitting, the knees should not be crossed, for this practice reduces the circulation of blood to the feet. In severe cases, special exercises or appliances may be prescribed by the orthopedic specialist.

HERNIAS

A hernia is a protrusion of a loop of the intestine or of some other organ through a weak place in the supporting tissues of the abdominal wall or of some other supporting tissue within the body cavity. When the weakened area is in the abdominal wall, the protrusion tends to stretch the skin, causing a corresponding bulge.

Hernias are discussed in chapter 17, volume 2. We mention hernias here to indicate that the fundamental cause is a weakening of the connective tissue (fascias) which provide support.

CARPAL TUNNEL SYNDROME

This is a condition in which severe pain sometimes described as a "bursting sensation" develops in the hand. This may awaken a person during sleep. The fingers feel numb and clumsy. As the day advances, the symptoms improve.

These symptoms are caused by pressure on the median nerve as it passes from the wrist into the palm of the hand. Here it lies among nine of the tendons on their way to the fingers. This area in which the tendons and the median nerve are crowded into a small space is called the carpal tunnel. An increase in the tissue fluid in this area or an increased pressure from conditions such as arthritis or an old fracture produces enough pressure on the median nerve to account for the symptoms.

Care and Treatment

The treatment consists of a minor surgical operation in which the connective tissues bounding the carpal tunnel are partially released. The symptoms disappear when this release is accomplished.

DUPUYTREN'S CONTRACTURE

This is a curious situation in which there develops a tightening of the connective tissues beneath the skin in the palm of the hand. Susceptibility to this problem becomes greater with age. There seems to be a hereditary factor, and the condition is more frequent among persons of European descent. As the connective tissues tighten, they tend to involve the tendon sheaths on their way to the fingers, with the possible complication of pulling the ring finger into a position of flexion toward the wrist.

Care and Treatment

Dupuytren's contracture usually progresses slowly and in most cases is not particularly handicapping. Surgi-

cal treatment, when necessary, consists of releasing the tight fibers of connective tissue in the palm of the hand.

C. Involvements of the Joints

DISLOCATIONS

In a dislocation of a joint, one of the bones which forms part of the joint becomes displaced. For example, in a ball-and-socket joint, the ball portion slips out of the socket portion. The bones that form a joint are normally held in place by the fibrous capsule of the joint and by ligaments that span the joint. In a dislocation the capsule and one or more of the ligaments are either stretched or torn.

TRAUMATIC DISLOCATION

As a result of such injuries as falls, automobile accidents, or athletic injuries, a joint may be moved beyond its normal range of motion, with the result that the joint is pulled apart and normal motion becomes impossible. It is often difficult to tell the difference between a dislocation and a fracture. When in doubt, it is wise to treat the injury as though it were a fracture and await the time when a physician can make an examination. Any one of several joints may be dislocated: the ankle, the elbow, the finger, the thumb, the toe, the hip, the jaw, the knee, the shoulder, or the wrist. For details on the handling of each of these dislocations, see chapter 23, volume 3.

CONGENITAL DISLOCATION OF THE HIP

In an occasional case a baby may possibly develop a dislocation of the hip joint (usually on just one side) at the time he begins to stand and walk. When this occurs, the head of the femur (thighbone) slips out of its socket and remains in this abnormal position. Such a dislocation, when untreated, causes a serious crippling defect. The fundamental cause is a tardy rate of development of the joint structures.

It is possible to examine a two-week-

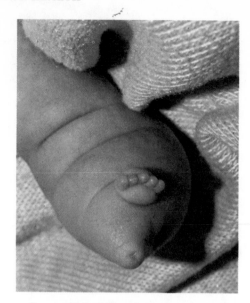

Congenital deformity of arm and hand.

old baby's thigh movements to determine whether the development of his hip joints has progressed normally. Those cases in which the development is retarded can be given a simple treatment at this early age which will prevent the later occurrence of a dislocation.

The examination consists of observing the range of hip motion while the baby is lying on his back. The baby's knees are flexed and then drawn up part way toward his shoulders. In this position the knees are then gently moved sideways (away from the midline). If the hip joints are normally developed at this age of two weeks the flexed knees can be easily moved away from each other until they both nearly touch the bed. If one of the hip joints is not normally developed as yet, the flexed knee on this side will move only part way in the sidewise direction. Of course this observation should be evaluated by a physician, preferably a pediatrician or an orthopedic specialist.

Care and Treatment

Early recognition and early treatment (beginning at two weeks of age) of a potentially troublesome hip joint can prevent the later development of this type of dislocation of the hip. The treatment consists of having the baby wear a jumperlike device which keeps his thighs spread apart, and yet allows continuous motion. The harness need not be removed and reapplied whenever the baby's diapers are changed. When started early, the wearing of this device needs to continue for only a few weeks.

SYNOVITIS

Synovitis consists of an inflammation of the synovial membrane which lines a joint, together with the accumulation of fluid within the joint space. Synovitis is usually caused by some injury to the joint, often a relatively minor one. Synovitis occurs quite commonly in athletes at the beginning of their seasonal activities before they have gained sufficient muscle strength to prevent injury to the joints.

Synovitis is recognized by swelling of the joint, caused by excess fluid within the joint space. There may be moderate pain when the affected joint is moved. In some cases the fluid within the joint consists partly of blood.

Care and Treatment

The fluid within the affected joint should be withdrawn by the use of a needle and syringe. The joint should be kept at rest during the early phase of recovery. When synovitis is the result of an injury, cold application to the joint, as by a padded ice bag, should be used during the first day or so. Thereafter, contrasting applications of hot and cold applied three times a day will increase the local blood supply and thus hasten the healing. See chapter 25, volume 3, under subheading "Hydrotherapy" for the use of hot and cold. As healing proceeds, an elastic bandage applied to the injured area serves to give temporary support. Motion should be progressively resumed as decreasing pain permits.

SEPTIC ARTHRITIS

In septic arthritis one or more of the joints are involved with an actual infection caused by bacteria, viruses, or fungi. In some cases the causative organism enters the joint directly, as in war wounds or other traumatic injuries in which the joint is torn open. Occasionally germs migrate into a joint from infection of an adjacent bone (as in osteomyelitis). Most commonly the causative organisms travel by the blood from some other part of the body, as from a boil, an abscess, a skin infection, an infection involving the heart's lining (endocarditis), the lungs (as in pneumonia or tuberculosis), the middle ear (as in otitis media), the intestines, or the urinary organs (as in gonorrhea).

Typically, just one joint is affected. Usually it is one of the larger joints, such as hip, knee, or shoulder. In gonorrheal arthritis the knee is involved in more than 50 percent of cases.

The symptoms of septic arthritis are those of a general infection (such as chills and fever), along with the symptoms that now develop because a joint is affected. The area of the joint feels warm. It is swollen and painful. The patient automatically guards against any contact or movement that would increase pain.

Care and Treatment

Septic arthritis deserves prompt treatment in order to prevent permanent damage to the joint. First attention should be given to the identification and treatment of the systemic infection. Appropriate antibiotic medication should be given.

During the first day or two of the joint involvement, cold applications to the joint either by a cold compress or a padded ice bag will help to minimize the inflammation and swelling and will reduce pain. Such cold applications can be used about 30 minutes out of each hour.

Inasmuch as fluid and purulent material usually accumulate in the joint cavity, it is advisable for the fluid to be removed by a needle and syringe at least once a day. In the acute phase it is sometimes helpful to support the joint by the use of a splint. This support should not be continued throughout the healing process, however, lest it interfere with the return of full function. Massage and graded exercises are helpful, once the acute phase is passed.

TUBERCULOUS ARTHRITIS

Tuberculous arthritis is a form of septic arthritis caused by the migration of the germs of tuberculosis from some other focus in the body, such as in the lungs or the intestines. Tuberculous arthritis affects children more commonly than adults. Fortunately, with the general reduction of the incidence of tuberculosis, this form of arthritis has become correspondingly rare. The symptoms of swelling, pain, and stiffness in the joint, with some wasting of adjacent muscles, develop gradually. The hip is most frequently affected, with the pain usually referred to the knee. The child limps and tends to hold the hip in a position of flexion.

Care and Treatment

Tuberculous arthritis should be treated promptly so as to reduce the

prospect of future deformity. The treatment consists essentially of the use of antituberculosis medications. These may need to be continued for as long as two years.

ARTHRITIS OF RHEUMATIC FEVER

Involvement of the joints is one of the principal manifestations of rheumatic fever. The arthritis of rheumatic fever is not caused by germs in the tissues of the joints but, rather, by an increased sensitivity of the tissues to the toxins produced by the streptococcus germs which established themselves in the pharynx.

Care and Treatment

The arthritis of rheumatic fever is but one manifestation of the systemic disease. The pain in the joints will subside as the patient's general condition improves. The treatment is therefore that of rheumatic fever, as presented in chapter 17, volume 1.

OSTEOARTHRITIS (HYPERTROPHIC ARTHRITIS)

Osteoarthritis is what elderly people used to call "rheumatism." Some physicians specialize in the diagnosis and

Diagrammatic representation of osteoarthritis.

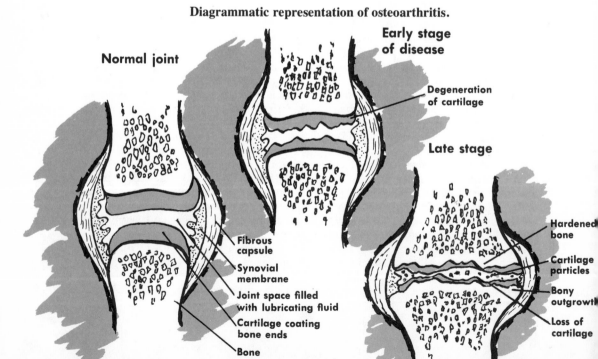

Normal joint

Early stage of disease

Degeneration of cartilage

Late stage

Fibrous capsule

Synovial membrane

Joint space filled with lubricating fluid

Cartilage coating bone ends

Bone

Hardened bone

Cartilage particles

Bony outgrowth

Loss of cartilage

treatment of the various forms of arthritis, including osteoarthritis. These specialists are called rheumatologists.

Osteoarthritis usually develops slowly and gradually in the latter half of life. In a sense, it is part of the aging process. Impaired circulation is possibly a causative factor. Injuries, excessive body weight, and overexertion of a sort that brings increased pressure on the joint cartilages have their influence. The joints of the spine, hips, knees, and fingers are most commonly affected.

There is a thinning of the bone in some parts of the joint, with an overproduction of bony tissue in other parts. It is this overproduction that gave origin to the name hypertrophic arthritis. The disease takes the form of "spurring" or "lipping" around the joint's margins. It may reduce the range of joint motion or, in time, prevent motion entirely. Usually adjacent bones do not actually grow together, even when the vertebrae are involved. The joint may be irregularly enlarged, but it is rarely inflamed. Many cases continue for years without any symptoms other than limitation of motion. Attacks of pain are usually brought on by sudden strain, injury, or a direct blow that causes an inflammatory reaction of the local area.

A surprising degree of osteoarthritis, even in the spinal column, may exist without causing any distress; but bony overgrowths along the posterior margins of the vertebrae may press on nerve trunks—one of the causes of sciatica in elderly people. Much can be done through physical therapy and/or orthopedic surgery to relieve distress and restore activity for the osteoarthritic individual, but there is no real cure for the disease.

Care and Treatment

In addition to the specific things listed below that can be done to help a person with osteoarthritis, the patient should give attention to his mental attitudes. Such a person typically fears, even though still young, that he has passed the prime of life. He resents this; therefore he disregards the symptoms as much as he can and tries to keep up his usual pace of activities. But he needs to establish a new lifestyle consistent with his reduced physical capacities. By living more moderately, he may prolong his period of productive usefulness even to the normal life-span. The following are specific recommendations:

1. When the joints are painful, apply dry heat in any form for half an hour or more at least three times a day.

2. Avoid injury to the involved joints and avoid bending them to the point of causing pain. Correct faulty posture as far as possible. Give massage and passive exercise with caution, taking care not to cause pain. In some cases splints or casts may be needed to prevent pain-producing motion.

3. Avoid fatigue and overexertion, especially in activities that involve use of the affected joint.

4. If overweight, reduce the weight to normal.

5. If the joints of the lower spine and hips are involved, lying down for more hours of the day than usual may help bring relief by taking pressure off the affected joint surfaces.

6. Pay attention to all habits that influence the general health, including such correction of posture as will improve body mechanics, also such exercise as will increase muscle power.

7. The use of appropriate drugs helps to relieve the symptoms of osteoarthritis but does not alter the course of the disease. The most commonly used drug, the one which carries the least hazard and is the cheapest, is aspirin. It should not be used indiscriminately, however. It is most effective in doses (for an adult) of 0.6 to 0.9 grams (10-15 grains) taken four times a day (total of 2.4 to 3.6 grams for the day), after each meal and with milk at bedtime. The reason for taking the medicine after meals or with milk is to reduce the ir-

ritating effect of the aspirin on the stomach's lining membrane. The patient should report to his doctor periodically for a checkup on possible side effects from the aspirin. Some physicians prefer to prescribe the more potent drugs, but these carry greater risks of side effects and therefore must be more carefully supervised.

8. Each affected joint should be put through its full range of motion daily, actively or passively.

RHEUMATOID ARTHRITIS (ARTHRITIS DEFORMANS)

Rheumatoid arthritis is a chronic inflammatory disease in which the principal manifestation is an inflammatory process involving many joints. The disease develops as a combined result of several factors. An infectious factor may be superimposed on a background of malnutrition, disorders of endocrine glands, or maladjustments to life. Physical or emotional shock, injuries, fatigue, exposure to cold and dampness, and, especially, hereditary predisposition may prepare the way for the development of this disease. It is more common in women than in men in a ratio of about three to one.

Rheumatoid arthritis usually makes its appearance after childhood and before the age of 40. Occasionally it appears as late as the sixties and seventies. Its onset may be rapid but is more often gradual. At first there are low-grade fever, headache, and a general feeling of debility. The knees and fingers are usually affected first, then the shoulders, wrists, ankles, and elbows. In extensive cases, nearly every joint in the body may finally be attacked. The joints are swollen because of active inflammation. The pain is often severe.

Large joints, when affected, are likely to be red, tender, and warm to the touch; and there may be an increase in the quantity of the joint fluid. Contractures and atrophy of muscles and tendons may cause the joints to bend in unnatural ways or may cause dislocations, giving rise to extensive deformity. In some cases the bone ends grow together, making the joints permanently stiff. The affected limbs, aside from the joints, are cold and clammy. The victim tends to be thin and anemic.

Especially in the early stages of the disease there may be one or more remissions; but as a rule the symptoms recur and the disease becomes more chronic with each recurrence. Modern methods of treatment usually enable the afflicted person to live productively, even though handicapped.

So much individual variation from case to case makes it impractical to recommend a detailed plan of treatment that will fit every patient. The physician who cares for a person with rheumatoid arthritis must plan the treatment to benefit the particular case.

Certain specific remedies work well for one case but not for others. Unfortunately, the most effective medicines often carry the greatest possibilities of side effects. The physician must therefore use his professional judgment in balancing the advantages of a certain medicine against its possible unfavorable complications.

Even though there may be times of remission, rheumatoid arthritis tends to run a progressive course. At the early stage, destruction of the joint tissues takes place, and during the later chronic stage the patient retains whatever handicap he acquired during the early stage. The treatment of a given case will therefore be directed first toward preventing or at least reducing the amount of damage that occurs during the first stage and, later, toward rehabilitating the patient and restoring his lost functions as far as possible.

Care and Treatment

This basic program of treatment for the early stages of rheumatoid arthritis will benefit all cases—whether severe or less severe. In the less severe cases, this basic program, by itself, may give adequate control of the disease for long periods of time. It consists of six items:

1. *Rest*. This requires that the pa-

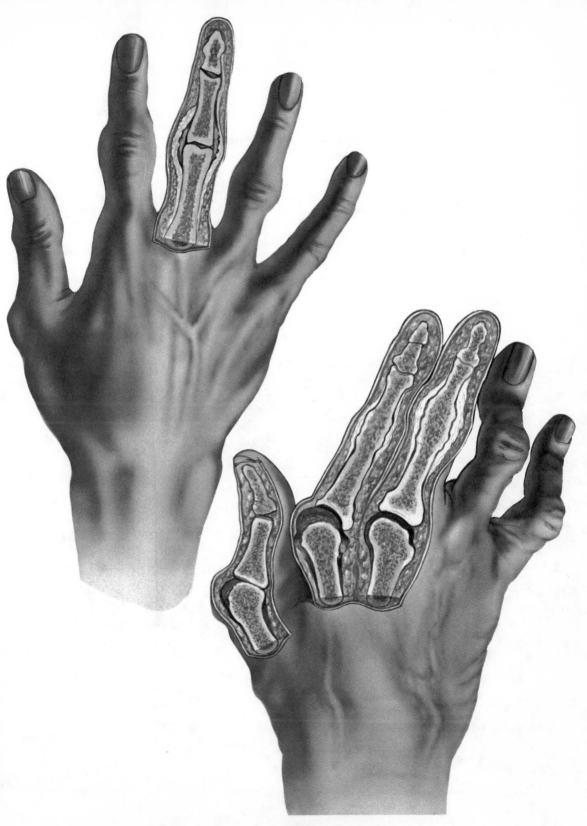

Rheumatoid arthritis. Note swelling of joints caused by synovitis and effusion. Right: Advanced case, showing deformity from stiffness and partial dislocation of joints.

tient avoid straining the joints presently involved and also that he reduce his general activities so as to conserve his quota of vitality.

2. *Psychological Adjustment.* The patient should be provided with a fund of information regarding his disease so that he knows what to expect. He should receive encouragement to become reconciled to the handicaps which his disease produces. On the positive side, he should plan his future so that he can be productive and can experience the rewards of success. Appropriate literature may be obtained from The Arthritis Founda-tion, 475 Riverside Drive, New York, NY 10027.

3. *Relief of Pain.* This is accomplished, in part, by the use of dry heat to the affected parts of the body and otherwise by pain-relieving medicines, as recommended by the doctor. The commonly used medicines are the salicylates, of which aspirin is the most popular and the least harmful. The use of pain-relieving medicine introduces the danger of anemia, for these medicines may have a damaging effect on the blood-forming tissues of the body.

4. *Measures to Combat Anemia.*

Modern methods of treatment enable many arthritic patients to carry on normal activities and live useful lives.

D. TANK

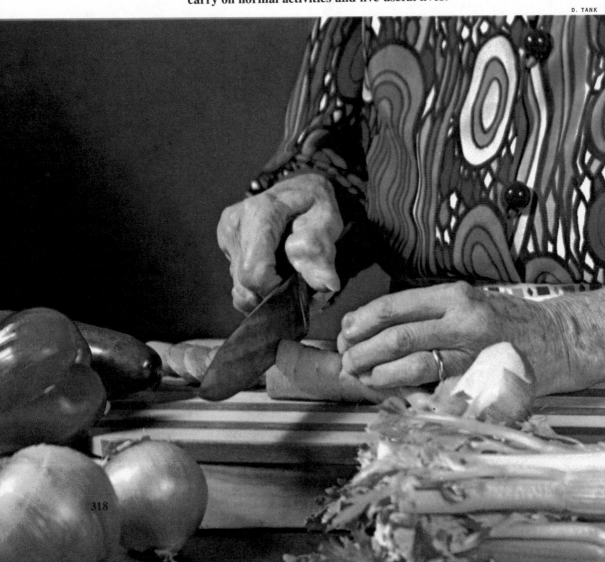

The physician in charge of the case will arrange for frequent blood tests to determine whether anemia is developing and, if so, to what degree. Based on this information he may recommend corrective measures.

5. *Therapeutic Exercise*. An exercise program should be adapted to the particular case, with the motives of keeping the muscles in good condition, preventing or reducing deformities, and helping the patient to maintain his general vitality.

6. *A Well-Balanced Diet*. It is important for the person with rheumatoid arthritis to maintain his general health and vitality. His diet should be simple but liberal, with plenty of vitamins from vegetables and fruits.

With severe and rapidly progressing cases, a more drastic program of treatment must be added to the basic program outlined above. It includes the following:

1. *Intensive Physical and Occupational Therapy*. This should be prescribed by the physician and administered by a paramedical person trained in these techniques.

2. *Orthopedic Devices*. Splints and other aids may be used to prevent or minimize deformities.

3. *Potent Drugs*. The more powerful anti-inflammatory and analgesic medicines are often used to arrest the destruction of tissue and to relieve severe pain. Certain other medicines are also used effectively in some cases. Included in this combined group are the corticosteroids, phenylbutazone, indomethacin, some of the antimalarial drugs, and certain gold salts. These more powerful medicinal agents carry the risk of toxic reactions and other unfavorable side effects. Their use must therefore be carefully directed by the physician.

4. *Orthopedic Surgery*. It is now recognized that the early use of orthopedic surgery in selected cases helps to prevent devastating deformities and disability.

5. *Rehabilitation*. In the later stages of rheumatoid arthritis efforts are directed toward restoring the functions lost earlier. The patient needs to be taught to carry on his activities in spite of his particular handicap. Many cases are greatly benefited by appropriate reconstructive surgery in which the affected joints are replaced or reconstructed and in which tendons may be transplanted in a way to restore lost functions.

GOUT

Gout is a systemic disease characterized by an inherited fault in the way the body handles uric acid. In most persons, uric acid is readily eliminated by the kidneys. But in a person with a tendency to gout, the uric acid is not eliminated as quickly as it should be, and the body's fluids and tissues thereby contain more than normal. This excess of uric acid in the body's fluids (hyperuricemia) is present in 5 to 10 percent of American men above the age of 30, but in only about one tenth as many women. Many persons with hyperuricemia have no symptoms and do not know that they have this condition. But in a minority of this group (about three persons per thousand population), crystals of uric acid become deposited in certain of the body's tissues.

We consider gout in this chapter because one of the locations in which the crystals of uric acid are deposited is in the joints. This condition of gouty arthritis occurs in attacks which come unannounced; and, if untreated, each runs a course of one to two weeks. The pain in such an attack is very severe and, if it be the first attack, usually emanates from just one joint—classically the joint at the base of the big toe. The joint becomes swollen, warm to the touch, and extremely tender. The skin over the joint is tense, shiny, and red.

There will usually be a series of attacks, successively more severe and more frequent. Various joints may be affected, such as those of the ankle, the knee, and even those of the hands and arms. With recurring attacks, often more than one joint at a time becomes involved.

For a further discussion of gout as a systemic disease and also for a description of the plan for care and treatment of this disease, see chapter 13, volume 3.

BUNION

A bunion is a tender and painful enlargement of the joint tissues, including bone, at the base of the great toe. The enlargement appears greater than it really is because the entire great toe is now inclined in the direction of the little toe. Bunions usually develop at the same time on both feet.

A bunion is caused by wearing a shoe which is too narrow, too short, or too pointed. There is sometimes an inherited tendency. The narrow shoe subjects this joint to increased pressure and friction during walking. The short or pointed shoe does the same by bending the end of the great toe toward the others, thus making the joint more prominent and more subject to pressure irritation. The longer the irritation continues, the greater the deformity. In severe cases, the second toe is virtually dislocated from the corresponding bone of the foot by the great toe deformity.

Care and Treatment

Wear shoes of such size and shape as to allow the great toe to assume its normal straightforward position. Then, by using soft padding between the great toe and the second toe, try to push the great toe into its normal position. Night splints are available commercially.

Rest and hot foot baths will bring relief in most cases. Afterward, the calloused skin may be pared away and the area protected by a bunion plaster. Surgery is sometimes necessary.

WORN-OUT JOINTS

Several of the diseases which affect the joints tend, in the long run, to destroy the joint's usefulness. The attempted processes of healing leave the joint stiff or otherwise unsatisfactory. The problem is the greatest in cases of hip and knee joints, although crippling deformities of the fingers also pose serious problems.

Within recent years, orthopedic surgeons have been increasingly successful in the replacement of certain joints with metal and plastic materials. Perhaps the greatest success has come in the replacing of hip joints. Success in a fair percentage of cases has attended the replacement of knee joints and of joints in the fingers.

Surgical replacement of joints is considered by some to be still in the experimental stage. However, in spite of the complications that develop in some cases, the percentage of successful replacements has been increasing year by year.

D. Collagen Vascular Diseases

The collagen vascular diseases, sometimes called connective tissue diseases, are classed as a group because they involve widespread inflammatory changes in the body's connective tissues and blood vessels.

SYSTEMIC SCLEROSIS (SCLERODERMA)

Systemic sclerosis is a chronic, slowly progressive disease of unknown cause which first affects the skin, causing it to become thick and inelastic. Later it produces scar-like changes in certain of the internal organs. It is at least twice as frequent in women as in men. It may begin at any age, but typically it appears first in persons between 25 and 55 years of age. The changes in the skin usually begin in the hands and the feet. The skin becomes tight, smooth, and shiny. This condition interferes with movement and causes deformities and ulcer formations. The affected face becomes masklike.

The eventual involvement of the internal organs affects the organs of digestion most frequently. The esophagus or the intestine may become so narrow as to interfere with their functions. The lungs, the heart, and the kidneys may become involved, as connective tissue encroaches on their functioning tissues.

Although there may be periods of remission, the disease is usually fatal within four to twenty years.

Care and Treatment

There is no known cure for this disease. Various medications have been tried, but so far none have altered the progressive course of the illness. The goal of treatment is to preserve normal functions and to prevent injury to the vulnerable hands. Passive and active exercises of the hands are helpful. Local skin infection should be treated promptly before the ulcers have time to develop. Complications, as they appear, should be treated appropriately as directed by the physician.

SYSTEMIC LUPUS ERYTHEMATOSUS

Lupus erythematosus is the most prevalent of the collagen vascular diseases. It occurs in two forms: (1) The cutaneous (discoid) form, which affects the skin primarily and is discussed in chapter 25, this volume, and (2) the systemic (disseminated) form, discussed here.

Systemic lupus erythematosus may first appear at any age, but most commonly between the ages of 20 and 40. It is five to ten times more frequent in women than in men. The manifestations vary from case to case. Typically it produces fatigue, pain in certain joints, skin rash on the areas exposed to the sun, and fever. Beyond this the symptoms depend on which of the internal organs is affected: the kidneys, the heart, the lungs, the digestive organs, or the nervous system.

Although the cause of this disease is not known, it is described as an autoimmune disorder in which the normal balance between tolerance and immunity has become altered. Affected persons seem to have developed antibodies to some of the constituents of their own cells. The rate of progress of the disease varies from person to person. Usually there is a series of remissions and relapses. In the occasional, fast-moving case, death may occur within a few weeks. In the more usual case the illness becomes chronic, with long periods of remission.

Care and Treatment

The aim of treatment is to hasten a remission when symptoms are present and to avoid or postpone a relapse when the patient is free from symptoms. Certain things which seem to predispose to a relapse should be avoided if possible: exposure to sunlight, use of drugs, especially the antibiotics and sulfa drugs; immunizations; blood transfusions; and elective surgery. The patient should follow an easy pattern of living, as free as possible from stress and extremes. Complications involving the various organs should be treated appropriately by a physician. The use of corticosteroid medication adapted to the circumstances of the individual patient is often helpful.

POLYARTERITIS NODOSA (PERIARTERITIS NODOSA)

In this disease it is primarily the small and medium-sized arteries that are affected in various locations throughout the body. Inflammation and destruction of the arterial tissue occurs in a particular spot along the course of each of the affected arteries. This accounts for the development of nodules (lumps) that can be felt by the examining finger, hence the term *nodosa*.

In the course of the attempted healing at the site of destruction of an arterial wall, the artery becomes closed to the flow of blood, or it may rupture. In some cases an aneurysm develops at the site of tissue damage.

An affected artery is no longer capable of conveying its usual quota of blood. Therefore the part of the body which the artery normally supplies is now deprived of blood. It is this com-

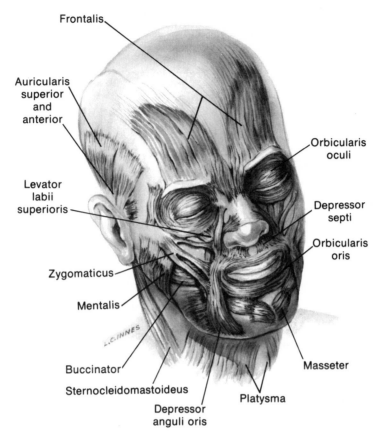

Frontalis

Auricularis
superior
and
anterior

Levator
labii
superioris

Zygomaticus

Mentalis

L.C.INNES

Buccinator

Sternocleidomastoideus

Depressor
anguli oris

Orbicularis
oculi

Depressor
septi

Orbicularis
oris

Masseter

Platysma

The muscles of facial expression.

fully, depending on the need of the moment. You use the same muscles to lift a ten-pound package of flour as to lift a piece of paper. In the latter case the muscles simply exert less power.

As explained previously, a muscle consists of many muscle fibers, and, in the case of skeletal muscle, each of these fibers is caused to contract by a tiny nerve branch. The nerves that control skeletal muscles originate either in the brain or in the spinal cord. It is here that the bodies of the nerve cells are located. Extending from the brain or spinal cord to the skeletal muscles are many nerve fibers, one fiber for each nerve cell body. As one of these nerve fibers approaches the muscle that it serves, the fiber divides into branches—sometimes only eight or ten but in other cases as many as 200.

Thus, one nerve cell in the brain or spinal cord controls as many muscle fibers as the nerve fiber has branches.

In the case of the muscles which move the eyes, the nerve fibers have about eight branches, which means that one nerve cell has only eight muscle fibers to control. This specialization explains a person's precise control over the movements of his eyes. In the case of the large muscles in one's back, however, the fiber from one nerve cell may have as many as 180 branches. Here precise control over the muscle fibers is not necessary, only approximate regulation.

The muscle fibers controlled by a single nerve cell are called a motor unit. When a particular nerve cell sends out a contraction impulse, only the muscle fibers of its motor unit respond.

331

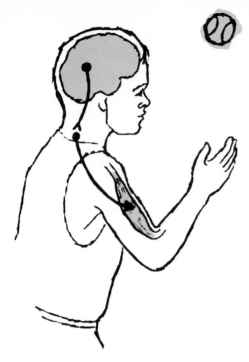

Nerve connections are like electric wires to a motor. A nerve impulse originating in the brain goes to the skeletal muscles, causing them to contract.

Every muscle abounds with motor units, with the muscle fibers belonging to a particular motor unit scattered throughout the muscle. Because of the scattered distribution of the muscle fibers of a motor unit, the contraction impulse emanating from a particular nerve cell causes a mild tightening of the muscle rather than a local twitch.

Now we can see that the relative power which a muscle exerts depends on how many of its motor units contract at the same time. When a muscle remains taut as a matter of readiness for action, only a few of its motor units are in operation—just enough to pull gently on the muscle's tendon. When this same muscle has a moderate amount of work to do, a greater number of motor units receive contraction impulses. When it must exert maximum power, all its motor units go into action.

Because of the element of fatigue, a muscle cannot maintain maximum activity for long. But it can do a reason-

Diagram of skeletal muscle showing three nerve fibers branching to supply scattered muscle fibers.

Tendons carry the power generated by the forearm muscles right to the hand's tiny bones, as needed.

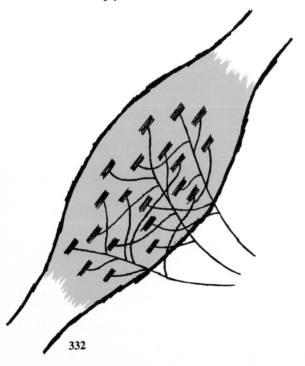

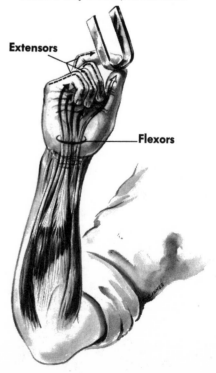

Extensors

Flexors

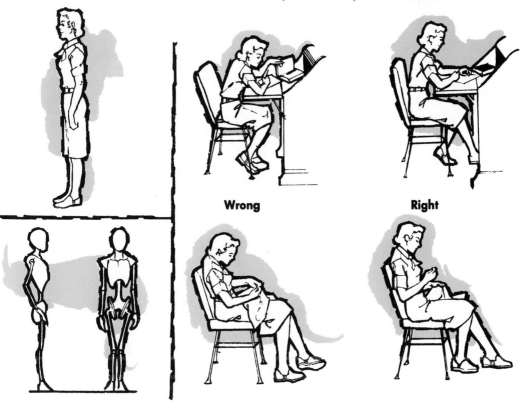

Wrong   Right

Incorrect and correct posture.

able amount of work hour after hour by a provision for certain motor units to rest while others are working.

Fortunately, you do not have to give conscious attention to the various motor units of your body's muscles. You do not even have to decide which muscle to use in order to flex your arm or extend a finger. Your brain and the related parts of your nervous system are organized in such a marvelous manner that the right combination of muscles is activated automatically at the right time. Even a provision exists by which the muscle group that would extend your elbow relaxes gradually as the opposing muscle group causes your elbow to bend. When certain motor units become fatigued, others are brought into play without your knowledge. All that you have to think about is the motion that you desire to perform, and your brain and spinal cord take care of the details.

Posture

A great deal of the power that the body's muscles produce is used in offsetting the force of gravity. It is only by the use of your muscles that you can rise from bed and stand upright. If, while standing, you were to relax all of your muscles, the force of gravity would pull you promptly to the floor.

It is the large muscles of your thighs and legs that stabilize these parts of your body, enabling you to use your legs as pillars on which to rest the weight of your body. Also, the large muscles of the back, located on either side of the spinal column, do a great deal to help you resist the pull of gravity. Even the muscles of your shoulders, arms, and neck play an important part in helping you to maintain a proper position.

A person's body build has something to do with his posture. The person with a heavy frame will have a posture different from that of someone naturally slender. The amount of fat also influences the posture. Perhaps the greatest determiner of posture, however, is habit. A person may either allow his muscles to become so limp that he stoops and slumps, or he may accustom himself to stand erect and move gracefully.

Posture is important for two reasons: (1) it has a definite relationship to a person's general appearance, and (2) it exerts an influence on the functions of his body.

The person who maintains a graceful, erect posture feels optimistic and courageous. Such a person influences others favorably, for when he appears erect with a spring in his step, people admire and welcome him.

As for the influence of posture on the body's functions, it is the digestive organs and the organs of breathing mostly affected. Of course, poor posture also influences the general circulation of blood throughout the body. The person who allows his shoulders to droop is thereby crowding the organs within his chest—particularly his lungs. When portions of the lungs are not allowed freedom of movement, the blood in these parts tends to stagnate. This favors disease. With good posture and good muscle tone, the food which has been eaten moves along the digestive tract easily and promptly. But with poor posture, the digestive organs become sluggish.

The accompanying chart, "Steps to Good Posture," lists ways to improve your posture while standing, sitting, and walking. But conscious attention to the way you hold your head, direct your feet, and balance your body does not constitute the whole of good posture. Developing general health rates high in this matter. The person habitually vigorous and healthy finds it natural to walk with firm step, head up, and shoulders raised. Also, the person who uses his muscles regularly and who therefore has strong, firm muscles will be more able to hold his body erect

Steps to Good Posture

A. Standing
1. Feet parallel, about 6 inches apart.
2. Head high, as if balancing a book on the head.
3. Chest out.
4. Stomach and hips firm.
5. Weight slightly forward, over the balls of the feet, and distributed evenly on each foot.
6. Knees very lightly flexed—NOT LOCKED.
7. Abdomen and back as flat as possible.

B. Sitting
1. Sit back in the chair, so that hips touch the back of the chair; feet flat on the floor.
2. Sit tall.
3. Rock forward from the hips when writing.
4. Keep chest out, and neck in line with upper back.

C. Walking
1. Knees and ankles limber, toes pointed straight ahead.
2. Legs close together—DON'T WALK LIKE A DUCK.
3. Swing legs forward from hip joints.
4. Lift feet off the ground—DON'T SHUFFLE.
5. Head and chest high.
6. Shoulders free and easy—NO PULLING OR TENSION.
7. The heel touches the ground first—in each step, the progression is: HEEL, OUTSIDE OF FOOT, TOES.

(Reprinted from the November 1947, issue of "SCHOOL LIFE," official journal of the Office of Education, U.S. Department of Health, Education, and Welfare.)

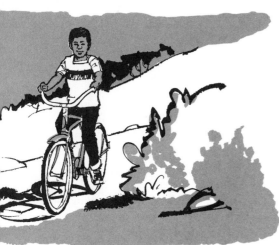

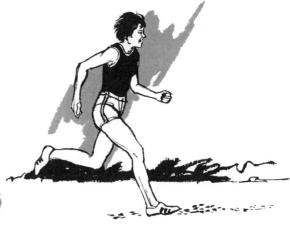

Some of the exercises that help to build good posture.

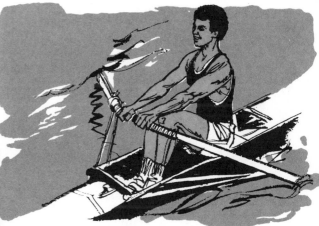

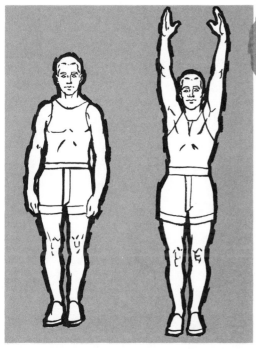

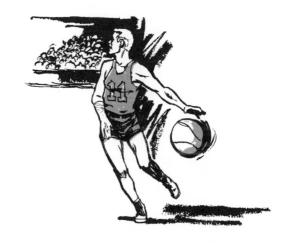

than one whose muscles are so flabby and weak that they permit the body to slump into bad positions.

One of the greatest handicaps to good posture is the wearing of poorly designed shoes. Usually it is women who suffer most on this account. High-heeled shoes throw a person off balance. In ordinary mechanics, when one factor tends to throw a weight forward, there must be some other factor to counterbalance it, else the center of gravity will be shifted. So, shoes with high heels force the wearer to compensate by assuming unnatural body positions.

B. Disorders of Muscle and Related Structures

Poor Posture

Some cases of spinal curvature in which the spinal column deviates to one side or the other are the result of an imbalance between the muscles of the right and left sides of the spine. Such imbalance may be caused by long-continued faulty posture. Lack of strength in the muscles in the back and even in the abdominal wall may result from a lack of proper exercise. Also, poor habits of sitting and standing may contribute to this condition.

Two posture faults are especially prone to develop during middle life—round shoulders and sagging abdomen. To prevent these defects requires active attention and personal effort. Fortunately, this endeavor need not take time away from the day's program. Simply by keeping the danger in mind and by following consistently the routine suggested here, you can sidestep the danger. Here is the routine: (1) several times a day, throw your shoulders back firmly, draw in your chin, and hold the position while you slowly and silently count to twenty. (2) Draw your abdomen in and keep its muscles firm, also to the count of twenty. As you become proficient, you can perform both parts of the routine at the same time.

In extreme cases of poor posture, es-

336

pecially when this occurs in an adolescent, a physician who specializes in orthopedics should be consulted.

WRYNECK (TORTICOLLIS)

In wryneck the head is held in an abnormal position, inclined more to one side than to the other. This abnormality is due to a shortening or a spasm of the muscles in one side of the neck. Wryneck frequently develops in infancy and may even be the result of some injury to the neck muscles at the time of delivery. In such a case the actual inclination of the head to one side may not be noticed until the child is old enough to hold his head up as he tries to walk. In the severe cases originating in infancy, there may be a one-sided development of the face—a condition called facial curvature.

Wryneck may develop at later periods of life as the result of injury to the nerves supplying muscles on one side of the neck. In some cases developing

A typical case of chronic torticollis of muscular origin.

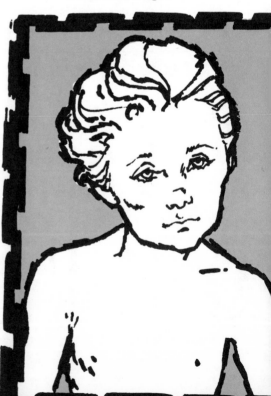

in adulthood, wryneck may be a hysterical manifestation of a deep emotional conflict.

Care and Treatment

Prompt treatment is particularly important in the cases which begin in infancy, for, if uncorrected, the deformity tends to become more severe. In mild cases, the condition is often benefitted by manipulations in which the mother stretches the child's affected muscles gently but firmly by overcorrecting the position of the head while massaging the stretched muscles for a few minutes. Such a procedure should be repeated about five times a day. In severe cases, the contracted muscle or muscles may need to be released by a surgical procedure. Following such a procedure, correction of the position of the head is temporarily maintained by the use of a plaster cast applied to the neck.

Muscle Cramps

Muscle Cramps at Night. A harmless type of distressing pain may occur in the calf of the leg or perhaps in the sole of the foot in persons of any age while lying in bed. The pain is extreme, and the individual tends to grasp the affected part and massage it vigorously in the hope of relieving the cramping of the muscles. In most cases, the spasm can be relieved by getting out of bed, standing erect, and bringing pressure on the ball of the foot by rocking up and down. The condition is harmless, and the symptom is caused by a reflex action of the muscles when, in the process of relaxation, they lose their normal muscle tone. The symptom typically occurs when, because of the weight of the bedclothes, the foot is allowed to drop forward.

There are two possible means of preventing these cramps that occur at night. One is to support the feet, while the individual lies in bed, by the use of a "foot cradle" or by a pillow so placed as to serve as a backdrop for the feet so that the foot does not drop forward. The second is to stretch the muscles of the calf of the leg, accomplished by the individual leaning far forward while standing in his stocking feet, keeping the heels in contact with the floor. He should lean so far forward that a pulling sensation is noted in the muscles of the calf of the leg. This position is held for ten seconds and then repeated after a five-second interval of rest. This exercise should be performed two or three times a day, or less often as relief from the cramps at night is accomplished.

Swimmer's Cramps. A type of leg cramp similar to the above may occur among swimmers, particularly among those who kick with their toes sharply pointed. This position of the foot while swimming favors the reflex spasm of the muscles in the calf of the leg. The same method of periodically stretching the calf muscles as described above will usually prevent the occurrence of swimmer's cramps. Otherwise, the swimmer should avoid keeping his toes sharply pointed while kicking in the water.

Claudication. This is a condition in which muscle cramps occur in response to exercise. The pain often occurs in calf muscles while walking hurriedly, especially when hurrying upstairs. The painful cramping is caused by a reduction in the blood supply to the muscles currently active and therefore in need of a more abundant supply of blood. Claudication occurs in persons who have neglected sufficient exercise to keep their vascular system in good condition or, in other cases, when the process of arteriosclerosis has reduced the volume of blood available to the affected muscles.

The remedy for claudication requires that the blood supply to this part of the body (usually the legs and feet) be increased. This is accomplished either by a consistent program of exercise or by the use of hot-and-cold-contrast leg baths.

FIBROMYOSITIS (MUSCULAR RHEUMATISM: LUMBAGO)

Fibromyositis is a distressing and

poorly understood ailment which consists of aching, pain, and stiffness in certain parts of the body. The neck, the lower back, the shoulders, and the thighs are the areas often affected. The discomfort is aggravated by movement. The victim may describe the problem as a stiff neck, as lumbago, or as rheumatism. In some the symptoms may last for a few hours, a few days, or even a few weeks. They may disappear as mysteriously as they began. In the meantime, however, the patient is incapacitated by being unable to carry on the usual movements of his body.

Care and Treatment

The usual methods for providing a degree of comfort consist of rest; local application of heat, either by a heating pad, heat lamp, or fomentations; or the moderate use of aspirin. In some cases it is possible to locate a particular spot from which the pain seems to emanate. The discomfort is sometimes relieved in such a case when the physician injects an anesthetic solution into the troublesome spot.

MUSCULAR DYSTROPHY

Muscular dystrophy is an inherited disease characterized by progressive weakness caused by degeneration of the component fibers of muscle tissue. No satisfactory treatment exists, and the outlook for a person with this illness is progressively unfavorable.

Child Type (Duchenne Form). This affects only boys. The weakness starts in the muscles of the hips, causing the boy to walk with a waddling gait. Sometimes the victim walks on his toes; he falls frequently and has difficulty in getting back to the upright position. The calf muscles often become enlarged and present the false appearance of being strong. In this form of the illness, the life expectancy is about 25 years.

Adolescent Type. In this form of the

illness, the weakness usually begins during adolescence and affects both sexes equally. The weakness is usually first noted in the shoulders and then in the face and upper arms. Eventually muscles in the hands, feet, and back may become involved. There is a resulting tendency for the back to become swayed and for the arms and legs to assume abnormal positions. Occasionally the disease becomes arrested spontaneously and the patient becomes no worse. The diagnosis is best confirmed by having a small sample of muscle tissue removed and examined microscopically.

Care and Treatment

There is no curative treatment. The aim in caring for the patient is to prolong the time during which he can move about and engage in routine activities. The use of appropriate braces and the performing of surgical procedures to correct deformities may help to keep the patient active.

POLYMYOSITIS AND DERMATOMYOSITIS

In polymyositis, the muscles are primarily affected and in dermatomyositis the skin as well as the muscles are involved. The cause of these diseases is not known, and they are often classed with the collagen vascular diseases. They are characterized by an inflammatory and degenerative process which causes weakness of the muscles, principally those of the limb girdles (shoulders and hips). These diseases usually run a progressive, downhill course. In some cases there are long periods of remission and, in a few, apparent recovery.

Care and Treatment

In the effort to find a satisfactory treatment, corticosteroid medications have been used, but with doubtful benefit. The care of the patient consists mostly of the use of physical therapy and of mild medications to make him as comfortable as possible.

How the Body Derives Its Energy

A. Food Constituents

In order to understand the source of the body's energy, we must first review the basic constituents of food. An apple, for instance, contains considerable water, some fruit sugar, a trace of protein, a trace of fat, some calcium, some iron, and several of the vitamins. The digestive organs have no formula for handling apples as apples. Rather, they handle various constituents contained in apples and in other articles of diet.

Take whole-wheat bread as another example. This product is 36 percent water. Each slice contains approximately 2 grams of protein, 1 gram of fat, 11 grams of carbohydrate, 35 milligrams of calcium, half a milligram of iron, and small amounts of several vitamins. As far as the digestive processes are concerned, the constituents of bread are handled separately, and in the same manner as those from any other item of food.

All foods are composed of proteins, carbohydrates, and fats, in varying proportions, along with minerals and vitamins. One food differs from another in the proportions of these various constituents and in the kinds of proteins, kinds of fats, carbohydrates, et cetera.

Milk is an excellent food, because it contains many essential nutrients. However, it is deficient in iron and vitamin C and has a high amount of saturated fat. Most other foods contain liberal amounts of one or two constituents and smaller amounts of the others. If a person were to try to live permanently on apples, for example, his diet would be deficient, because apples lack certain elements essential to good health. For this reason a person needs to eat a variety of foods each day so that the constituents of one food will make up for the deficiencies of others.

It is not possible, in selecting one's food for a particular day, to select just the exact amount of each food constituent which the body needs for that day. But as long as a person eats a reasonably adequate diet, his body's tissues will receive proper nourishment.

Carbohydrates

Carbohydrates are the body's principal energy food, providing, on the average, one half of the calories needed for heat production and muscle action. For the most part, carbohydrates occur in the form of starches and sugars. We have abundant supplies of carbohydrates in fruits, vegetables, cereal products, and milk. The molecules which compose carbohydrates are

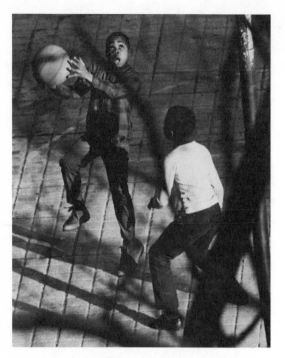

For muscle action the principal energy food is carbohydrates.

made up of chains of carbon atoms to which atoms of hydrogen and oxygen are attached. During the process of digestion the long chains of the large molecules of complicated carbohydrates are broken down into shorter chains and, thus, simpler molecules. One large molecule of starch, for example, can be broken down by chemical transformation to produce several smaller molecules of simple sugars.

The small molecules produced by the process of digestion are small enough to pass through the lining of the small intestine and to be transported by the blood to the various tissues where needed. When carbohydrates are used in the tissues for the production of heat and energy, their simple sugar molecules are further dismembered until only carbon dioxide and water remain. In principle, this is the sort of chemical reaction that occurs when any fuel, even in a mechanical device, undergoes combustion for the sake of producing energy.

Fats

Fats in our foods help to make them palatable. Fats along with carbohydrates provide readily available energy; and the amount of energy available in fats is slightly more than twice as much, for a given weight, as in carbohydrates.

The amount of fat contained in the diet of the average American has increased through recent years, fat now providing more than 40 percent of his food calories. This abundant use of fat is unfortunate, for too much solid fat in the diet (so-called saturated fat) is harmful in that it favors the development of arteriosclerosis, which sets the stage for coronary heart disease and stroke.

The chief sources of fat in our diet are dairy products, margarines, oils and salad dressings, nuts, and various kinds of meat.

The molecules of fat are composed of the same three chemical elements—carbon, hydrogen, and oxygen—as occur in the molecules of carbohydrates. When fat is used in the body to produce heat and energy, the final products are carbon dioxide and water, just as in the complete oxidation of carbohydrates.

A fat molecule is a curious combination of a molecule of glycerine with three molecules of fatty acids. The difference between one kind of fat and another lies in what particular fatty acids occur in their molecules. There are many kinds of fats, some solid, others liquid.

Certain of the fatty acids are essential to the body's nutritional needs. These fatty acids or their precursors must be obtained from the foods in the diet. One of the most important of these essential fatty acids is linoleic acid, which is necessary for growth and reproduction and which aids in the transport and utilization of fats in the body. Linoleic acid is one of the "unsaturated" fatty acids, and the fats in which it is contained in generous amounts are usually oils rather than solids. It is the saturated fats (solid fats), by contrast, which, when eaten to excess, seem to favor the development of arteriosclerosis.

Proteins

What is protein? Someone has said you get the best answer by looking in the mirror. The human body is essentially a package of protein, for protein is the predominant constituent of the body tissues. If the water were subtracted from the human body, half of the remaining weight would consist of protein. Skin, muscles, hair, fingernails—all of these are composed largely of protein. Even the bones and the teeth contain some of this interesting constituent. The blood contains many kinds of protein. Hormones and enzymes consist of molecules of protein.

Protein contains the elements of carbon, hydrogen, and oxygen, just as carbohydrates and fats do. But in addition protein contains nitrogen. Other elements such as sulfur may also occur in protein molecules.

Protein molecules have to be made by living cells, either plant or animal cells. Plants, with the aid of energy they get from the sun, are able to draw nitrogen out of the soil and use it in building protein molecules. Human beings, as well as most animals, are dependent upon the foods they eat for the proteins their tissues need.

Protein molecules are very large and are composed of smaller amino acid molecules linked together somewhat like railroad cars are coupled to form a train. There are about 22 kinds of amino acids and one protein differs from another in that it contains different kinds and combinations of amino acids. Certain amino acids are necessary to maintain healthy body tissues. Some amino acids must be obtained in the diet; others may also be made in the body. This emphasizes again the need for a variety of food in the diet so a person can be sure of obtaining all of the amino acids his body requires.

During the process of digestion the large protein molecules are broken down into their component amino acid molecules, just as the large molecules of carbohydrates and fats are broken down into their constituents so that they can penetrate the wall of the small intestine and then be transported by the blood. Once the amino acid molecules arrive in the liver or other tissues they are reassembled to form protein molecules. This time there is a precise selection of the particular amino acids that will make just the kinds of protein each tissue requires.

Proteins are necessary for growth and for the repair of worn-out tissues. Proteins are not stored, except as they are built into the tissues. In order to supply the body's needs, a person must include a reasonable amount of protein in each day's food.

Other Food Constituents

In addition to the carbohydrates, fats, and proteins, our food contains other needed substances. Among these are minerals, vitamins, and fiber (or roughage).

Calcium and phosphorus are constituents of bones and teeth. Iron is important as a part of the hemoglobin molecule which conveys oxygen and carbon dioxide. Sodium, potassium, iodine, and certain trace elements are important to various body functions.

Vitamins are essential for many reactions involved in protein synthesis, bone formation, the production of energy, reproduction, and the body processes.

Fiber (roughage) consists largely of cellulose and other complex carbohydrates which are found in fruits, vegetables, nuts, legumes, and coarse cereals. Fiber is relatively inert and is not affected by the chemical processes that normally occur in the digestive tract. It therefore passes through the small intestine unchanged and has a mild laxative action by adding bulk to the feces. It is important to include in the diet a reasonable amount of foods each day which provide fiber. One of the disadvantages of using large amounts of animal foods and highly refined vegetable products is that they are deficient in fiber.

Recent research has shown dietary fiber to play other important roles besides relieving constipation. It lowers blood cholesterol, decreasing the risk of coronary heart disease. Fiber aids in preventing obesity by providing more bulk, thus decreasing overeating. It is protective against adult onset diabetes by decreasing the rate of the digestion and absorption of starches and sugars. High fiber eaters have less cancer of the colon because intestinal wastes are eliminated more rapidly from the intestine.

B. The Body's Fuel

The cells of the body are living units and require a continuous supply of fuel in order to carry on their activities. When we think of the body's energy production, we think first of muscle cells and the work they perform. True, muscle cells produce a great deal of energy, and their fuel requirements exceed those of other cells. But the body's other cells also require fuel in order to perform their activities.

The principal fuels from which cells derive energy are glucose (blood sugar) and fatty acids. In order for these nutrients to provide energy, they must first combine with oxygen, very much as fuel in an engine must be mixed with air in order to produce power. Oxygen is brought to the cells throughout the body by the hemoglobin molecules contained in the red blood cells.

The chemical action by which glucose is oxidized to produce energy is not an instantaneous process. But the action of certain cells (particularly muscle cells) must be very rapid—so rapid that there is no time at the moment of action for glucose molecules to combine with oxygen molecules.

The rapid action of a muscle cell is made possible by the presence in the cell of a high-energy compound. This is adenosine triphosphate (commonly called ATP), a compound built up within cells by the oxidation of glucose.

When a muscle contracts, it is because the ATP within its cells suddenly releases its energy by being converted to adenosine diphosphate (ADP)—a low-energy compound.

Continued action of a muscle tends to use up its immediate supply of ATP. It is replenished, somewhat at leisure, by a reverse process in which the oxidation of glucose and fatty acids provides energy to convert the ADP back to ATP. About 60 percent of the energy for muscles and other organs at rest and during moderate exercise comes from the burning or oxidation of fatty acids.

When a muscle or muscle group is being used over and over again, as in active physical exercise, ATP has to be replenished almost as fast as it is being consumed. This need makes it necessary for the amount of blood flowing through an active muscle to be much greater than the amount flowing through a resting muscle.

The liver is the body's chemical laboratory. It is in the liver that many transformations of molecules take place. It should be noted, as in the accompanying illustration, that the liver receives blood through the portal vein, which provides transportation for food materials after they are absorbed through the wall of the small intestine. Thus the liver has first access to the constituents of carbohydrates, some fatty acids, and amino acids that are being carried by the blood.

There is a remarkable provision for converting some excess fat and some amino acids from proteins into glucose so that these nutrients can be used by the cells as fuel. So, even though the proportions of food constituents in a person's diet may vary from day to day, the liver is capable of transforming food constituents into those most needed at the moment.

These processes of chemical transformation can operate in either direction, depending upon the body's present needs. That is, when there is a large demand for fuel, molecules of fat and portions of the molecules of pro-

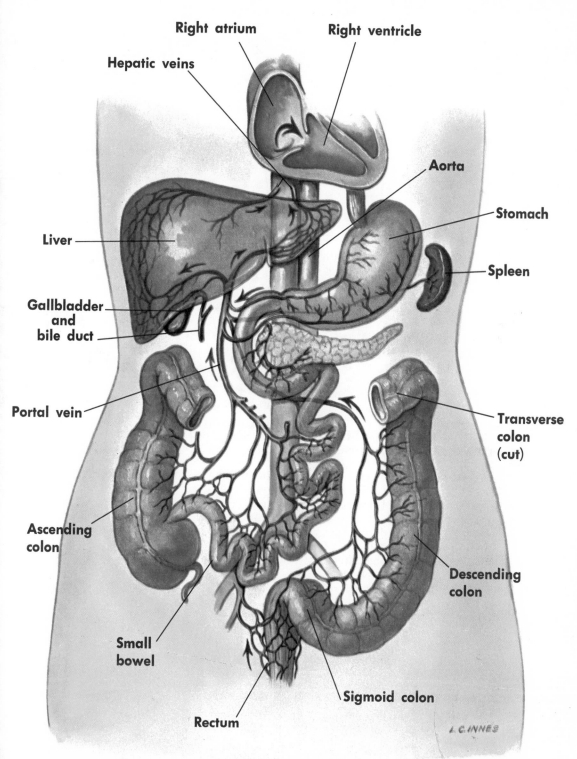

Right atrium

Right ventricle

Hepatic veins

Aorta

Stomach

Liver

Spleen

**Gallbladder
and
bile duct**

Portal vein

**Transverse
colon
(cut)**

**Ascending
colon**

**Descending
colon**

**Small
bowel**

Sigmoid colon

Rectum

I. C. INNES

The liver receives through the portal vein the blood that comes
from the intestines (shown in blue) laden with newly absorbed food.

tein can be converted into energy. But when the amount of glucose and fatty acids in the circulating blood is greater than the body's present needs require, these excess nutrients can be converted into fat, which is then stored in the fatty tissues throughout the body. Then, when a person fasts for a few hours or even for a few days, the fat stored throughout his body becomes the source of fuel.

C. Body Heat

The chemical processes by which the molecules of food constituents are broken down into smaller molecules also produce heat. This is the source of the heat that keeps the body warm. The most active cells produce the most heat.

Muscles make up about half of the body's mass, so it is not surprising that even during rest they produce about 25 percent of the body's heat. When very active, muscles may produce up to 50 times as much heat as when at rest. The process of shivering when a person is cold is the body's automatic way of activating the muscles to produce more heat.

Calories

It is customary when speaking of the body's energy production to measure the activities in terms of calories. A calorie is the amount of heat necessary to raise the temperature of a liter (about 1.1 quarts) of water one degree Centigrade (1.8° F.). This is the large calorie. (In certain scientific calculations not concerned with the body's energy production, the small calorie is used. A thousand small calories equal one large calorie.)

A person's energy requirements vary a great deal, of course, according to his muscular activity. An adult resting quietly in bed for 24 hours needs only 1200 to 1700 calories to provide for his body heat and to maintain the minimal activities of his tissues. This same adult, when doing long-continued, heavy work may need as much as four or five thousand calories during each 24-hour

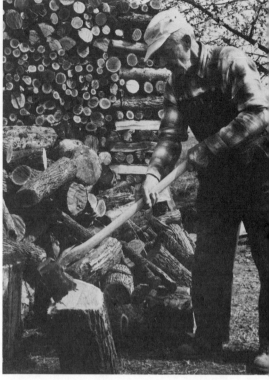

A person working hard requires more calories than a person at rest.

period. A person's need for calories varies also with his size and with his need for producing body heat. (The calorie requirement is greater in cold weather.)

Metabolism

The word *metabolism* refers to the various processes of cell activity occurring throughout the body. These processes require the expenditure of the body's fuel. And the rate of fuel consumption is measured in calories. When the body's cells are exceptionally active, we say that the metabolic rate runs high. When the activity of the cells is at slow pace, we say the metabolic rate runs low. Even when a person lies quietly in bed, the activity of his cells throughout the body requires a certain minimum consumption of fuel. Although the muscles are not being used in exercise, the body's metabolism proceeds at a certain minimum rate which we call the basal metabolic rate.

Factors That Affect the Metabolic Rate

Exercise. Of the various factors that influence the rate at which the body's cells carry on their activities, exercise is the most dramatic. Its influence depends largely, of course, on the activity of the skeletal muscles. Vigorous, sustained exercise by a physically fit person can increase his metabolic rate by as much as 20 times. The accompanying chart (page 346) which indicates the number of calories consumed per hour in various types of exercise gives convincing evidence that the more vigorous the exercise, the greater the body's demands for energy-producing fuel.

Thyroxine. Thyroxine, the principal hormone produced by the thyroid gland, has the effect of stimulating the metabolic processes in all of the body's cells. In cases in which the production of thyroxine is greater than normal, the metabolic rate is correspondingly higher than usual, a condition called hyperthyroidism. Conversely, in case of a deficiency of thyroxine, all of the body's cellular processes are carried on at a slow rate, and we speak of the condition as hypothyroidism. For a further discussion on the function of thyroxine, see chapter 2, volume 3.

Norepinephrine and Epinephrine. These hormones, the latter commonly called adrenaline, are produced in response to stimulation by the sympathetic nervous system, and their effect is to increase the metabolic rate suddenly. These hormones are produced in automatic response to emergency situations, and their proper effect is to whip up the functional activities of all cells throughout the body.

D. Body Temperature

Mechanical devices, for the most part, consist of mechanisms which convert the potential energy of fuel into kinetic energy, which performs work. In the process of this conversion, a certain amount of heat is produced.

In the human body the food processed in the digestive organs possesses enormous amounts of potential energy. Within the cells of the body, glucose and fatty acids combine with oxygen as the potential energy within these nutrients is converted to the kinetic energy needed to perform the cells' activities. And in the process of this transformation, heat is produced.

When certain parts of the body are more active than others, the greatest amount of heat is produced in the active parts. But all parts of the body are bathed continuously by flowing blood. This flowing blood returns to the heart and lungs on an average of about once a minute and is then redistributed to all parts of the body. As the blood circulates through an active part of the body it is warmed and carries this heat with it as it flows. And as the warmed blood flows through less active parts, the heat is shared with the cooler portions of the body. Thus, under usual circumstances, all parts of the body are warmed to about the same degree.

The remarkable thing about the temperature of the body is that under usual circumstances it remains nearly constant. Even when in a cold room, the actual temperature of a person's body tissues is about the same as when he is out of doors on a hot day. He may feel cold when in a cold room and he may feel warm on a hot summer day, but the actual temperature of the tissues of his body is very nearly the same under both circumstances. It is as though the human body were equipped with a thermostat such as turns on more heat in a building when it becomes cold and reduces the heat when it becomes too warm, even activating the cooling system.

Furthermore, the body contains automatic regulating mechanisms which reduce the amount of blood flowing to the hands and feet when the surroundings are cold. It is a means of conserving the body's heat. The body's

Burning calories through exercise

Activity	Calories
Bicycling (5$\frac{1}{2}$ mph)	210
Walking (2$\frac{1}{2}$ mph)	210
Gardening	220
Canoeing (2$\frac{1}{2}$ mph)	230
Golf	250
Lawn mowing (power mower)	250
Lawn mowing (hand mower)	270
Rowboating (2$\frac{1}{2}$ mph)	300
Swimming ($\frac{1}{4}$ mph)	300
Walking (3$\frac{3}{4}$ mph)	300
Badminton	350
Horseback riding (trotting)	350
Square dancing	350
Volleyball	350
Roller skating	350
Table tennis	360
Wood chopping or sawing	400
Tennis	420
Water skiing	480
Hill climbing (100 ft. per hr.)	490
Skiing (10 mph)	600
Squash and handball	600
Cycling (13 mph)	660
Scull rowing (race)	840
Running (10 mph)	900

The average adult man burns between 2400 and 4500 calories a day depending upon the amount and kind of exercise he gets. Active persons such as workers and athletes may consume as many as 6000 calories a day and yet not gain weight. This chart indicates the probable calorie expenditure per hour for a 150 pound person engaged in various activities.* It was prepared by Robert E. Johnson, M.D., Ph.D., and colleagues at the department of physiology and biophysics at the University of Illinois.

*Note: Softball, fishing and hunting were not included in this study.

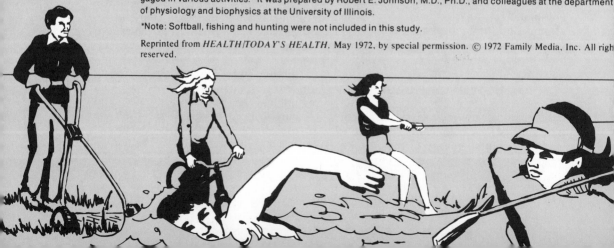

temperature, when measured by either an oral or a rectal thermometer, remains surprisingly constant, even though the hands and the feet may be cold.

The usual, normal body temperature is 98.6° F. (37° C.), and it varies not much more than one degree Fahrenheit, even under external circumstances of heat or cold or extremes of physical activity.

Control of Body Temperature

The body's thermostat is located in that portion of the brain called the hypothalamus. This area receives signals from nerve receptors located in various parts of the skin which indicate the hot or cold condition of these parts. Also, there are nerve cells within the hypothalamus sensitive to changes in the temperature of the blood that flows through these parts.

The hypothalamus is a part of the autonomic nervous system, which functions automatically and which sends controlling nerve signals to all parts of the body. When the hypothalamus receives nerve impulses indicating that the body is becoming overheated, it operates through the autonomic nervous system to decrease the amount of heat production and to activate the body's cooling system. When nerve impulses indicate that the tissues of the body are becoming cold, nerve signals go out to increase the production of heat and to conserve what heat is already present.

When the body becomes cold. When the amount of heat produced within the body is not as great as the amount of heat being lost (as when the individual is in cold surroundings), the heat-control center in the hypothalamus functions in two ways: (1) It reduces the amount of heat being lost from the body, and (2) it increases the amount of heat being produced.

Heat loss is reduced by an automatic constriction of the blood vessels in the skin so as to reduce the amount of blood flowing through the capillaries.

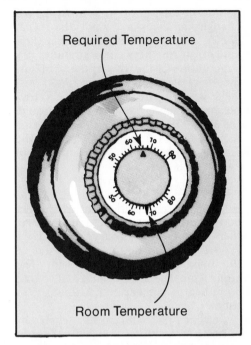

Temperature within the body is automatically regulated by a thermostat-type of mechanism located within the brain.

Inasmuch as the blood is the conveyer of heat, not as much heat will be lost from the body surface when the blood flow in the skin is thus reduced. This adjustment largely accounts for a person's cold hands and feet when he is in cold surroundings.

At the same time that the amount of blood in the skin is reduced, the tone of the skeletal muscles is increased. This adaptation causes shivering, which generates more heat. Another means by which the body's heat production is increased is by the liberation of more norepinephrine and epinephrine, produced by the adrenal glands. These hormones increase the rate of metabolism in all of the body's cells, and thus the circulating blood becomes warmer.

When the body becomes too warm. When more heat is being produced than is necessary to maintain a normal body temperature, the control center in the

347

hypothalamus brings about two changes in the skin. First, the sweat glands are stimulated to pour out their secretion on the skin's surface. By evaporation of the sweat, the skin surface is cooled. Second, the blood vessels within the skin dilate, thus permitting more blood to flow through the skin. The heat which the circulating blood conveys is thus dissipated by the cooling effect of the evaporation of sweat.

Fever

Fever is a condition in which the body's temperature rises to higher level than normal. It is brought about by a resetting of the body's thermostat in the hypothalamus of the brain. The control mechanism is readjusted so that more heat is present in the tissues than usual.

Certain toxic substances, when circulating in the blood, cause the thermostat in the hypothalamus to demand a higher body temperature. These toxic substances may be produced by germs, or they may be released when tissues are damaged, as in a serious injury, or in dehydration, when the body's supply of water becomes deficient.

Inasmuch as fever is associated with some serious condition, the physician looking after a patient with fever often judges the seriousness of the condition by the degree and the duration of the fever. Body temperature of 104° F. (40° C.) indicates a serious illness of some kind. Persons can even tolerate temperatures up to 106° F. (41° C.) for short periods of time. Body temperatures above this usually terminate in death.

It is interesting to notice that the development of fever is usually accompanied by the patient's feeling of chilliness, often associated with shivering. This is brought about because a resetting of the body's thermostat to a higher level produces the same reactions as are necessary to conserve heat and increase heat production. It is as though the patient were suddenly reacting to being placed in a cold room.

Heatstroke

Heatstroke is the most severe disorder that may occur as the result of exposure to excessive heat. In heatstroke the usual mechanisms for getting rid of body heat no longer suffice to hold the body's temperature within normal limits. It occurs in situations in which the circulation of air is inadequate. The body's temperature rises to dangerous levels, and the rate of the heartbeat increases to 160 per minute or above. This increased rate of heartbeat is the automatic attempt of the body to circulate the blood through the skin fast enough to dissipate the excess heat.

Heatstroke requires emergency means of reducing the temperature of the body. For instruction on administering first aid for heatstroke, see chapter 23, volume 3.

The Skin and Its Diseases

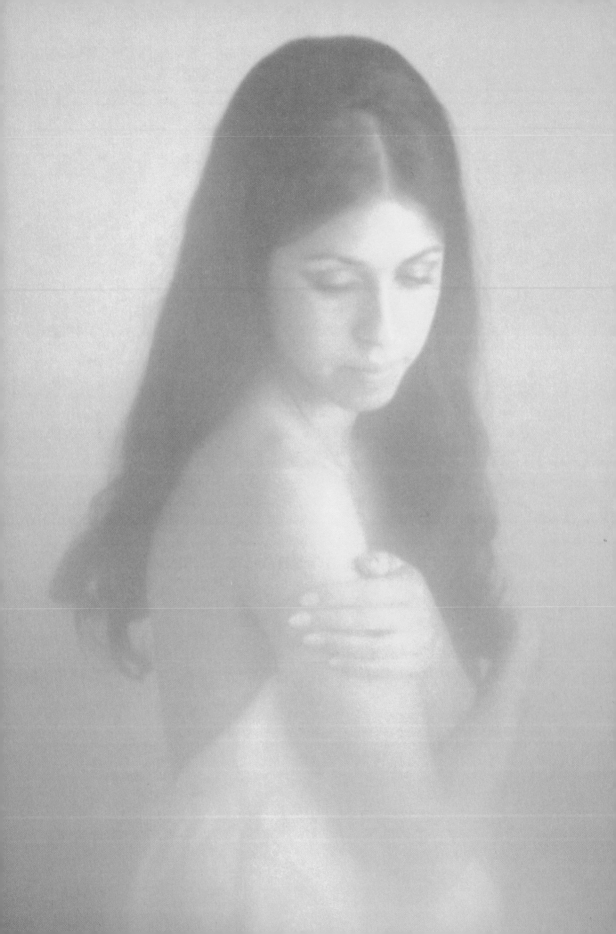

The Body's Covering

When the teacher asked Johnny the purpose of the skin, he responded, "The skin keeps the body from looking raw." And Johnny was right.

The skin serves as a barrier between the atmosphere that surrounds the body and the tissue fluids within. Being on the body's surface, the skin prevents the movement of fluid in either direction. It also prevents the entry into the body of irritating dusts, chemicals, and germs.

But the skin is more than a tight-fitting envelope. It helps control the body's temperature. It contains the sense organs for touch, for heat and cold, for pain, and for the feeling of pressure. The skin contains many small glands which discharge their fluid or oil onto the body's surface. Furthermore, the skin can repair itself following injury.

No single description applies to the skin of all parts of the body. Its features in one location differ from those in another. It is modified for protection against heavy friction on the palms of the hands and soles of the feet, for flexibility around the joints and parts of the body which move freely, for remarkable sensitivity around the face and other parts of the body where sense perception is important, and for the growth of hair in those areas where hair provides added protection or im-proves a person's appearance.

In all parts of the body, however, the skin has two principal layers—a surface layer of closely packed cells (the epidermis) and a deeper layer of strong fibers arranged in a feltwork (dermis or corium).

The epidermis contains no blood vessels—just layers of closely packed cells. The deepest of these cells are very much alive and keep producing more cells just like themselves. As new cells develop, they crowd their way toward the surface, meanwhile moving farther away from their source of nourishment and undergoing chemical changes which make them horny and scalelike. When they reach the surface, they are no longer alive and eventually rub off by friction with the towel after bathing or by coming in contact with some unyielding surface. The thickness of the epidermis is greatest in those parts of the body exposed to wear and tear. A person walking barefoot develops a thick epidermis on the soles of his feet. A person whose shoe pinches develops thick areas (calluses) at the points of friction with his shoe. A violinist forms a thick epidermis on the parts of his fingers that press against the strings. The skin of the eyelids has such a thin epidermis that it is very sensitive to touch.

The deeper layer of the skin, the

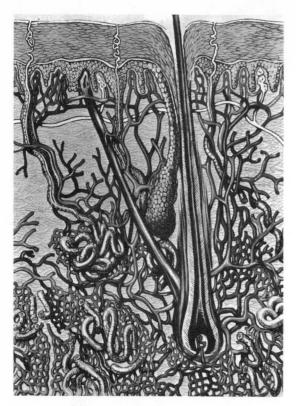

Microscopic view of a section of skin. The skin's surface is at the top.

through the epidermis but also allows some of the fluid portion of the blood to seep into the epidermis and thus nourish its cells.

The Skin's Color

The color of the skin depends on two things: (1) the amount of pigment in the skin and (2) the amount of blood momentarily present in the dermis. The skin's pigment is called melanin. It is produced by a special kind of cells called melanocytes situated at the junction between epidermis and dermis. They produce tiny granules of dark pigment which find their way into neighboring cells of the epidermis.

The skin of a light-complexioned person contains a small amount of pigment, whereas that of a dark-complexioned person contains so much pigment that most of the cells of the epidermis contain granules of melanin. Even in the same individual, some areas of skin contain more pigment than others. The skin of a very dark-complexioned person does not appear "rosy" because the large amount of pigment does not permit the blood's red color to be seen.

Fingerprints

The boundary between the dermis and the epidermis does not follow a straight plane. The underlying dermis has many hills and ridges which fit into corresponding pockets and grooves on the undersurface of the epidermis. This arrangement provides a firmer attachment for the epidermis than if it were merely placed over the dermis like one sheet of paper on another. These hills and ridges account for fingerprints and footprints. Their particular pattern— unique for each idividual—serves as a means of personal identification and provides a non-skid quality, increasing the firmness of a person's grip with his fingers and the surety of his step when walking barefoot. A person leaves fingermarks on a pane of glass or on a polished surface because the sweat glands pour out their secretions through tiny openings located along the ridges of the fingerprint pattern.

dermis, is composed mostly of strong connective tissue fibers. Many of these run in various directions, but some are in bundles that run parallel to each other to provide strength in the line of greatest mechanical stress. This accounts for the tiny folds that appear in the skin, more prominent in some areas than in others.

The dermis contains the structures that provide the skin's "utilities." Here are nerve fibers and blood vessels of various sizes. The dermis and the loose connective tissue just beneath it hold the skin glands, the receptor organs for the various sensations, and the functioning portions of the hair follicles which produce and maintain the hair shafts. Many capillaries lie close to the boundary between the dermis and the epidermis. This proximity not only permits the color of the blood to shine

Subcutaneous Tissues

Just beneath the dermis is a layer of very loose tissue called subcutaneous tissue. Even in a slender person this contains considerable fat. It is this loose, underlying layer that permits a fold of the skin to be grasped by thumb and finger and pulled out of its usual shape. The subcutaneous layer is thicker in some places than in others. That is, it fills in the hollows of the deeper structures so that the skin covers these smoothly and beautifully. It is the fat in the subcutaneous layer that increases when a person puts on weight. It thus serves as a depository for the body's fat which, in time of need, can be used as a source of body fuel. It also helps to insulate the body and thus retard heat loss in cold weather.

Age Makes a Difference

During childhood the skin is soft and smooth. Most of a child's skin is covered by fine, inconspicuous hair; but only on the scalp is hair thick enough to be noticed. As a child reaches adolescence the output of the skin glands increases, and the growth of hair on certain parts of the body becomes conspicuous. The production of oil may be so copious that the skin, especially that of the face, becomes oily. This condition increases the tendency for blackheads to form and for infections to occur in the ducts of the oil glands, producing acne pimples. Within the next ten years, however, the activity of the oil glands usually quiets down and the skin clears itself, in most cases, of these unsightly blemishes.

As a person becomes older, the production of skin oil is further reduced and the skin becomes less elastic. The decreased elasticity largely accounts for the appearance of folds and wrinkles. Habits of facial expression such as squinting, frowning, and drawing down the corners of the mouth have their influence in producing wrinkles, even before old age arrives. A person may delay the drying and wrinkling of

Skin sections showing how a blackhead forms in relation to a hair follicle and how it can develop into an infected cyst.

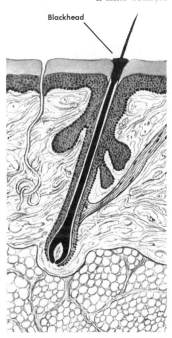
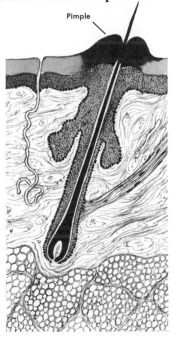
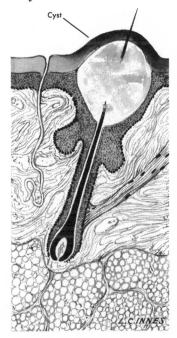

Blackhead

Pimple

Cyst

L. C. INNES

his skin by avoiding too much exposure to sunlight and wind.

Moles

A mole (nevus) involves a limited area of skin, sometimes large and sometimes small, in which there is an unusual cluster of melanocytes—cells that produce melanin pigment. Virtually every person has several moles, there being an average of about 15 per person. Some are noticeable during childhood, and others become apparent at the onset of adulthood. Some are flat, some are elevated; some contain hair, others have no hair; some are the color of the surrounding skin, while others vary in color from light pink to almost black.

Occasionally a mole undergoes a transformation in which it develops into a dangerous form of cancer (melanoma). It is not possible to predict in advance that a certain mole may undergo this tragic transformation. For a list of the danger signs that indicate such a transformation, see the item on "Melanoma" in chapter 25, volume 2.

The Glands of the Skin

The skin's sweat glands are shaped like tiny coiled tubes. Each gland has one opening to the surface through which its watery secretion escapes. The deeper, coiled portion of a sweat gland is surrounded by small blood vessels. From the blood flowing through these vessels water and salt, the principal constituents of sweat, are extracted.

Certain parts of the body, such as the armpit and the groin, have large sweat glands associated with the roots of hairs. Slight discoloration and a distinctive odor mark the secretion of the sweat glands in these locations.

Along the margin of each eyelid a single row of highly specialized sweat glands secrete oil. The film of oil produced here serves two important purposes: First, it seals the eyelids during sleep to prevent the evaporation of the fluid produced by the tear glands. Second, it prevents the overflow of the fluid which normally keeps the membranes of the eye moist.

The majority of the skin's oil glands (sebaceous glands) are located in relation to the roots of hairs. These produce an oily substance that keeps the skin pliable and prevents the hairs from becoming dry.

The sweat and the oil produced by the skin's glands tend to dry on the surface of the skin, forming a film that becomes rancid and offensive. This film collects dirt, and the mixture of oil and dirt may clog some of the outlets of the glands. One good reason for periodic bathing is to remove this film.

Sense Organs in the Skin

In the dermis, near where it contacts the epidermis, are located many tiny sense organs from which delicate nerve fibers carry nerve impulses to the brain. There are several kinds of these sense organs, each one being adapted to registering a particular sensation, such as touch, heat, cold, pressure, and pain.

Perhaps a person can best appreciate how the skin provides important sensations by noticing what happens when he prowls about the bedroom in the dark. He cannot see because of the darkness. He hears nothing because all is silent. But the sense organs in the skin provide him with the information he needs at such a time.

He gropes his way from one piece of furniture to another by making contact, usually with his fingertips, with familiar objects. If he tends to fall, pressure produced by the side of the bed or by the arm of a chair stimulates his sense organs for pressure, thus informing him about the object he needs to avoid. If, carelessly, he stubs his toe, sensations of pain quickly reprimand him for moving too quickly. If the room is cool the receptor organs for cold notify him, and he arranges for another blanket on the bed. After his prowling, he returns to the warmth of his bed, and the organs for heat, as they are moderately stimulated, give him a sense of comfort. But if, in the meantime, he has

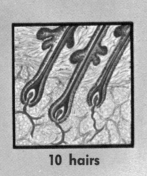

10 hairs

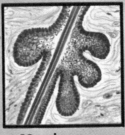

12 sebaceous glands

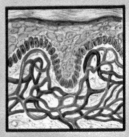

1 yard of blood vessels

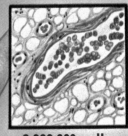

3,000,000 cells

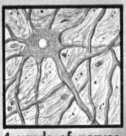

100 sweat glands

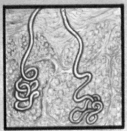

4 yards of nerves

1 square centimeter of skin contains:

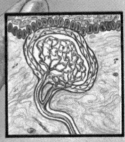

12 sensory apparatuses for heat

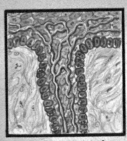

2 sensory apparatuses for cold

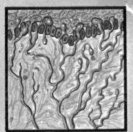

3,000 sensory cells at the ends of nerve fibers

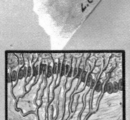

200 nerve endings to record pain

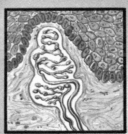

25 pressure apparatuses for the perception of tactile stimuli

L. C. INNES

turned on the electric blanket, the same organs will warn him if overheating threatens.

Heat Regulation by the Skin

When the weather is warm or when a person is exercising vigorously, the skin becomes flushed through increased blood circulation in it, and the sweat glands become particularly active. This reaction develops promptly when excess heat is produced by the body's activities or when the temperature of one's surroundings runs high. The body's heat-regulating mechanism is so efficient that a healthy person's body temperature varies only slightly, night or day, cool weather or warm, during work or rest.

The skin reacts to prevent too great a loss of heat when the surroundings are cold. The skin's blood vessels contract, thus reducing the flow of blood and decreasing the radiation of heat from the body. There is little or no perspiration. The oil glands pour out more oil, which spreads on the skin and decreases evaporation.

Tattooing

Tattooing involves the injection of insoluble, colored dyes into the dermis of the skin. Tattooing is usually performed by a tattoo artist who uses various colors of dyes to make a design. Inasmuch as the dyes are insoluble and inasmuch as they are injected into the dermis rather than into the epidermis, most of these dyes remain in place for the remainder of life.

Two problems arise in connection with tattooing. The first is the danger of infection. The process of tattooing involves the use of needles inserted into the dermis in order to carry the dye. Many serious infections have resulted from the use of needles not properly sterilized. The second problem is that tattooing, once performed, is difficult to remove. Many persons who have been tattooed desire later that the design be obliterated. But this is practically impossible without leaving a scar.

Skin Grafting

In cases in which large areas of skin have been destroyed by burns or destructive accidents, healing is often greatly hastened by the use of skin grafts (skin transplantation). When the epidermis of the skin is completely absent from an injured area, the skin can replace itself naturally only by growing in from the margins of the wound. When a large area is involved, the long time required for the epidermis to grow in from the margins makes it easy for infection to develop. Furthermore, the scar that develops in an area in which healing was long delayed tends to contract and cause disfigurement.

When skin is transplanted from another person the same problems of tissue rejection occur as when any other tissue or organ is transplanted from a donor to a recipient. Therefore, in skin grafting, the preferable method is to take a sample of skin from some other part of the patient's own body. This is not a difficult procedure, for the samples of healthy skin used in skin grafting are usually thin—so thin that the area from which the sample is taken heals quickly.

Exposure to the Sun

It is now recognized that excessive exposure to the sun is damaging to the skin. It produces premature wrinkling, thinning of the skin, and favors the development of skin blemishes (solar keratoses) which lay the foundation for the later development of skin cancer. These damages occur especially in those areas of the skin exposed to the sun. They are most noticeable in persons whose occupation requires them to spend much time in the sun.

It is the ultraviolet portion of the sun's spectrum that damages the skin. But it is these ultraviolet rays that stimulate the production of pigment in the skin and are thus responsible for the suntan so much desired by persons who feel that suntan is an aid to personal attractiveness.

The same type of radiation (in the

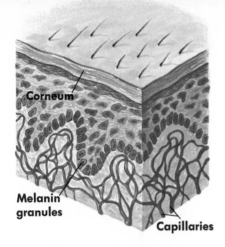

Corneum

Melanin granules

Capillaries

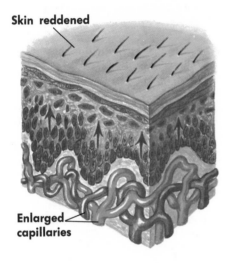

Skin reddened

Enlarged capillaries

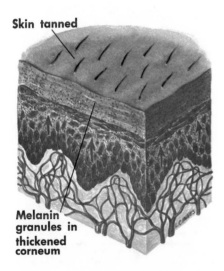

Skin tanned

Melanin granules in thickened corneum

Effects of exposure of skin to sunlight: upper, normal skin; middle, twenty-four hours after exposure (redness from blood-filled capillaries); lower, one week after exposure (tan coloration due to increase in granules of melanin).

ultraviolet range) is produced artificially in the popular suntanning salons. It is just as damaging to the skin as the ultraviolet portion of sunlight. Persons of blond complexion, persons living in areas where the sunlight is intense (as Arizona, Texas, and Florida), and those who work continuously outdoors are the most susceptible to the skin damage caused by the ultraviolet component of sunlight.

Physicians who specialize in care of the skin recommend caution regarding exposure to the sun. They advise against patronizing the suntan salon, and they urge those who must be in the sun a great deal to protect the skin of the exposed areas by the use of a sunscreen ointment. Sunscreen ointments are available at the drugstore and do not require a prescription.

Dry Skin

Soaps, solvents, and some disinfectants have the effect of removing the natural oil from the skin. When such are used excessively or continuously, the skin becomes dry and chapped. Exposure to dry air or to cold winds also removes the natural oil from between the surface cells of the epidermis.

Avoiding the excessive use of soap when washing the skin or bathing helps to prevent such drying. For persons living in cold climates, protective clothing (including scarves, gloves, and mittens) plus the use of humidifiers in living quarters will help to prevent dry and chapped skin.

Once the skin becomes dry because of the loss of its natural oil, the best treatment consists of soaking the involved area in warm water for five to ten minutes, following which a greasy ointment, such as petrolatum (Vaseline) or lanolin, should be rubbed into the skin. Creams and lotions for the treatment of dry skin are also available at the drugstore. Some of these consist of an emulsion designed to leave a thin film of oil on the skin.

Hair and Nails

Each individual hair is the product of

357

a small organ, the hair follicle, located within the skin. Cells at the depth of the follicle are continuously active in producing more of the cells out of which the root and shaft of the hair are composed. This continuous production of new cells causes the hair to increase in length at the rate of from three eighths to three quarters of an inch (10-20 mm.) per month. The cells composing the shaft (the visible part) of the hair are no longer living cells but are comparable to the cells on the surface of the epidermis of the skin.

The color of a hair depends on the quality and quantity of pigment contained in the cells of the hair shaft.

After growing for a period of a few years, a hair tends to fall out, leaving its follicle dormant for a while; but later the follicle becomes active again and produces a new hair. It has been estimated that a person loses 50 to 100 scalp hairs every day and that about 10 percent of the hair follicles are dormant at any given time, except on scalps be-coming bald, where more may be permanently dormant.

Gray hair grows at approximately the same rate as pigmented hair. Some people turn gray at an earlier age than others. Nobody knows why. It is not the result of ill health or malnutrition, but seems to be the result of some hereditary factor.

Some people are troubled because of the excessive growth of unwanted hair (hirsutism). Usually this overproduction is a manifestation of an hereditary tendency and is harmless except for the embarrassment it may cause. In an occasional case, an unusual growth of hair is the result of abnormal activity of the endocrine organs.

Effective methods of removing unwanted hair include plucking, shaving, the use of depilatories, and removal by electrolysis. Plucking is painful but effective. Shaving is a simple, effective method of removing unwanted hair and, contrary to the opinion of some, it does not cause the

The shape of the individual hairs is the determining factor as to whether a person's hair is straight or curly.

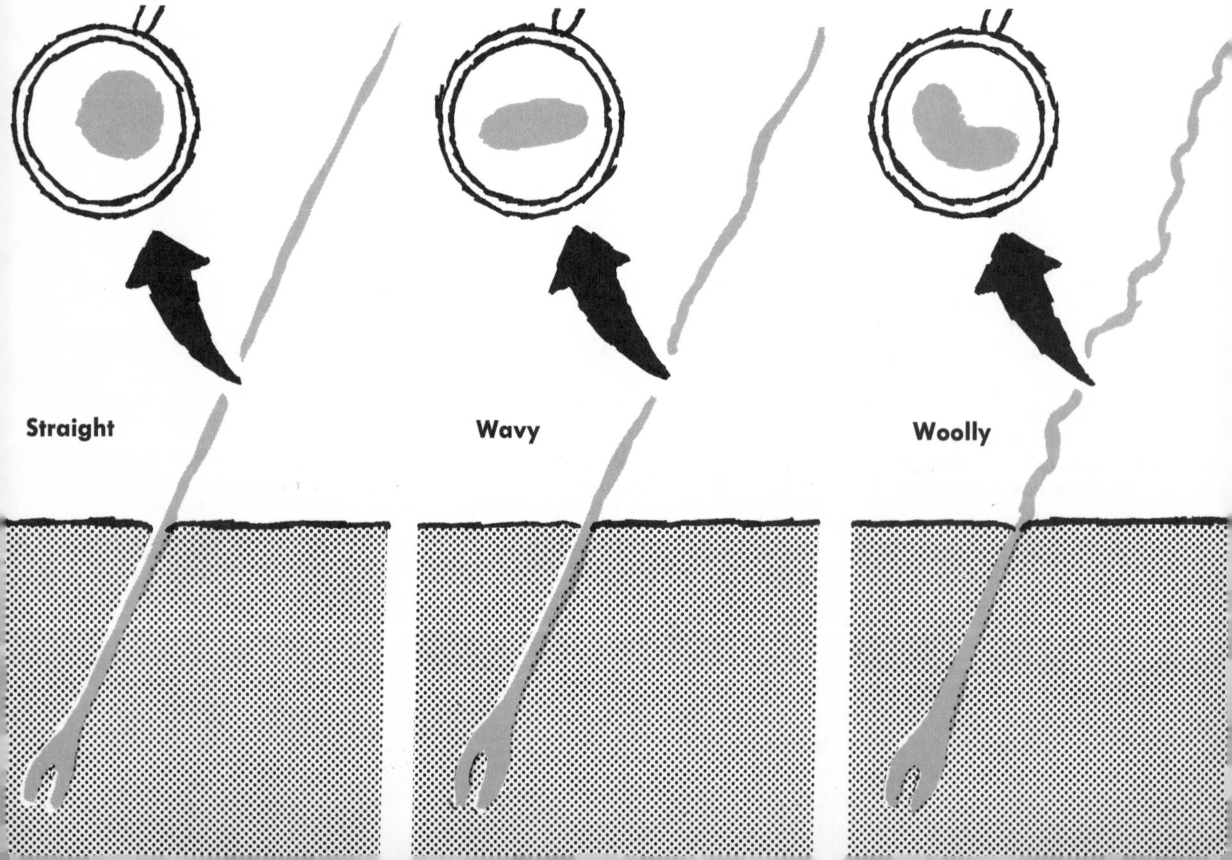

Straight

Wavy

Woolly

unwanted hair to become stiff or more abundant. Depilatories such as may be purchased at the drugstore contain chemical ingredients which cause the hair to disintegrate, but depilatories do not affect the roots of the hairs. Therefore, the hairs will continue to grow as though they had been removed by shaving. The disadvantage of depilatories is that the chemicals which they contain may be irritating to the skin. In electrolysis the root of the hair is destroyed by an electric current. This prevents the regrowth of the hair, but the procedure may produce temporary irritation and may result, later, in small pitlike scarring.

Fingernails and toenails are produced by specialized cells of the epidermis of the skin. They grow by the activity of cells at their roots, much as a hair grows in length through the activity of cells in the hair follicle. However, the cells which produce nails do not contain or transmit pigment. Therefore the nail plates are translucent.

The most important consideration in the care of nails, as also in the care of hair, is to make sure of an abundant circulation of blood in the skin. Tight hatbands may reduce the circulation of blood in the scalp, impairing the nourishment of the hair-forming cells. An impoverished diet, almost any acute illness with fever, and distorted action of certain glands may make the nails brittle or malformed. Anemias and hypothyroid conditions may cause the hair to fall out or leave it lusterless.

Brittleness of the nails may be caused by the excessive use of soap or detergents or by contact with solvents. It is advisable for persons whose work requires them to use detergents or solvents to use rubber gloves. If gloves must be worn for long periods of time, simple cotton gloves may be worn underneath the rubber gloves. Brittleness of the nails may be somewhat relieved by applying Vaseline to the nail before retiring at night. After the Vaseline has been carefully worked into the skin surrounding the nails, the fingers may be wrapped with light bandages left in place until morning, or cotton gloves may be worn throughout the night.

Skin Diseases

The skin is commonly affected in ways that bring discomfort and concern. It is estimated that 10 to 15 percent of patient visits to physicians are prompted by some skin ailment.

Because of its exposed position as it covers the body's surface, the skin is commonly damaged by trauma and by contact with various physical agents. It often becomes involved by infections caused by bacteria, fungi, yeasts, parasites, and viruses. It is susceptible to inflammations, to allergic reactions, and even to the development of cancer. The skin may be involved by certain systemic diseases. Some skin diseases are caused by inherited predisposi-

tions, and for some the cause has not been determined.

It is the purpose of the present chapter to systematize the present knowledge on skin diseases so that the reader can find answers to his questions on the characteristics of the common skin ailments, their causes when known, and the most successful procedures for treatment. The chapter is organized according to the following outline. Each subdivision includes detailed discussions of the individual skin diseases belonging to each respective category. To locate the discussion for a particular disease consult the index following the outline or use the General Index.

Outline of the Chapter

Index of Skin Disorders

Skin Lesions

Physicians have an advantage in dealing with skin diseases, as compared with diseases of the internal organs, in that the skin is readily available for examination. Recognition of a disease that affects the skin depends in large measure on the characteristics of the skin lesion that the disease produces. By definition, a skin lesion is an alteration in the appearance and/or structure of the skin. There are various kinds of skin lesions, depending on the particular ailments. Large areas of skin may be uniformly involved (as in erythema), or there may be multiple blemishes appearing in certain areas of the body (as with the rashes of measles or chickenpox). Some forms of skin disease consist of just one lesion, as with a boil or a tumor. The lesions of some skin diseases consist of irregular blotches of involvement.

In order to understand the descriptions of the various skin diseases the reader must be familiar with the following terms:

1. *Macule.* A macule is a discolored spot not elevated above the skin's surface. Examples are freckles or the rash of measles (rubeola).

2. *Papule (Pimple).* A papule is a small, circumscribed elevation of the skin which contains no accumulation of fluid (no blister). Papules appear in some drug eruptions and in some phases of solar keratoses.

3. *Vesicle.* A vesicle is a small, circumscribed elevation of the skin with a tiny blister containing serous fluid at the apex. Vesicles appear in some insect bites and in herpes simplex (cold sore).

4. *Pustule.* A pustule differs from a vesicle in that it contains pus rather than serous fluid. A boil is a large pustule. Pustules appear commonly in cases of acne.

5. *Rash.* A rash is a temporary eruption of the skin consisting of visible lesions characterized by redness or elevation or both. Skin rashes occur in some of the communicable and infectious diseases as, for example German measles (rubella). A rash occurs in the deficiency disease of pellagra, in reaction to certain drugs, and in some allergic manifestations. A rash may consist of a combination of the lesions already mentioned; and we can then speak, for example, of maculo-papular lesions.

6. *Erythema.* Erythema consists of a reddening of the skin which may appear in a small area or may be widespread. It is caused by a dilatation of the blood capillaries in the skin which permits a larger volume of blood to be present there. The pressure of a finger against such an area of skin will cause the redness to disappear momentarily because the pressure pushes the excess

blood out of the dilated capillaries. Erythema occurs typically as the result of some irritation of the skin as by heat or by exposure to the sun. Erythema develops as a part of many skin ailments.

7. *Wheal (Welt)*. A wheal is a small area of elevated skin produced by swelling (edema) of the skin's tissues. Wheals occur commonly in connection with insect bites and other manifestations of allergic reaction.

8. *Bulla (Blister)*. A bulla is a large blister (larger than a pea) which contains serous fluid or serous fluid mixed with pus. The wall of a bulla is usually thin and is easily ruptured. Bullae occur typically in such skin diseases as pemphigus.

9. *Nodule*. A nodule is a solid lesion (not a blister) larger than a papule and smaller than a tumor. A small fatty tumor (lipoma) would qualify as a nodule.

10. *Erosion*. An erosion consists of a loss of part or all of the surface layer of the skin (the epidermis) in a localized area. It may be caused by scuffing or scratching and may occur as part of the damage caused by the skin disease pemphigus.

11. *Ulcer*. An ulcer is a lesion deeper than an erosion and involves part of the dermis as well as the epidermis of the skin. An ulcer may be caused by physical trauma in which part of the skin is torn away, or it may occur as the result of the death of an area of skin deprived of its usual blood supply (varicose ulcer). A trophic ulcer (bedsore) occurs as a result of continuous pressure against an area of skin. The pressure prevents the normal circulation of blood in the involved area.

12. *Scar*. A scar is the final product of healing of a skin injury or a skin lesion. Scars vary in size and shape, depending on the size and shape of the original skin lesion. A scar is more or less conspicuous, depending upon its size and location. A simple erosion of the skin, in which only the surface layer (epidermis) has been damaged, heals without the formation of a scar.

But a deeper lesion in which the dermis of the skin has been involved, results in the formation of a scar. Acne, among other skin diseases, tends to form scars as the lesions heal.

13. *Tumor*. A tumor is an abnormal mass of tissue which, by definition, is larger than a nodule. A tumor may be soft or firm. It may cause an elevation of the skin, or it may be deep-seated. A tumor may be harmless in its effect on the surrounding tissues, or it may increase in size until it outgrows its source of blood supply and its component tissues break down. Some forms of cancer develop as tumors, but not all tumors are cancerous. Examples of harmless tumors are large lipomas and sebaceous cysts.

14. *Pigmentary Disorder*. Normal skin contains a certain amount of pigment (coloring material). The exact amount depends upon the individual's complexion, whether he be blond or brunette or black. There are certain skin ailments in which the amount of pigment in the skin is either increased or decreased. Albinism is an extreme example in which, because of a hereditary defect, the skin lacks pigment in all parts of the body. Vitiligo (leukoderma) is a skin ailment characterized by loss of pigment in certain patchy areas. Melasma is a skin ailment characterized by a blotchy increase in pigment in certain areas of the skin.

A. Ailments That Itch (Pruritus)

GENERALIZED ITCHING

Itching (pruritus) is an uncomfortable sensation which creates the desire to rub or scratch the affected area of skin. It may be limited to a small area, or it may be generalized.

Itching may occur as a symptom in many diseases. It occurs in parasitic infections of the skin such as pediculosis and scabies. It occurs in eczema (atopic dermatitis). Pinworm infection can cause intense itching (see chapter 20, volume 3). It occurs commonly as a symptom of some systemic diseases not primarily related to the skin.

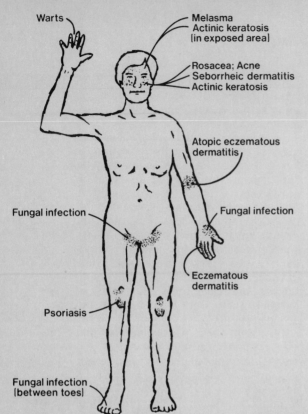

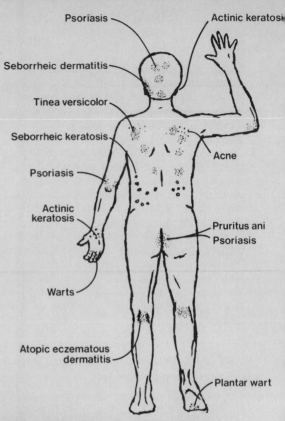

The typical areas of the body in which some of the common skin ailments occur, front view.

The typical areas of the body in which some of the common skin ailments occur, rear view.

Among these are diabetes, obstructive liver disease, certain kidney diseases, and some instances of internal cancer. Itching may occur also in certain endocrine disturbances, at the time of menstruation, and in connection with the menopause. It often occurs in elderly persons in whom the skin glands are not as active as they were formerly (see chapter 40, volume 1).

Care and Treatment

1. Bran, starch, vinegar, or a cupful of table salt should be added to the bath water. Following the bath, the skin should be dried without harsh rubbing. Baths should not be more frequent than necessary for cleanliness.

2. Wear underclothing that will not irritate the skin. Launder underwear with care, making sure that all traces of soap or detergent are rinsed out.

3. Apply a 1 percent phenol in calamine lotion three times a day to the itching areas. If this proves too drying to the skin, use a lotion prepared by the pharmacist as follows:

Menthol	3
Phenol	2
Glycerine	15
Alcohol 35%, q.s.ad.	240

4. Try to determine the cause of the itching and avoid, treat, or correct it. This may call for the aid of a physician.

5. For soothing the itching that is too troublesome in some elderly persons, commercial preparations may be used such as Nivea Creme or Nivea Skin Oil, Keri Lotion, or Cetaphil Lotion.

ITCHING IN THE ANAL REGION (PRURITUS ANI)

Pruritus ani is a persistent itching,

frequently with redness, maceration, and fissuring of the skin, occurring in the skin around the rectal outlet. The itching sometimes becomes very distressing. It tends to be worse at night. There are many possible causes, but the most common is an infection of the skin by a yeastlike organism called monilia (*Candida*). The constant moisture between the buttocks lessens the normal firmness of the skin. Germs in the yeastlike organisms, being always present, grow easily in this softened skin.

Care and Treatment

The most important factor in controlling itching in the anal region is to keep the skin clean and dry. It may be advisable to keep a pad of dry absorbent cotton between the buttocks.

Avoid the use of soap, but keep the skin around the rectal outlet clean by washing it gently but thoroughly with warm water after each bowel movement and drying after each washing. Repeat at other times, if necessary, to a total of at least two bathings a day. Cotton rather than toilet paper should be used as an aid in washing and drying.

After washing and drying, apply a lotion made as follows:

Phenol	1
Glycerine	15
Rosewater q.s.ad.	120

After the lotion has dried, apply a generous amount of powder, and repeat the application of powder every two hours. A good powder is made as follows:

Salicylic acid	2
Talcum powder	58
Mix thoroughly.	

CAUTION: *Preparations containing salicylic acid, as in this and the following item, should not be used by a person who has diabetes.*

Each night at bedtime apply a small amount of salve made as follows:

Salicylic acid	1
Sulfur ppt.	2
Cold cream q.s.ad.	60

If the above treatment does not bring relief within one week, have a physician make special studies to determine the underlying cause of the condition and prescribe appropriate remedies.

B. Dermatitis

By definition dermatitis is a superficial inflammation of the skin. There are several types of dermatitis and many possible causes, now to be considered under their respective subheadings:

CONTACT DERMATITIS

Contact dermatitis consists of an inflammation of the skin caused either (1) by direct contact with some irritating chemical substance or (2) by an allergic reaction in which the skin becomes reddened, swollen, and itchy because of contact with some substance to which the individual has become sensitized.

It is often difficult to determine just what is irritating the skin or causing it to react unfavorably. Patience coupled with intelligent sleuthing are often necessary. Individuals react differently, and what bothers one person may have no detrimental effect on another. Once the offending substance is identified, the prevention and treatment consists, of course, of avoiding contact with this substance.

Many preparations useful around the house contain substances to which some people become sensitive. Common offenders are certain kinds of soap, detergents, bleaches, toilet bowl cleaners, oven cleaners, drain pipe cleaners, lye, and various ammonia preparations.

For persons who work in industry the list of things that may cause irritation of the skin is long.

Prominent among substances that may cause dermatitis are nickel and chromium. Nickel is contained in coins, jewelry, and watchbands, to

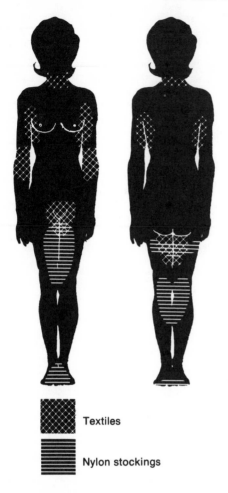

Textiles

Nylon stockings

Textured areas in the diagrams indicate location on the body where irritants contained in stockings and other garments may cause sensitive skin to react.

cases. Some rubber products, such as bathing caps, gloves, and the elastic components in stretch garments, contain chemicals irritating to some people. Often, in such cases, the particular area of the skin affected will suggest what article of clothing contains the offending substance.

The appearance of the skin in contact dermatitis may mimic that of several other skin ailments.

Care and Treatment

Use all reasonable means of discovering the substance to which the skin is sensitive. Physicians often use patch tests to help in this discovery. The patch test is performed by strapping to the skin sample substances that may possibly be responsible. These are left in place for 48 hours to determine whether the skin reacts unfavorably.

Once the responsible irritant has been discovered, ingenuity must be used to avoid contact with this substance or to protect the skin from it. Some persons must change employment in order to obtain relief. Others may benefit by switching to a different brand of clothing. In many cases it is necessary to solicit the help of a physician who specializes in diseases of the skin (a dermatologist). He will help to identify the offending substance and to find ways to prevent contact with it.

name a few. Skin contact with articles containing this metal, especially when the skin is moist with perspiration, may irritate the skin. Chromium is used frequently in the tanning of leather and can thus cause a dermatitis of the skin of the feet or of other parts of the body exposed to leather thus tanned.

Modern technology has multiplied the number of chemical substances used in preparing fabrics. Some people become sensitive to certain dyes. Durable press finishes cause trouble in other

POISON IVY AND POISON OAK

Some persons develop a serious inflammation of the skin after contact with the leaves of poison ivy or poison oak. The affected area of the skin becomes inflamed, swollen, and, in the early stages, covered with tiny blisters. The area itches intensely. The substance causing this skin reaction is a waxy or resinous material which can be dissolved by strong soapsuds or rendered harmless by strong oxidizing agents. Extracts of poison ivy or poison oak have been prepared for use as vaccines. These have proved beneficial in some cases, but not in all.

Care and Treatment

If contact with the offending substance is recognized within a few minutes, much of the poison can be removed or destroyed by washing the endangered skin areas with strong soapsuds or by bathing them in a salt solution or a solution of Epsom salt (1 tablespoonful of table salt or 1 tablespoonful of Epsom salt to the quart of water).

During the stage of blisters and oozing, use cold (never hot) wet dressings as much of the time as practicable. For the dressings, use 8 to 10 layers of gauze, fluffed and crumpled, then wet with one or the other of the following solutions: (1) saturated solution of aluminum acetate (Burow's solution) diluted 1 to 15, (2) saturated solution of magnesium sulfate (Epsom salt), or (3) 1 percent solution of zinc sulfate. Apply the wet dressings over the entire affected skin areas; cover with waxed paper, oiled silk, or plastic to keep in the moisture; and bind on snuggly with bandages. The dressings should be kept wet, and the room kept warm enough to protect the patient from chilling.

When the blisters have dried and the oozing ceased, apply 1 percent phenol in calamine lotion three times a day.

As a preventive measure, before going places where poison ivy or poison oak grows, apply to the skin a vanishing cream to which 5 percent of sodium perborate powder has been added. If you must stay in such a place very long, wash away the medicated cream and make a fresh application about every three hours.

ATOPIC DERMATITIS (ECZEMA)

Atopic dermatitis has some resemblance to contact dermatitis and some to skin diseases caused by allergy. It consists of an inflammatory reaction in the skin characterized by itching, burning, and redness. Its severity and its particular manifestations vary from person to person. It occurs in persons who have inherited a type of hypersensitive skin. It is most likely to occur during either infancy, childhood, or young adulthood. It may occur for the first time in any one of these three periods.

Specific information on this skin disease, including the treatment in each of the three age groups, is given in chapter 17, volume 1.

EXFOLIATIVE DERMATITIS (ERYTHRODERMA)

Exfoliative dermatitis is a serious, even life-threatening skin involvement which usually occurs as a complication of other illnesses. It consists of a scaling of the skin in which the superficial layer of the skin of almost the entire body is lost. This loss of the skin's protective layer increases the body's water loss and introduces the possibility of infection. Exfoliative dermatitis may follow a drug reaction, such skin diseases as atopic dermatitis or psoriasis, or systemic illnesses such as leukemia or lymphoma. About one third of cases end fatally. Survivors usually recover in about nine months.

Care and Treatment

The patient should be placed in a hospital. The first attempt is to discover and treat the possible underlying cause. The patient's discomfort can be partially relieved by the application to the skin of emollient ointments and by the use of starch or oatmeal baths. Corticosteroid medications by mouth may be life saving in severe cases.

SEBORRHEIC DERMATITIS

Seborrheic dermatitis is a common scaling disease which affects areas of the skin in which there are large sebaceous (oil-producing) glands. The scalp is the area primarily and most commonly affected, and here the scales are recognized as dandruff. Other skin areas that may be affected in the more severe cases include the face, neck, chests, armpits, groin, and genital regions.

When seborrheic dermatitis affects areas other than the scalp, the eruption is characterized by oily crusts instead of dry scales. The skin beneath the crusts is thickened and mildly inflamed. The only unpleasant sensation is that of itching.

A hereditary tendency, hormone imbalance, unfavorable nutritional status, and emotional stress are possible causative factors. Seborrheic dermatitis tends to persist for a matter of years, though it may occur in successive attacks, each lasting possibly weeks or years.

Care and Treatment

For dandruff on the scalp shampoo three times a week for four weeks— afterward once a week until a satisfactory cure is accomplished. Once a week at bedtime, after a shampoo, apply Pragmatar ointment, which contains salicylic acid and sulfur and is available at any drugstore. Next morning, wash away all traces of the ointment with mild soap and warm water, massaging the scalp well. After the washing and massage, rub into the scalp a little of the following lotion:

Phenol		5
Castor Oil	1	5
Salicylic acid	2	
Alcohol, 70% q.s.ad.	120	

CAUTION: *This preparation, which contains salicylic acid, should not be used by a person who has diabetes.*

For oily dandruff, proceed as above but make the morning washing brief and avoid all massage. Though the condition is not primarily infectious, germs may be present and may make the condition worse, so sterilize the comb at least once a week. Use no hairbrush, because a hairbrush cannot be sterilized.

When the skin of the face or the body is affected, on alternate nights at bedtime, rub into the involved skin a 5 percent sulfur ointment. On the in-between nights, apply lotio alba.

For those cases which do not respond to the above procedures, the physician may recommend the use of a cream containing a corticosteroid medication.

STASIS DERMATITIS

Stasis dermatitis involves a deterioration of the skin of the legs, in which the skin itches, becomes reddened, is susceptible to minor injuries, and heals slowly with scarring and brown pigmentation following such injuries. This ailment is the result of a slackening of the flow of blood through the veins of the legs. The condition usually develops slowly over a period of years, often as a consequence of varicose veins or thrombophlebitis. In the more extreme cases, the skin actually breaks down with ulcer formation as described in Section L of the present chapter.

Care and Treatment

Avoid standing in one position for long periods of time. When seated, elevate the legs to the level of the hips. In stubborn cases, elevate the foot of the bed about four inches above the level of the head of the bed to facilitate the return of blood from the legs during sleep. If the veins of the legs are prominent, use an elastic bandage or elastic hose to minimize the stagnation of blood in these veins.

Engage in exercise requiring the use of the legs as the general condition permits. Use leg baths with contrasting hot and cold water (three minutes of hot followed by a few seconds of cold, then repeat, up to 15 minutes per treatment) two or three times per day. Take precautions against bumps and injuries to the skin of the legs.

C. Bacterial Infections

The normal skin is an important barrier to protect the body's deeper tissues from invasion by disease-producing germs. But the skin is a living tissue, and sometimes it becomes infected by germs. Several kinds of germs can involve the skin, but the ones usually responsible for skin infections are the staphylococci and the streptococci. The seriousness of bacterial infections of the skin varies all the way from incidental, relatively harmless infections to those so serious as to threaten life. The types of germ causing the infection and the resistance of the individual in whom the infection occurs are variables which determine how serious the infection is.

FOLLICULITIS

Folliculitis consists of an infection with pustule formation involving one or more hair follicles. The infection is caused by a staphylococcus germ. It is most common in men and tends to involve the bearded area of the skin, but may attack any area in which hair follicles are present. The skin around the affected follicles becomes reddened and crusted. Symptoms are not usually acute, being limited to mild burning and itching, with pain only when an involved hair is pulled. Contamination of other skin areas by pus from a pustule is likely to lead to infection of other hair follicles. If not properly treated, folliculitis may become chronic and persist for months or even years.

Care and Treatment

Gentle cleansing of the affected area with an antiseptic solution such as is available at the drugstore may prevent the spread of the infection. The use of an antibiotic cream, such as Neosporin-G, applied to the affected skin may help to control the infection. In persistent cases, it may be necessary for the physician to determine just what type of germ is causing the infection and then prescribe an appropriate antibiotic to be taken by mouth.

BOILS (FURUNCLES)

A boil is a hard, red, painful, localized infection which usually begins in relation to an infected hair follicle and may thus be considered as a complication of folliculitis. A boil tends to in-

crease in size and develop a core in its center. As is true in folliculitis, a boil is caused by a staphylococcus germ. The core of a boil consists of a collection of innumerable bacteria surrounded by and interspersed with white blood cells. This core tends to soften and form thick liquid pus, which eventually escapes when the boil ruptures. When this occurs, the pus, containing living germs, tends to spread the infection and cause other boils if it comes in contact with unprotected skin.

There is danger in squeezing or picking at a boil. The collection of germs in the forming core may be broken up and spread into the surrounding tissues, thus making the boil larger than otherwise. The germs may even spread into the bloodstream, causing septicemia.

The most dangerous spot for a boil to be located is the area marked out by the bridge of the nose, the corners of the mouth, and the outer corners of the eyes. This area includes the inside of the nostrils. Cases of fatal septicemia or meningitis have resulted from the squeezing of boils or pimples in this area.

In some cases, boils tend to recur, with new lesions developing even while the older ones are in the process of

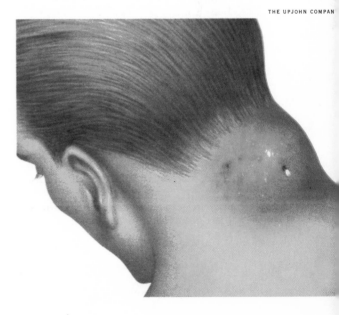

healing. In such instances, the infection is either spread by allowing the infected pus from the original boil to contaminate other skin areas, or else the individual's body contains a reservoir of infection from which the germs are spread by the bloodstream to other skin areas. This turn of events requires investigation by the physician as he searches out the possible source of the germs causing the problem. In some instances an unrecognized condition of diabetes favors the development of recurrent boils. The doctor should therefore check for this possibility.

Care and Treatment

The skin that covers the center of a boil tends to soften and then to rupture, allowing the pus contained at the center of the boil to escape. Once this occurs, the pain is relieved and healing occurs. It is helpful to hasten the process by treating the boil several times a day with warm, moist compresses consisting of several thicknesses of gauze wrung out of hot water or a hot solution of table salt or Epsom salts. The use of these warm compresses will shorten the time until the boil "points" and discharges its contents of pus onto the surface.

Many physicians in caring for a patient with a boil prefer to lance the boil rather than allowing the skin to break in a ragged fashion. This minor surgical procedure of lancing a boil is performed only after the center of the boil has become softened by the accumulation of pus.

For cases in which boils tend to recur, careful attention should be given to preventing the spread of the infection from one skin area to another. Clothing and bedding should be disinfected or boiled before being reused. The physician caring for such a case may prescribe the use of an antibiotic medication as a means of controlling the infection.

CARBUNCLE

A carbuncle may be compared to a multiple boil. It develops in the deeper layer of the skin and in the subcutaneous tissue and is composed of several abscess cavities which connect with one another and which become filled with pus. As with a boil, the surface tissue tends to soften so that the pus can break through at one or more "points." The staphylococcus germ is responsible for such an infection.

Care and Treatment

The person with a carbuncle should be kept quiet so that the defense mechanisms of his body can have the best opportunity to combat the toxemia that results from this type of infection. Warm, moist compresses (as for the treatment of a boil) help to soften the surface tissue so that the pus contained in the underlying abscess cavities can be more readily discharged. As soon as "pointing" occurs, it is time for the physician to make an incision through the surface tissues so as to allow the underlying pus to escape. Antibiotic medication suitable for combating the staphylococcus germ should be administered.

CELLULITIS

Cellulitis is a spreading infection usually caused by the staphylococcus germ which affects the tissues beneath the skin as well as the skin itself. Because it involves the deeper tissues, the borders of the affected area are not distinct. It is particularly serious when it occurs on the face or in a person who has diabetes. The germs usually gain entrance through a break in the skin. Usually the lymph nodes which serve the affected area of the body become enlarged and tender. The affected skin is hot, red, and painful. Without proper treatment, the condition is persistent and tends to recur even after the infection subsides.

Care and Treatment

The effective treatment consists of the use of a proper antibiotic medication administered by mouth or even by injection. The application of heat to the affected area, plus keeping the part elevated if it involves an extremity, serves to decrease the swelling and reduce the pain.

ERYSIPELAS (SAINT ANTHONY'S FIRE)

Erysipelas is a serious, rapidly spreading infection of the skin and the tissues beneath it. It can be confused with cellulitis; but, by contrast, erysipelas involves the tissues closer to the skin surface, is usually caused by a streptococcus germ, and produces systemic symptoms of general illness, including high fever. The face is the area most commonly involved. The affected area is red, swollen with a glazed appearance, and produces sensations of itching and burning. The swollen area feels firm and hot to the touch and may display small blisters. The involvement tends to spread in all directions from the original site.

Care and Treatment

Erysipelas is a serious illness and deserves prompt and adequate treatment. The patient should be bedfast and under the care of a physician. The application of cold compresses or the intermittent use of an icebag will help to relieve the discomfort. The effective treatment consists of the administration of the proper antibiotic medication, using large doses and continuing the medication for at least two weeks.

ERYTHRASMA

Erythrasma is a skin infection caused by a particular bacterium, *Corynbacterium minutissimum,* which typically occurs in adults in locations where two skin surfaces come in contact, such as the toe webs and the region of the genitalia. Irregular pink patches develop which later become brown and produce a fine scaling of the skin. Erythrasma often occurs in persons who have diabetes mellitus.

Care and Treatment

Erythrasma in mild form usually responds favorably to the use of anti-

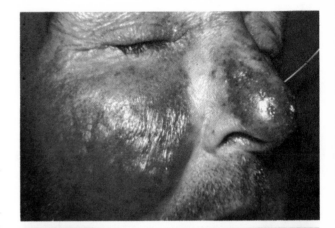
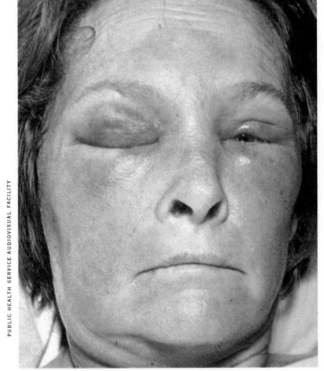

PUBLIC HEALTH SERVICE AUDIOVISUAL FACILITY

Typical manifestations of erysipelas.

bacterial soap. In the more persistent cases, antibiotic medication by mouth clears up the infection.

IMPETIGO

Impetigo is a troublesome, superficial skin infection which may be caused either by streptococci or staphylococci

371

of mild virulence. The disease occurs principally in children. Because of its predilection for children, it is described in chapter 17, volume 1.

D. Fungal Infections

Fungal diseases may attack various tissues of the body, but probably they attack the skin most often. Fungi are a more complex form of vegetable organisms than bacteria. They usually multiply by means of spores. Diseases caused by fungi tend to be persistent. They seldom cause fever or result in true pus formation unless complicated by a secondary bacterial infection.

Generally speaking, the ordinary antibiotic medications are not helpful in treating fungal infections. In fact, fungal infections sometimes develop in persons who have been taking antibiotic medications over a period of time. Fortunately, there is one exception, the antibiotic griseofulvin taken by mouth. Griseofulvin should be taken only under the supervision of a physician because it occasionally produces some uncomfortable side reactions.

We consider here two types of fungal infections of the skin: (1) ringworm infections (the dermatophytosis) and (2) the yeast infections.

1. Ringworm Infections
(Dermatophytosis)

Ringworm infections are especially common among children and they are therefore also discussed in chapter 17, volume 1. They are spread from person to person or from animals (pets) to per-

sons. The infections may be acquired either by direct contact or by contact with infected towels, combs, or other objects in common use. Scratching the lesions tends to spread the infection to other parts of the skin. Ringworm infections are not caused by a worm, as the name would suggest, but by fungi. The name ringworm stems from the observation that the lesions tend to heal at their centers and continue to spread in a widening, ringlike fashion.

ATHLETE'S FOOT (TINEA PEDIS)

This is probably the most common fungal infection of the skin. The organisms which cause athlete's foot are spread from contaminated shoes and from contaminated floors in public places, such as areas surrounding pools. The skin between the toes is most frequently attacked, but the disease may spread to any part of the feet. As the infection develops, blisters and cracks appear in the skin, which softens, turns white, and tends to peel away and flake. Pustules and ulcers may form in severe cases, accompanied by itching and burning—occasionally pain.

The infection can be transferred to the hands by contact with the affected areas of the feet. Usually, however, what appears on the hands is caused by absorbed toxins which circulate in the blood.

Care and Treatment

Most cases respond favorably to local treatment of the affected skin. In a severe case in which the affected skin

Athlete's foot between fourth and fifth toes, the view on the right being the same lesion, only under Wood's light. The orange color fluoresced by the secretion from the organisms identifies the disease.

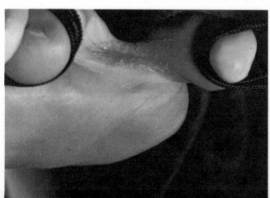
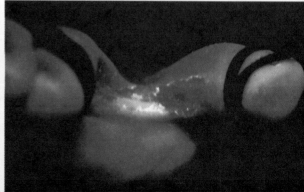

is oozing fluid, wet dressings wrung from a 1:20 dilution of a saturated solution of aluminum acetate (Burrow's solution) may be applied three or four times a day for 15 minutes each time. Loose skin should be removed gently. In all cases one of the following medicated creams should be worked into the affected skin areas night and morning: Halotex cream, Lotrimin cream, or MicaTin cream. In obstinate cases it may become necessary also to use a prescribed medication by mouth: micronized griseofulvin (marketed as Fulvicin P/G tablets). For an adult, a 250 mg. tablet in the morning and again in the evening, continued for four to eight weeks, is the accepted procedure. For a child the dosage is proportionately less. Precautions should be taken to avoid the spread of the infection to other persons.

RINGWORM OF THE SCALP (TINEA CAPITIS)

Ringworm of the scalp appears first as small, round, reddish, scaly spots with blisters. The spots enlarge rapidly, become grayish in color, show definite boundaries, and generally cause loss of hair. Fungal infection of the scalp occurs amost exclusively in children and adolescents. Baldness, when it occurs, is not likely to be permanent.

Care and Treatment

Ringworm of the scalp is best treated by the use of micronized griseofulvin (Grisactin) by mouth continued for at least six weeks. For an adult, a 125 mg. tablet of Fulvicin P/G (micronized griseofulvin) taken in the morning and again in the evening is recommended. For a child, the dosage is proportionately less. When secondary infections develop, appropriate antibiotic medication should be prescribed.

RINGWORM OF THE BODY (TINEA CORPORIS)

Ringworm of the body is a mildly contagious disease which affects the skin of the face, neck, body, arms, and legs. It is characterized by reddened patches, round or irregular in shape, and usually scaly. The patches are pea-sized at first, but grow rapidly. They heal at the center, thus forming rings. The outer edges of the ring consist of tiny papules and a few small blisters. This disease causes no feeling of general illness and only a mild itching.

Care and Treatment

This is treated by the same procedure as recommended above for athlete's foot. When medication by mouth is used it may be usually terminated at the end of three or four weeks.

RINGWORM OF THE BEARD (TINEA BARBAE: BARBER'S ITCH)

Ringworm of the beard begins with an inflammation in and around the hair follicles of the beard. It is more persistent than either ringworm of the scalp or ringworm of the body. Fortunately, it is not a common ailment.

Small superficial nodules appear, which grow and become deep-seated. Inflammation is general over the skin of the affected areas, but more marked over the nodules, which have a tendency to occur in groups. Usually a brittle hair projects from the center of each nodule.

The follicles may discharge thin pus. The disease causes itching and discomfort and is sometimes mildly painful.

Care and Treatment

This is best treated by the use of micronized griseofulvin (Grisactin) by mouth continued for four to six weeks. A 250 mg. tablet of Fulvicin P/G (micronized griseofulvin) in the morning and again in the evening is recommended. A 10 percent ammoniated mercury ointment may be applied to the affected skin twice daily. The beard may be clipped during the period of treatment, but all instruments should be sterilized after each use.

RINGWORM OF THE GROIN (TINEA CRURIS; JOCK OR CROTCH ITCH)

Ringworm of the groin manifests itself as brownish-red scaly patches with tiny blisters at the spreading edges. It affects the inner surfaces of the upper thighs and the genital and anal areas. Heat, moisture, profuse sweating, and chafing by clothing are aggravating factors. There is mild itching or smarting.

Care and Treatment

Treatment is the same procedure as recommended above for athlete's foot. When medication is used by mouth, it may usually be terminated at the end of three or four weeks.

RINGWORM OF THE NAILS (TINEA UNGUIUM)

This fungal infection causes the nails (either fingernails or toenails) to become thickened, brittle, broken, white, and often ridged. It seldom causes pain, itching, or other discomfort. Frequently, only one nail is affected.

Care and Treatment

This is a persistent infection and may require continuous treatment over a period of many months. The preferred medication (prescribed by a physician) is Fulvicin P/G tablets. For an adult the dosage is two 250 mg. tablets taken in the morning and again in the evening.

2. Yeast Infections

CANDIDIASIS (MONILIASIS)

Candidiasis is an infection caused by the yeast organism *Candida albicans*. The skin areas most commonly involved by this infection are the corners of the mouth, fingernail folds, body folds, and the regions around the anus or vagina. The affected areas become red, raw, and beefy in appearance, but may have whitish, curdlike deposits on their surfaces. There may be mild burning sensations and itching. Warmth and moisture make the condition worse.

The *Candida albicans* is the same organism that causes thrush in the mouths of babies. It may also affect the mucus membranes of the digestive tract or those of the interior of the vagina in debilitated people or those who have been taking antibiotics by mouth for a long period of time. Obese people, those who sweat freely, and those who have diabetes mellitus are particularly susceptible to this infection.

Care and Treatment

Certain fungicidal preparations usually prove effective in the treatment of candidiasis. These contain nystatin (Mycostatin or Nystaform) or amphotericin B (Fungizone).

TINEA VERSICOLOR

Tinea versicolor is a curious skin ailment which typically affects young adults who perspire freely. The lesions are small, rounded, velvety flat spots which appear on the chest, shoulders, armpits, and abdomen. It is caused by a yeast organism which has an unusual effect on the pigment-producing cells of the affected areas. Thus the flat spots contain less pigment than the surrounding skin areas. This contrasting color is particularly noticeable in the summertime or whenever normal tanning occurs, for the flat spots caused by this disease do not tan. The lesions itch slightly; and when scratched, slight scaling occurs.

Care and Treatment

The affected area of skin should be washed vigorously twice a day with soap and warm water. After thorough drying, a 20 percent solution of sodium thiosulfate is applied to the affected area and allowed to dry. Tinver lotion is a commercial preparation that may be used in place of the sodium thiosulfate solution.

E. Parasitic Infections

Parasites such as the itch mite and the several kinds of lice, when they gain access to the human skin, damage the skin and cause tremendous itching. The infestations tend to persist if untreated. Furthermore, the ready pos-

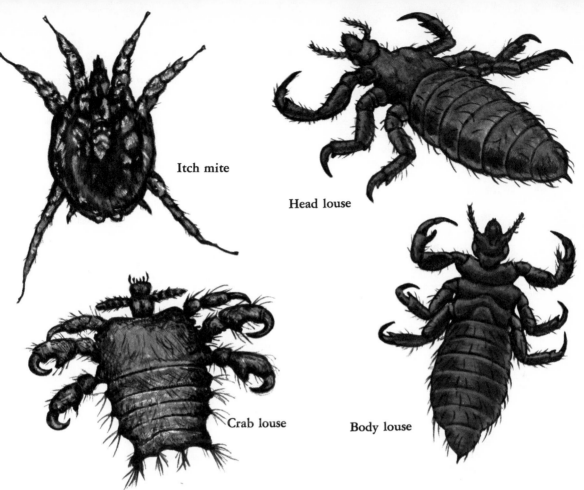

Itch mite

Head louse

Crab louse

Body louse

sibility exists that the parasites will be transmitted to other persons through contaminated bedclothing and wearing apparel.

SCABIES (THE ITCH)

Scabies is a contagious skin disease caused by the itch mite, which bores beneath the surface of the skin, forming burrows. The disease is characterized by intense itching, especially at night, and by a form of eczema caused by scratching. The mite is yellowish white and barely large enough to be seen by the unaided eye. The female, typically larger than the male, burrows into the skin to lay its eggs. The burrow may be either straight or crooked, is an eighth of an inch (3 mm.) or more in length and looks somewhat like a very narrow and light pencil mark.

The itch mite prefers the tenderest parts of the skin, such as the webs between the fingers; the inner surfaces of the forearms, thighs, and legs; the armpits, the breasts; the buttocks; and the navel. When one member of a family is infested, other members are likely to become so.

Severe inflammation, with the development of papules, blisters, pustules, and crusts, may come as a result of infection from scratching. The disease may become fully developed within two weeks; the eggs hatch in about six days, and the parasites grow very rapidly. The infestation may persist for months or even years if not recognized and properly treated. It is transmitted by body contact with others suffering from it or by sleeping in an infested bed or wearing infested clothing.

Care and Treatment

Usually, by the time scabies is recognized for what it is, the afflicted person has scratched the skin so much in some places that it has be-

come infected with ordinary bacteria. In caring for such a case the first effort must be to treat this ordinary infection. For this purpose, Neosporin ointment rubbed into the affected skin four or five times a day is the remedy of choice.

The treatment of the scabies as such requires that a precise routine be followed for the double purpose of killing the itch mites that still reside in the patient's skin and also of killing those that may be lying dormant in the patient's clothing and bed linen. The procedure is as follows:

1. Every night for three nights apply an ointment (to be specified below) to the entire body from the level of the mouth and earlobes downward. Make sure that all areas of the skin receive an application of the ointment. Apply it beneath the fingernails and toenails and on the skin of the genital area. Two suitable ointments for this purpose are Eurax and Kwell.

2. Use the same underclothes, nightclothes, and sheets throughout the three- to five-day course of the treatment.

3. The first night, before applying the ointment, scrub the entire body with soap and warm water. Each night, apply new ointment without washing off the old ointment. If it is impossible to leave the ointment in place during the daytime, wash it off each morning, but continue the treatment for five nights instead of three.

4. The next night following the nights of the treatment, take a thorough hot bath and change to clean sheets, clean nightclothes, and clean underclothes for the next day. All clothes used before and during the treatment should be disinfected by drycleaning, or by washing in cleaning solvent, or by sending them to a laundry, or by boiling them before placing them in the clothes washer.

5. After completing the course of ointment treatment, apply to the skin a 1 percent phenol in calamine lotion four or five times a day. This is for the purpose of soothing the skin.

6. One week after completing the treatment program, if it seems that the condition is not entirely cleared up, repeat the treatment with ointment as described above.

HEAD LICE (PEDICULOSIS CAPITIS)

In this condition a particular kind of louse *Pediculus humanus capitis,* establishes itself at the base of the hairs of the scalp. This louse is dark in color and large enough to be seen with the unaided eye. During the short space of six days, a female head louse can lay as many as 50 eggs. These are glued to the hair shafts and can be seen easily, being white in color. The eggs hatch in three to eight days, and the young lice are able to reproduce within two weeks. Infestation is spread from one person to another by personal contact or by the wearing of infested headgear.

The presence of head lice on the scalp causes severe itching. Continuous scratching of the infested area causes the oozing of fluid, watery at first but later pussy or bloody. This fluid dries and forms crusts, which remain sticky and mat the hair and give off an offensive odor.

Care and Treatment

1. Shampoo the scalp with an ordinary shampoo preparation to remove oil and dirt. Rinse thoroughly. Then apply Kwell shampoo and rub vigorously for four minutes. Rinse thoroughly and dry.

2. Comb the hair with a fine-toothed comb to remove all remaining ova (nits). Brushes and combs should be treated with Kwell shampoo after each use.

3. Shampoo the scalp again, as above, in seven days.

4. If the scalp becomes infected with ordinary bacteria, the physician should prescribe an antibiotic medication to control the infection.

BODY LICE (PEDICULOSIS CORPORIS)

A body louse, *Pediculis humanus*

corporis, is slightly larger than a head louse and is usually grayish in color. It lives in the seams of the underclothing most of the time, particularly in the regions of the back, the chest, and the waistline, laying its eggs there. The eggs hatch in about six days, the young being ready to reproduce in about two weeks. They invade the skin of the body only when they wish to feed.

The presence of body lice causes severe itching. If the clothing has recently been changed, the lice may be hard to find on the body. However, the itching, the bloody streaks which result from scratching, and the location of these are enough to indicate the nature of the condition. The lice can usually be discovered in the seams of underclothing that has been worn for a few days. The infestation is spread by body contact, by wearing infested clothing or by sleeping in an infested bed. In addition to their damage to the skin, body lice are known to transmit several infectious diseases.

Care and Treatment

1. Do not sleep in underwear worn during the daytime. Underwear, hose, and bedclothes that will not be harmed by boiling should be boiled for ten minutes in soapsuds. Pressing the seams of clothing with a hot iron will kill many of the lice and their eggs.

2. Every seven days until the condition is cured, lather the entire body for four minutes in a shower with Kwell shampoo. Rinse very thoroughly at the end of the four minutes.

3. If the skin continues to be inflamed, the physician may prescribe antibiotic medication or ointments.

CRAB LICE (PEDICULOSIS PUBIS)

The crab louse, *Phthirus pubis,* is smaller than either the head louse or the body louse, is translucent in appearance, is nearly round in form, and usually infests the hair-covered part of the pubic region. The bite of this louse causes a sensation like a sharp pin-prick. It produces intense itching and often a skin eruption, which may become severe enough to resemble eczema. The infestation is spread by body contact as a rule—most often at the time of sexual intercourse—though sometimes by means of infested toilet seats.

Care and Treatment

1. Shave or clip the hair from the infested region, then burn this hair.

2. Wash the area daily with soap and warm water. After washing, apply Kwell lotion each morning for three mornings. This kills the nits by dissolving them off the hair stumps.

3. Other persons who may have been exposed should be treated in the same manner. Clothing, toilet seats, and bedsheets should be sterilized.

4. If the skin continues to be inflamed, apply Eurax ointment.

F. Viral Infections

HERPES SIMPLEX

Herpes simplex is caused by the herpes simplex virus, of which there are two types, Type I and Type II. The herpes simplex viruses are transmitted from one person to another by close personal contact. The symptoms, when they occur, appear between two and twenty days (average of six days) after the virus enters.

The illness occurring when the virus first enters a person's tissues is called primary herpes simplex. Later manifestations are caused by a reactivation of the virus which has remained latent in this person's tissues since the time it first entered. These are called recurrent herpes simplex.

a. *Primary herpes Simplex.* Primary herpes simplex may affect the skin or the membranes of any part of the body. It is an approximate rule that involvements occurring above the waist are caused by Type I virus, while those below the waist and those involving the hands and fingers are caused by Type

II virus. Type I virus may affect the lining of the mouth, the skin around the mouth, the eyes (even involving the cornea), or the skin of the body (above the waist). In some serious cases it may even produce encephalitis. Type II virus affects the delicate tissues of the genital organs of either male or female. The illness caused by Type II virus is called genital herpes simplex and is considered specifically in chapter 31 of this volume.

Primary herpes simplex is ordinarily a self-limited involvement with a short duration of perhaps two weeks. It is typically characterized by the appearance of tiny blisters on the membranes or skin. But it may produce no symptoms and thus pass unnoticed. Even so, the body produces antibodies in response to this primary infection.

b. *Recurrent Herpes Simplex*. The herpes simplex virus, once it enters a person's tissues, survives there for the rest of life. After the primary manifestation, the virus remains latent, only to produce recurring symptoms from time to time from then on. There are several conditions which may set the stage for recurring attacks. For the lesions that occur on the lips or around the face, an overexposure to sunlight or a stretching of the tissues around the mouth such as may occur when a dentist repairs a tooth may be a sufficient stimulus to cause reactivation. Undue emotional stress or some systemic disease which reduces the individual's general resistance may cause a recurrent attack.

Cold Sores (Fever Blisters). Lesions which occur from time to time on the lips and exposed parts of the face are caused by a reactivation of the Type I virus. The lesions consist of small vesicles which develop on a slightly inflamed base. Within a few days these form a yellowish crust and usually disappear within about ten days.

Care and Treatment

Inasmuch as herpes simplex is caused by a virus, there is no specific cure. Medical researchers are still trying to find some medication that will rid the body of the virus.

For cold sores (fever blisters) the use of some drying lotion or spirits of camphor applied to the lesions may be of some help. In any case in which the lesions become secondarily infected with ordinary germs, the infection should be treated by the use of antibiotic medications. Persons subject to recurrent attacks of cold sores on the lips and face will do well to protect the skin of the area by the use of a sunscreen ointment.

VIRAL TUMORS OF THE SKIN

1. *Common Warts (Verruca)*. Warts are caused by viruses. They appear most frequently in the early years of life and may persist for years. They are firm, possibly elevated, sharply demarcated tumors, $1/16$ to $3/8$ inch (2 to 10 millimeters) in diameter, which may or may not be pigmented. They commonly appear on the hands and may develop on other areas, including the neck and eyelids.

2. *The Plantar Wart (Verruca Plantaris)*. The plantar wart, occurring on the sole of the foot, is among the most distressing of warts because of pain when compressed by the body's weight. Plantar warts often occur in groups, and their removal is followed by two or three weeks of discomfort as healing takes place slowly.

Care and Treatment

The most satisfactory treatment for common warts is by the use of the electric needle or by freezing the wart. Such procedures are simple and are performed easily in the doctor's office. For larger warts and, particularly, for plantar warts, the surgical removal by a physician is the best procedure.

3. *Genital Warts (Condylomata Acuminatum)*. Genital warts are caused by a virus and are usually trans-

mitted by sexual contact. They develop in one to six months after exposure and occur most commony on the moist surfaces of the genital areas in males and females. They may be skin-colored or gray, and the lesions may occur separately or in a compound accumulation. Treatment by a physician consists either of the repeated application of a 25 percent tincture of podophyllum (which must be handled with great caution) or by the use of electrocautery. In very severe cases it may be necessary to remove the involved area of skin by a surgical procedure.

G. Disorders of Hair Follicles and Sebaceous Glands

ACNE VULGARIS

Acne vulgaris is a troublesome skin ailment which occurs commonly during the adolescent years of life. This skin disease is therefore discussed in chapter 26, volume 1.

ROSACEA (ACNE ROSACEA)

Rosacea is a chronic skin ailment in which prominent areas of the face appear flushed. It is not a life-threatening disease but a cosmetic problem. The color varies from pink to a deep red to a purplish red. The areas affected are the nose, cheeks, brow, and chin. Except in severe cases, the affected area of the skin is cool to the touch and fades easily under pressure. There may develop a permanent enlargement of the blood capillaries in the skin. Dimples, plaques, and thickening of the skin may appear in the more advanced cases, which accounts for the comparison with acne as indicated by the synonym acne rosacea. The ailment is most common in women between the ages of 30 and 50; but when it occurs in men, the skin of the nose may thicken, causing the nose to appear distorted.

The exact cause of rosacea is unknown, but it is observed that agents such as alcoholic drinks, which dilate the blood vessels of the skin, serve to aggravate the condition.

Care and Treatment

A 5 percent precipitated sulfur ointment applied to the affected skin area one or two times a day is helpful. A more specific treatment requires the supervision of a physician and consists of the use of one of the tetracycline antibiotic medications in moderately heavy dosage for about one month, following which the dosage is gradually reduced to a smaller amount, administered each day and continued indefinitely, such as is sufficient to control the flushing of the skin. In severe cases in which the skin becomes thick the physician may find it advisable to pare away the overgrown tissue, thus allowing the surface layer of the skin to regenerate in normal fashion.

BALDNESS, FALLING HAIR (ALOPECIA)

There are about 100,000 hair follicles in the scalp of a young adult. The number of follicles decreases with age. Hair follicles pass through functional cycles, with an active phase in which hair is produced continuously for about four years and a resting phase of about four months during which the hair is shed. Following the resting phase, a new hair grows from the same follicle. Of course the functional cycles of the various hair follicles are staggered so that at all times the majority of hair follicles are in their functional phases. A person normally loses up to 100 scalp hairs per day as this many follicles reach their resting phases.

The rate of loss of hair from the scalp increases under certain conditions: following childbirth; following a high fever, major illness, or a surgical procedure; following blood loss or severe emotional stress; as a result of taking certain drugs; and in some cases of thyroid disease, cancer, and diabetes.

Progressive thinning of the scalp hair is very common in men and occurs also in women about 15 to 20 years later than in their male relatives. The timing and extent of baldness depend in large part upon hereditary factors.

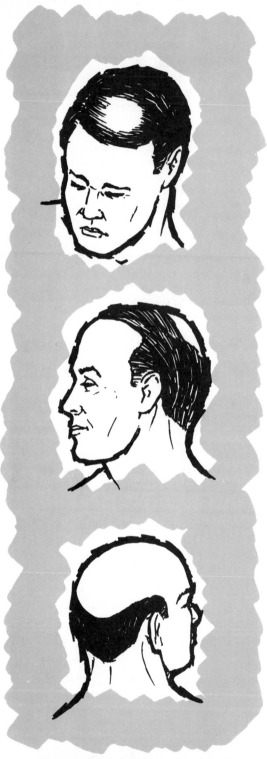

Development pattern of common male baldness: First, hair recedes from forehead and becomes thin around the crown (top and center); then the two balding areas merge (bottom), leaving a fringe.

Dealing with Baldness

Baldness, as it occurs in some people, is a progressive thing, with no remedy. Many commercial preparations and certain procedures such as injections, radiation, and physical treatments are promoted as cures for baldness. None of these are effective except as they may involve massaging the scalp, which increases the circulation of blood through these tissues and may delay the baldness. No foods or vitamins have specific stimulating effects on the growth of hair.

Sutured hairpieces and fiber implantation are sometimes promoted as means of restoring hair to the scalp area. In each of these procedures a foreign substance is actually introduced into the living tissue of the scalp. Thus a real danger of infection threatens, which can become destructive to the scalp tissues, with the final result of scar formation. Probably the only satisfactory procedure for restoring hair to a bald area is by the surgical procedure of hair transplantation, in which tiny plugs of hair-bearing skin are taken from the rear scalp and transplanted to the bald area. The procedure requires about 200 such plugs to be transplanted to the receding hairline. When the transplantation is properly performed, most of the plugs of hair-bearing skin grow into their new location, and each plug bears perhaps three or more hairs.

ALOPECIA AREATA

Alopecia areata is a condition in which a spotty loss of hair occurs, so that oval or round areas are devoid of hair. Usually the hairless areas appear in the scalp, but in 10 percent of cases hairless areas appear on other parts of the body. In a minority of cases of alopecia areata affecting the scalp, the hairless areas enlarge until the entire scalp becomes bald. Recovery occurs in many cases, but the condition remains permanent in about one fourth of those affected.

The precise cause of alopecia areata is vague, but it often occurs in association with emotional stress, some forms of anemia, Addison's disease, ovarian failure, and diabetes. Curiously, when regrowth of hair in these bald areas takes place, the new hair may be white or gray.

Care and Treatment

The treatment of alopecia areata consists of attempting to find and remove the basic cause. It is observed, however, that in some cases hair will regrow in the affected areas within a few weeks even though no treatment is given, whereas in other cases the condition persists in spite of all attempts at treatment. Corticosteroid ointments are helpful in some cases.

H. Scaling Papular Diseases

PITYRIASIS ROSEA

Pityriasis rosea is a mild, self-limited, harmless skin disorder which occurs typically in young adults and for which there is no known cause and no urgent requirements for treatment. It is characterized by the appearance, usually on the trunk, of a single "herald" patch, oval in shape, salmon-colored, and slightly raised, with a firm, wrinkled, "cigarette paper" scale. The herald patch may be more than one inch (2.5 cm.) in its longest diameter. It is followed in a few days by the development on the body and often on the arms of similar but smaller lesions. Itching is troublesome in some cases. The larger patches may clear in their centers so that the lesions then appear ring-shaped.

Care and Treatment

There is no specific treatment for pityriasis rosea. The lesions usually disappear within six to eight weeks. To relieve the itching, starch baths (2 cups of starch to a tub of bathwater) may be used. Moderate exposure of the involved skin areas to sunlight may hasten recovery.

LICHEN PLANUS

Lichen planus is a skin disease characterized by an eruption which consists of violaceous, flat-topped polygonal papules with little or no observable scale. The lesions occur singly or in patches and appear chiefly on the flexor surfaces of the wrists; on the ankles, genitals, and lips; and on the mucous membranes of the mouth or vagina. In some cases the eruption may become generalized, but the face and scalp are rarely attacked. The outcropping of the eruption is usually symmetrical on the two sides of the body. Sometimes the mucous membranes only are affected. Spots on the mucous membranes are characteristically covered with a lacy network of white lines. The disease occurs most commonly in persons above 30 years of age.

Although the onset is sometimes gradual and the course chronic, in the typical acute phase of the disease the patient usually experiences a general feeling of illness immediately before the skin lesions appear. Then within one or two days the eruption is complete. The slightly raised, red or light-purplish spots usually cause intense itching.

The exact cause of lichen planus is unknown, but the illness often occurs in persons who have been under mental or physical strain or who are in a general run-down condition.

Care and Treatment

Measures for improving the patient's general health are indicated. For the mild cases, soothing baths to which Aveeno meal has been added are helpful. The use of soothing lotions and ointments applied directly to the affected skin may give some relief from the itching. Application to the skin of triamcinolone or betamethasone creams are also helpful.

For the severe cases with extensive involvement, the use of corticosteroid medication under a physician's supervision is indicated.

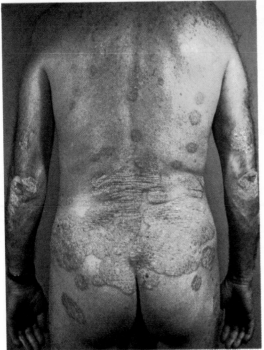
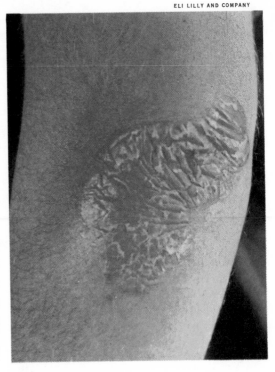

Reddish patches characteristic of psoriasis.

PSORIASIS

Psoriasis is a serious, chronic, relapsing skin ailment in which the involved skin areas produce enormous numbers of silvery scales. The areas usually affected are the skin of the elbows, knees, back, buttocks, and the scalp. The lesions consist of large red plaques covered with overlapping, shiny scales which are shed continuously.

It is estimated that no less than six million people in the United States are troubled with psoriasis in one degree or another. In about one half million, the disease is of a severe, incapacitating degree. In about 5 percent of cases there is an associated arthritis in which the joints of the fingers and toes and also those of the spine become painful.

The fundamental cause of psoriasis is vague. It appears that heredity is a factor in about one third of cases. The essential alteration in the skin is an overproduction of cells in the epidermis. The cells composing this surface layer of the skin are normally shed continuously at such a rate that the average life of a cell is about 28 days. In psoriasis the cells are produced and shed so rapidly that the average life of a cell is only three or four days. Taking this difference into consideration, the modern methods of treatment involve the use of strong chemical substances which inhibit the production of new cells. The ordinary drugs available at the drugstore are usually not effective in the treatment of psoriasis.

Acute attacks of psoriasis usually end spontaneously but with the probability that the ailment will recur later. The effective treatments bring only temporary relief, for no method assures a complete cure of the ailment.

The number of persons with psoriasis is so great and the disease is so persistent that a National Psoriasis Foundation has been formed with headquarters at Suite 250, 6415 S.W. Canyon Court, Portland, OR 97221.

This organization has literature available for those who make requests. Another helpful pamphlet entitled "You, Your Dermatologist and Psoriasis" may be obtained from the American Academy of Dermatology, 2250 N.W. Flanders St., Portland, OR 97210.

The severity of the illness varies a great deal from person to person. It cannot be known, in the early phase of the illness, just how severe it is going to be in a certain case. It is advisable to consult a physician early, however, even though the skin problem may not be very severe. Early in the course of the disease it is best to use the simpler forms of treatment, preserving the use of the strong medications for the future, if needed.

Care and Treatment

Give attention to building up and maintaining the patient's general health by obtaining adequate rest each 24 hours; by using a simple, nutritious diet; by taking care of other health problems; by following a program of conservative outdoor recreation; and by developing a mental attitude of confidence and courage.

Each day remove the scales from the affected skin areas by using soap and water and a soft brush. Following this daily cleansing, apply an ointment such as the doctor may prescribe. The following prescription serves satisfactorily as an ointment:

Sol. coal tar	**12**
Zinc oxide	**24**
Starch	**24**
Glycerine	**36**
Water q.s.ad.	**120**

For the more severe, obstinate cases, a dermatologist (physician who specializes in diseases of the skin) should be consulted. He may recommend and supervise some of the more potent medications that can be applied directly to the skin, or in stubborn cases he may use such medications as the antimetabolites or the systemic corticosteroids. These often **produce troublesome side effects, and their use must be professionally supervised.**

I. Inflammatory Skin Reactions

DRUG ERUPTIONS (DERMATITIS MEDICAMENTOSA)

Some persons develop an eruption of the skin or of the mucous membranes after they have taken a drug either by mouth or by injection. Many of the drugs in common use can cause such a response in persons who happen to be thus reactive. Some persons are reactive to one or more specific drugs, while other persons are reactive to entirely different drugs.

The skin eruptions that may follow

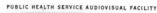

PUBLIC HEALTH SERVICE AUDIOVISUAL FACILITY

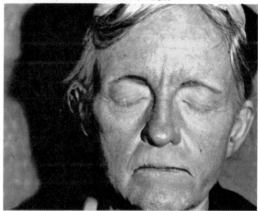

**Above: Rash caused by iodides.
Below: Rash caused by penicillin.**

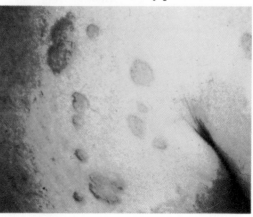

the use of drugs vary in severity from a mild rash to very severe conditions in which the skin is even partially destroyed. Skin eruptions caused by drugs may appear promptly after the taking of the drug, or the eruption may appears hours or even days later. Drug eruptions may appear in just a certain area of the body, as in a case where a drug causes the skin to be sensitive to the exposure to light, or the eruption may be generalized over major portions of the body. The types of skin lesions may resemble those of skin diseases not related to the use of drugs.

Some drug eruptions are caused by allergic mechanisms by which the individual becomes sensitive to a particular drug, such as penicillin. The initial dose of penicillin causes no difficulty. But subsequent doses cause a skin eruption, because in the meantime the body has built up an immunologic sensitivity to this particular drug. In other cases the changes in the skin are caused by the accumulation of a particular drug which now exceeds the tolerance of the person's skin. In still other cases, the skin eruption is caused by the chemical action of the drug itself.

Care and Treatment

The primary consideration in dealing with a skin eruption caused by a drug is to determine what drug has caused the problem. This may be difficult in a person taking several drugs or in a person whose condition of health requires that he continue to take certain drugs. It must be remembered that even a small amount of a drug can cause a skin eruption in a person sensitive to that particular drug. Furthermore, a skin eruption may develop even days after the last dose of a drug to which this person happens to be sensitive.

The practical procedure is for the patient to stop all drugs and medications that he may be taking. With the doctor's cooperation, it can be arranged for him to use alternate drugs if he is dependent for his health on one or more particular drugs.

In some cases of proved drug eruption, further treatment is needed after the drug is discontinued. No simple, general treatment will fit all cases. Many patients will be benefitted by the use of a corticosteroid cream or by a corticosteroid medication, taken either by mouth or by injection. This, of course, must be under a doctor's direction.

ERYTHEMA NODOSUM

Erythema nodosum is an acute skin disease, marked by tender red nodules which appear in successive crops, usually on the front surfaces of the legs but sometimes on the forearms, accompanied by intense itching and burning sensations. The nodules are from one half inch to two inches (1.2 to 5 cm.) in diameter. Their appearance is often accompanied by mild fever, a general feeling of lack of energy, and rheumatic or joint pains. On careful examination, a patient who develops erythema nodosum will usually be found to have an infection, such as by the streptococcus, in some other part of his body.

Care and Treatment

Bed rest is essential, even while the physician in charge is searching for the source of the infection responsible for this skin involvement. Once the infection causing the skin problem has been discovered, the treatment program is directed toward correcting this infection. The therapy may require the use of an antibiotic medication or whatever other treatment is indicated to combat the underlying disease.

ERYTHEMA MULTIFORME

Erythema multiforme, as the root meaning of the term implies, is characterized by reddish lesions of variable shape. It is an acute, self-limited disease with a tendency to recurrences. It affects all age groups but most commonly young adults. The lesions are about equally distributed on both sides of the body; they may be in a limited area or may be widespread. The lesions occur especially on the backs of the hands and feet, the palms, the soles, and the extensor surfaces of the limbs. The lesions vary all the way from macules and papules of red to purple color to vesicular lesions that may ulcerate.

Erythema multiforme rarely attacks a person in good health. Typically it occurs as an aftermath of some other disorder, especially in association with viral diseases such as those caused by

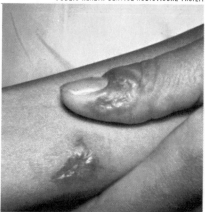

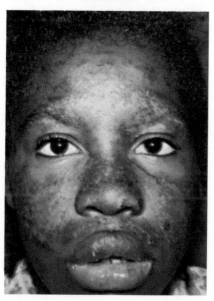

Cases of erythema: Above, erythema multiforme; below, erythema nodosum.

the herpes simplex or sensitivity to certain drugs.

Care and Treatment

In about 50 percent of cases, no specific cause can be found for erythema multiforme. When a cause can be found, primary attention should be given to treating or eliminating it. Otherwise, the treatment should be directed toward easing the patient's discomfort by the use of wet dressings, lukewarm baths, and soothing skin lotions such as calamine lotion. In stubborn cases, the physician may prescribe a corticosteroid medication.

CUTANEOUS LUPUS ERYTHEMATOSUS

Lupus erythematosus is an inflammatory disease of unknown cause. Its manifestations vary a great deal from one case to another. It may affect any organ of the body, either individually or in various combinations. Classically, two forms of the disease are described: (1) cutaneous or discoid lupus erythematosus, which primarily affects the skin and (2) systemic or disseminated lupus erythematosus, which affects the body's organs, one or more.

Only about 5 percent of the cases of cutaneous lupus erythematosus develop into the systemic variety of the disease, but 50 to 80 percent of the cases of systemic lupus erythematosus develop skin involvements at some time during the course of the disease. In the present chapter we are concerned only with the cutaneous type. The systemic type is described in chapter 21 of this volume.

Cutaneous lupus erythematosus is a chronic recurring disorder of the skin which most frequently begins between ages 20 and 30 and is more common in women than in men. The skin lesions are red, rounded, slightly raised, scaly patches which appear typically in a "butterfly" pattern involving the bridge of the nose and the cheeks. Other areas of the face and scalp are often involved. Occasionally the lesions

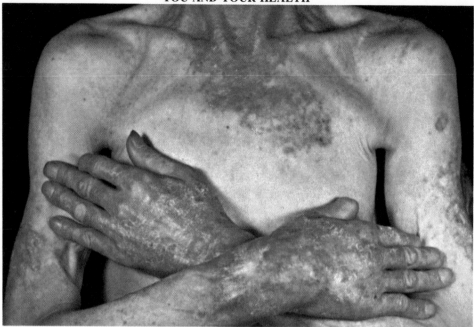

M. COUPERUS, M.D.

Lupus erythematosus.

may appear quite widely distributed over the trunk, arms, and legs. Often the lips and the membranes of the mouth are involved. The lesions tend to spread at their borders and heal at the center. The healing may involve the formation of conspicuous scars. The skin involvement may disappear, sometimes permanently. More commonly, however, it recurs from time to time. The condition is typically aggravated by exposure to sunlight.

Care and Treatment

Lupus erythematosus is a serious disease, and the treatment should be directed by a qualified physician. Excessive exposure to sunlight should be avoided. The patient should use a sunscreen ointment on the exposed portions of the skin whenever he is out of doors. The patient should avoid fatigue and should obtain adequate rest during each 24-hour period. The physician may advise the use of a corticosteroid cream applied to the affected skin areas. Some cases are benefitted by the use of the same medications used to control malaria.

J. Pemphigus

Pemphigus is an uncommon but very serious skin disease. Untreated cases are usually fatal within a few months. It is an autoimmune disease in which the body produces antibodies that bring about serious changes in the structure of the skin. In cases that end fatally, death comes either as a result of infection or of starvation because the involvement of the membranes of the mouth make it difficult to eat. The disease occurs in both men and women of all races. It usually begins after age 40.

Blisters develop on the skin and, in about 60 percent of cases, on the lining of the mouth. The blisters break easily, and the raw areas heal poorly and tend to spread.

Care and Treatment

Modern methods of treatment have greatly reduced the mortality rate and even permit those who develop this disease to continue to lead useful lives. But the medicines used in the treatment are powerful drugs and often produce unpleasant side effects.

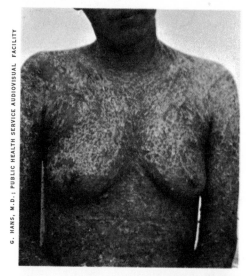

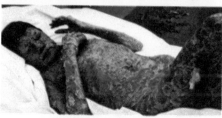

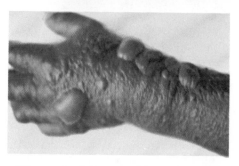

G. HANS, M.D.; PUBLIC HEALTH SERVICE AUDIOVISUAL FACILITY

Characteristic manifestations of
pemphigus.

The treatment program must be modified to suit the individual needs of each patient.

Best results follow when the disease is recognized and treated early. The treatment program, under a doctor's direction, requires the use of several medicines. A corticosteroid taken by mouth is the essential item. The reason for the other medicines is to prevent, as far as possible, the unfa-

vorable side effects of the corticosteroid. Oatmeal or starch baths often make the patient more comfortable. (Stir a cup of cornstarch or powdered oatmeal into the bathwater.) Local applications to the skin with corticosteroid ointments or wet (tapwater) compresses changed every four to six hours may help to heal the acute lesions and soften the crusts.

K. Disorders of Cornification

CHAFING (INTERTRIGO)

The rubbing together of two skin surfaces or friction caused by harsh clothing may cause a skin area to chafe, become red, moist, and raw in appearance. This condition produces smarting and burning sensations. Chafing often affects chubby children and overweight older people. Prevention of chafing by keeping likely skin areas clean, dry, and well powdered is preferable to cure after chafing has occurred.

Care and Treatment

Carefully clean the affected areas with a soft cloth and warm water. Use a small amount of mild soap at first, if necessary, but rinse the area after soap has been used. Dry thoroughly but gently and apply a suitable powder liberally. A powder made of equal parts of talcum and zinc stearate, or of starch and zinc oxide, will be effective. Powder acts as a lubricant and facilitates the movement of skin against skin. If the afflicted person is an infant or a young child, care should be taken to prevent inhalation of any of the powder used, particularly that containing zinc stearate.

CALLUSES AND CORNS

A callus consists of a patch of thickened and hardened epidermis (the surface layer of the skin), caused by long-continued pressure or friction.

A corn is similar to a callus in texture and has similar causes; but while a callus may be found on any one of several

387

ELSTON ROTHERMEL, D.P.M.

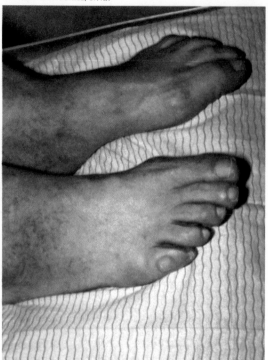

At bedtime apply a bit of the following mixture to the affected area only and cover the area with adhesive tape:

Salicylic acid	3
Lactic acid	3
Flexible collodion q.s.ad.	15

In the morning remove the adhesive and scrape off the softened skin tissue. Continue this procedure night by night until the callus has been reduced to the thickness of normal skin.

For the treatment of a corn, surround the corn with a close-fitting felt ring or corn protector (available at almost any drugstore). On each day, for three to five days, apply to the corn the salicylic acid preparation mentioned above. At the end of the three to five days, soak the foot for 15 minutes in warm water and then try to lift out the corn. If it cannot be completely removed from its bed, continue the application of the salicylic acid preparation for a day or two longer and try once more to remove the corn. If the use of the salicylic preparation causes extreme soreness, discontinue the treatment temporarily and repeat at a later time. If this treatment does not permit the corn to be removed, it may be advisable for it to be removed by a minor surgical procedure at the doctor's office.

different parts of the skin surface, a corn is almost always on a foot, and usually on a toe. A corn is smaller than a callus, and is conical in shape, with the apex of the cone directed inward. A corn produces pain when pressure is applied to its surface.

Care and Treatment

Inasmuch as both calluses and corns are caused by long-continued pressure or friction, the first effort in caring for them should be to relieve the pressure or friction causing them. This may require the wearing of a different kind of shoe or the covering with a circular pad of felt to distribute the pressure over a wider area.

For the immediate treatment of a callus, the application of salicylic acid in one form or another serves to soften and loosen the surface layer of the callus.

Caution: *A preparation which contains salicylic acid should not be used by a person who has diabetes.*

ICTHYOSIS (FISHSKIN DISEASE, XERODERMA)

Ichthyosis is a skin ailment characterized by dryness, roughness, thickness, and scaliness of the skin. The condition appears early in life and seems to run in families. It is therefore considered in detail in chapter 17, volume 1.

L. Ulcers

An ulcer of the skin is a lesion in which an area of skin and a certain amount of underlying tissues has been destroyed. It differs from an ordinary wound in that the vitality of the tissue is less than normal and healing is therefore retarded. Ulcers occur under many circumstances, but the fundamental reasons for the lowered tissue vitality center around a reduction in blood or nerve supply or the presence of infection.

BEDSORE (TROPHIC ULCER, DECUBITUS ULCER)

Bedsores may occur in persons confined to bed or otherwise unable to change the position of their body or some part of the body. The tendency is greatest in persons who have lost the normal skin sensation and who are therefore not impelled to make frequent changes in their position in bed. The ulcer develops because continuous pressure against an area (as from lying too long in the same position or because of a tight-fitting plaster cast) deprives the local tissues of their normal amount of blood. Bedsores occur in locations where parts of the skeleton are close to the skin, as over the bony prominences of the lower back, pelvis, upper part of the hips, and in the vicinity of the ankle. Prevention requires cleanliness of the skin, gentle massage of the vulnerable areas with application of skin lotion or talcum powder, and frequent turning of the patient to new positions in bed.

Care and Treatment

Under favorable conditions, a simple bedsore will heal spontaneously if the pressure causing the ulcer to develop is prevented and the ulcerated area kept clean and dry. For the more persistent and deeper bedsores, it becomes necessary to remove the fragments and strands of dead tissue from the base of the ulcer. This procedure can be aided by the preliminary use of wet dressings of normal salt solution. The devitalized tissue is then removed with forceps and scissors. Karaya gum powder sprinkled sparingly in the wound inhibits the growth of bacteria and thus promotes healing.

In the still more serious cases of bedsore, especially those that involve the layer of fat and underlying muscle tissue, it may become necessary for the surgeon to remove all devitalized tissue and then close the wound by the use of a full thickness skin flap graft. Antibiotic medications are useful for combating secondary infections at the ulcer site.

ULCERS RELATED TO DIABETES

Diabetes is often associated with arteriosclerosis (especially in persons above 40). The reduction of blood supply caused by the arteriosclerosis, plus the reduced vitality of the tissues caused by the diabetes, causes the areas in the most dependent parts of the body (as the feet and the legs) to become susceptible to ulceration. The ulcer usually develops after some local injury, often trivial.

Care and Treatment

Ulcers of the skin occurring in a person who has diabetes require primary attention to the diabetes, along with a careful secondary program of promoting the healing of the ulcer, as described in the previous item on bedsores.

INFECTED ULCERS

When wounds in the skin become infected by germs, the process of healing is retarded and the unhealed area is properly called an ulcer.

STASIS ULCER

In cases of reduced blood supply to the legs a tendency develops for areas of the skin of the leg to become devitalized. This deterioration results in the condition of stasis dermatitis as described earlier in this chapter, page 368. If the condition worsens, the skin breaks down and ulcers form.

Care and Treatment

The first aim is to increase the circulation of blood in the affected leg. This can be accomplished by a graduated program of physical exercise, by the use of gentle massage, or by the use of contrast leg baths, in which the affected leg or both legs are immersed

389

in a tank of hot water (within the patient's temperature tolerance) and
then suddenly immersed in cold
water, the time in the hot water being
three to five times as long as in the
cold water. For details of such treatment, see chapter 25, volume 3.

Other than the above, the treatment of stasis ulcer is the same as that
for bedsore as described in this section.

TROPICAL ULCER

In rural tropical areas ulcers of the
lower leg and foot are quite common.
Some of these are caused specifically
by the germs of yaws or leprosy. Others—the so-called tropical ulcers—
when once established, contain several
kinds of germs, no one of which appears to be actually responsible for the
destruction of tissue. A deficiency of
protein in the diet is an important con-
tributor to the development of tropical
ulcer because of the related reduction
in the vitality of tissues.

TUBERCULOUS ULCER

When a tuberculous abscess, either
of the soft tissues or of the bone,
breaks through to the surface, the resulting lesion is slow to heal, constitut-
ing an ulcer.

VARICOSE ULCER

Ulcers of the lower leg are a common
complication of varicose veins. In varicose veins there is a stagnation of
blood, with consequent reduction of
the vitality of the skin and subcutaneous tissues. See chapter 9, volume 2.

VENEREAL DISEASE ULCER

In syphilis and in chancroid there
usually develops a small ulcer at the
site where the germs of the disease enter the tissues. This site is usually on
the genital organs, although it can be on
other parts. In syphilis this initial ulcer
(the chancre) has a firm, buttonlike
base. By comparison, the initial lesion
in chancroid is soft in consistency.

Skin ulcers may also appear in cases
of untreated syphilis which progress to
the so-called second stage of the disease. See chapter 31, volume 2.

M. Pigmentary Disorders

ALBINISM

Albinism is a curious inherited metabolic disorder in which the skin and the
hair lack the melanin pigment which
skin and hair normally contain. Albinism is said to occur in one of 20,000 individuals. In addition to the lack of pigment in skin and hair, persons with albinism (albinos) have an intolerance for
light because of the lack of pigment
within their eyes. They are predisposed
to the development of skin cancer and
should therefore use sunscreen lotions
to protect the exposed areas of their
skin from the effects of ultraviolet light
when they are out of doors.

VITILIGO (LEUKODERMA)

Vitiligo is a condition in which areas
of the skin lose their normal pigment.
The cause is not known, but vitiligo
does appear more commonly among
relatives of those with this disorder. It
affects about 1 percent of the general
population. It occurs in otherwise normal individuals. When vitiligo affects
different areas of the scalp, the hair in
these areas may or may not lose its pigmentation. The white patches on the
skin are especially subject to sunburn,
and the person with this problem does
well to use sunscreen lotion, not only
to prevent sunburn of the areas which
lack pigment, but also to prevent tanning of the normally pigmented areas
which, if tanned, would make the white
areas more conspicuous.

Care and Treatment

Vitiligo does not endanger a person's general health, but it does constitute a cosmetic blemish. Skin dyes
are now available which, when applied to the depigmented areas of
skin, make them less conspicuous.
Dy-o-derm or Neo-dy-o-derm are
available in light and dark shades.

For large areas of affected skin, such cosmetic preparations as Covermark or Erace may be useful.

GRAY HAIR

Grayness of the hair is usually the natural result of aging, coming from a failure of pigment formation in the hair follicles. Graying of the hair begins at

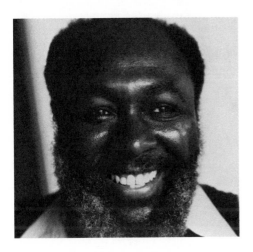

various ages in different family lines. It can result from disturbances of the endocrine system, most frequently those of the thyroid gland.

Concealing Gray Hair. The person who chooses to conceal grayness of the hair by using hair dyes needs to be cautious in what he uses. Dyes which contain silver nitrate, pyrogallic acid, or paraphenylenediamine may be dangerous to the health. Before hair dyes are used, they should be first tested for skin sensitivity in the person to be treated.

FRECKLES (EPHELIDES)

Freckles are considered in chapter 17, volume 1, relating to childhood.

MELASMA (CHLOASMA)

Melasma is characterized by pigmented blotches, brownish in color, which appear in women over the cheekbones, on the forehead, and frequently, on the upper lip.

Melasma often develops during preg-

nancy. It usually disappears a few months after delivering the baby, only to reappear with subsequent pregnancies. It sometimes appears, unrelated to pregnancy, in connection with some disorder of the ovaries. It is seen frequently among women taking birth control pills.

Care and Treatment

No satisfactory method exists for causing the darkened areas to disappear completely. Direct exposure to sunlight should be avoided by the use of sunscreen ointment on the exposed areas of skin. The use of a bleaching cream, such as 2 percent hydroquinone cream (Eldoquin), sometimes makes the blotches less conspicuous. The cream is rubbed into the involved skin areas twice daily. If skin irritation results, the cream should be applied less frequently.

LIVER SPOTS (SENILE LENTIGINES)

Liver spots consist of small darkened areas that appear on exposed areas of skin in middle-aged and elderly persons. They occur in greatest numbers on the back of the hands.

Care and Treatment

There is no completely satisfactory treatment. Protecting the exposed skin from exposure to sunlight is helpful. This can be accomplished by the wearing of gloves or by the use of sunscreen ointment on the exposed areas of skin. The use of a bleaching cream, such as 2 percent hydroquinone cream (Eldoquin), sometimes makes the colored areas less conspicuous. The cream is rubbed into the involved skin areas twice daily. If skin irritation results, the cream should be applied less frequently.

DIFFUSE HYPERPIGMENTATION

Certain systemic disorders such as Addison's disease, as well as the taking of certain drugs, such as the phenothiazine medications, may result in a rather generalized increase in the pigment in the skin.

N. Disorders of Sweating

ANHIDROSIS

Anhidrosis is an absence of sweating even when the body becomes overheated. This unfortunate condition may occur as a part of ichthyosis or of psoriasis. It can also occur in certain disorders of the nervous system in which the autonomic control of the sweat glands is deranged.

Care and Treatment

Usually the best that can be accomplished by way of relief is through care in adjusting to the weather so as to avoid overheating. Cocoa butter, lanolin, or some other soothing creamy application may be used to relieve the dryness and harshness of the skin which occurs in anhidrosis.

HYPERHIDROSIS AND BROMHIDROSIS

Hyperhidrosis is characterized by excessive perspiration due to overactivity of the sweat glands. There are two principal types: (1) thermogenic and (2) emotional. In thermogenic hyperhidrosis a disturbance occurs in the temperature regulating mechanism in the brain, causing the body's response to be the same as when the individual is in excessively warm surroundings. This type of hyperhidrosis occurs commonly in such diseases as tuberculosis, hyperthyroidism, gout, diabetes mellitus, and some forms of cancer.

In emotional hyperhidrosis the increased sweating occurs principally in the face, under the arms, and in the skin of the palms and soles.

In bromhidrosis the perspiration has a foul odor. The odor results from fermentation, bacterial infection, or a chemical change in the perspiration after it has escaped from the sweat glands. The offensive odor is most obvious on parts of the body where perspiration is free but cannot readily evaporate, such as the armpits or the feet, if confined in poorly ventilated shoes. Certain foods, drugs, and germs give the perspiration characteristic odors, and some of these are unpleasant.

Care and Treatment

Cleanliness is the first requirement in controlling the unpleasant features of either hyperhidrosis or bromhidrosis. A daily bath, with change of underclothing and hose, is recommended.

A 5 percent solution of alum or zinc sulfate in 70 percent alcohol, dabbed on the surface of the affected skin areas and allowed to dry on, may be helpful. Commercial antiperspirant preparations available at the drugstore (such as those containing compounds of aluminum) often work well when applied according to directions after a thorough cleansing of the skin. The use of such a preparation should be stopped, however, if skin irritation results.

A good powder for dusting on the skin of the feet and sprinkling into the socks or stockings can be prepared by the pharmacist as follows:

Salicylic acid	1
Aluminum chloride	1
Powdered alum	1
Starch	15
Talcum powder	15
Mix thoroughly.	

CAUTION: *This preparation, which contains salicylic acid, should not be used by a person who has diabetes.*

O. Skin Reactions to Light and Temperature

SUNBURN

Overexposure to the ultraviolet rays of the sun causes a more serious disturbance of the skin than many people realize. The actual damage varies from person to person, being greatest in fair-skinned persons and redheads. The

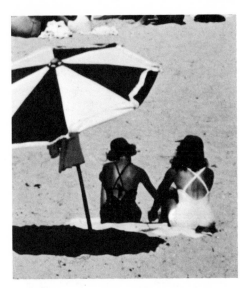

Capsule message of dermatologists gathered at the 1983 World Congress on Cancers of the Skin: Bring back the parasol.

damage is caused by sunlight even when it is reflected by glass or water or snow. It occurs even on cloudy days because the ultraviolet rays of the sun penetrate the clouds and fog.

Many persons are surprised at the degree of suffering caused by sunburn because the symptoms appear after the exposure. A person cannot, therefore, know his tolerance for exposure to the rays of the sun while the exposure is taking place. The symptoms may even increase in their intensity up to three days after the exposure.

In mild cases, the skin becomes red, and as the redness fades in a day or two a slight scaling of the surface layer of the skin takes place. In the more severe cases, the patient experiences pain and tenderness of the skin, with swelling and even with blisters. In the very severe cases, systemic symptoms of fever, chills, weakness, and shock appear.

Long-range effects of repeated exposure to the sun consist of premature aging and wrinkling of the skin. Actinic keratoses are skin blemishes that develop after years of exposure to the

sun. These are not only unsightly, but in some cases they also become transformed into a type of skin cancer. Actinic keratoses are described in the following subsection. It has been demonstrated statistically that the development of the various kinds of skin cancer is greatest in those geographic areas (such as the southwestern part of the United States) offering the greatest opportunity for exposure to sunlight.

Care and Treatment

Sunburn may be largely prevented by limiting one's exposure to sunlight to not more than 30 minutes a day between the hours of 10 a.m. and 4 p.m. Also, the application of sunscreen ointment to the exposed areas of the skin helps to prevent skin damage. Notice that the type of ointment to be used for prevention is not the type recommended for tanning the skin, but rather the type designed to prevent the penetration of ultraviolet rays into the skin.

For moderate cases of sunburn, keeping the affected areas of the skin covered with tapwater compresses helps to relieve the discomfort. A similar effect may be obtained by immersing the body in a lukewarm starch bath, prepared by stirring one or two cupfuls of Linit starch into a tub of bathwater. The use of anesthetic (pain-relieving) ointments is to be avoided in the treatment of sunburn. In the severe cases the doctor may prescribe corticosteroid medications by mouth.

ACTINIC KERATOSIS (SOLAR KERATOSIS)

This is a skin condition which develops on those areas that have been repeatedly exposed to the sun (principally on the face, nose, ears, and the backs of the hands). It occurs commonly in middle-aged and elderly persons, especially those of fair complexion. The skin lesions are patchy, poorly defined, slightly elevated, rough, uneven, dry, and often scaly. The lesions are skin-color or slightly red. Often the lesions itch and may bleed slightly when the scales are removed.

Actinic keratosis deserves serious consideration because of its tendency to develop into skin cancer.

Care and Treatment

A person may protect himself from the development or further development of keratosis by the use of a sunscreen lotion or cream such as is used for the prevention of sunburn.

Single lesions of actinic keratosis may be treated by the physician by the use of liquid nitrogen or solid carbon dioxide to freeze the involved area. For multiple lesions most physicians now prefer to prescribe a liquid preparation containing 5-fluorouracil (such as Fluoroplex) applied directly to the affected skin. Except where skin cancer has already begun, a course of this treatment usually restores the skin to its healthy condition.

If there is a question of whether a certain lesion is being transformed to skin cancer, the physician will arrange for a microscopic examination of a sample of the involved tissue.

PRICKLY HEAT (MILIARIA)

Miliaria is a condition in which the sweat glands in the skin become obstructed, and a skin eruption occurs as a result. The condition occurs in very warm climates or when a person is too heavily clothed. The involved skin areas are those in which two skin surfaces come together as at the bend of the elbow, the bend of the knee, beneath the breasts, and in the inguinal region. The condition sometimes occurs in infants.

Care and Treatment

The obvious remedy for miliaria is to wear lighter clothing, move to a cooler climate, or otherwise avoid overheating one's body. The immediate treatment of the involved skin areas involves the use of a soothing ointment such as calamine lotion.

PHOTOSENSITIVITY

Unrelated to sunburn, the skin of some persons reacts unfavorably to sunlight. The reaction may occur after an exposure of only a few minutes. These unusual cases of hypersensitivity to sunlight fall into three categories: (1) those related to other skin diseases, (2) those in which the taking of a certain drug has caused the skin to become sensitized, and (3) those in which the application of certain substances to the skin have made it sensitive to sunlight.

The skin diseases which should be considered when a person's skin reacts unfavorably to short exposures of sunlight are these: lupus erythematosus, ichthyosis, porphyria, and cold sores or herpes simplex. (See the General Index for page references to these diseases.)

Several drugs, when taken into the body either by mouth or by injection, may cause the skin to become hypersensitive to sunlight. This reaction occurs in only a small percentage of persons taking the drugs. The possible offenders include sulfonamides, tetracyclines, thiazides, and griseofulvin.

Substances which, when applied to the skin, may cause sensitivity to sunlight include certain toilet waters and perfumes, sulfonamides, coal tar, and certain medicated soaps.

The particular skin reaction that results from exposure to sunlight in a hypersensitive person may mimic any one of other skin manifestations. There may be a simple reddening of the skin, an actual inflammation, hives, large blisters, or thickened scaly areas.

Care and Treatment

Have your doctor check for the possibility of other skin ailments as mentioned above. Take note of any medications being used. If it seems urgent that these be continued, check with your doctor to see if any one of these may be causing the present skin problem. Discontinue any lotions, medications, perfumes, or medicated soaps recently applied to the skin. Sometimes the sensitivity of the skin persists for a matter of days, even after the offending chemical has been discontinued.

BURNS

Burns by heat, by electric current, by chemical agents, or by radiation typically damage or destroy portions of the skin or the mucous membranes lining the body passages. The severity of burns varies all the way from those which cause minor discomfort and heal promptly to those so severe and extensive as to cause the death of the victim. When healing occurs following severe burns, complications are often caused by the contraction of the resulting scars.

Burns cause a great deal of discomfort, and severe burns require precise and prompt treatment. The subject of burns is therefore treated in chapter 23 dealing with emergencies, volume 3.

Cold Injury

Human tissues are designed to function within a certain optimal temperature range, not too hot or too cold. The continuous flow of blood through all parts of the body tends to keep the tissues' temperature quite stable even though the temperature of the surroundings may be much hotter or much colder. But there is a limit to how much stabilizing of temperature can be performed when external temperatures become extreme.

We are concerned here with what happens when external temperatures become so low that the tissues of certain parts of the body can no longer be maintained in the temperature range that permits them to function normally. Obviously it is the exposed or distant parts of the body that suffer first: the feet, the hands and fingers, the ears, the cheeks, the nose.

CHILBLAINS

In this condition the involved tissues have not been frozen; there have not developed any spicules of ice among the cells. But there has been a continu-

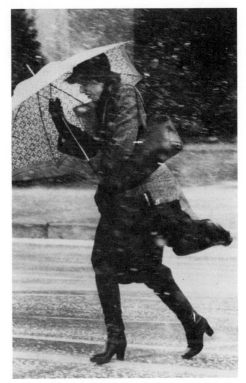

Exposure to extreme cold may cause injury to body extremities.

ing, off-and-on exposure to low temperatures. And the tissues of the exposed parts (especially hands, feet, ears, and face) have suffered. Spotty areas on these parts now appear bluish-red and swollen, and they itch and burn. With proper care the symptoms may clear up in a week or two, but a brownish color and a scaling of the skin may last for several weeks. In less favorable cases, the areas may become ulcerated or infected.

Care and Treatment

Avoid rubbing or massaging the affected parts. The parts should be kept dry and moderately warm. Adequate clothing and other methods of preventing further chilling should be used. The general circulation should be improved by regular exercise and by taking a hot shower followed by brief cold each morning. Just before

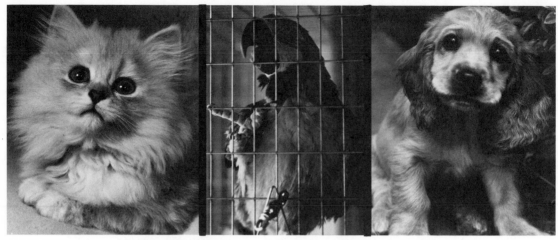

Hives may indicate an allergic reaction caused by
breathing animal dander or dust from feathers.

bedtime, alternate hot and cold baths or compresses to the affected parts should be administered for 20 minutes (see chapter 25, volume 3, for details). Following such a treatment, the skin should be gently but thoroughly dried and the affected parts anointed with warm oil. If the feet are affected, woolen socks should be worn throughout the night. Inasmuch as tobacco tends to decrease the circulation of blood to the extremities, the person with chilblains should abstain from all forms of tobacco.

FROSTBITE

Frostbite involves an actual freezing of the tissues of certain exposed parts of the body. Just before the tissues become frozen, they may appear violet-red in color. Once freezing has occurred, the color changes to gray-yellow.

The occurrence of frostbite constitutes an emergency. The care and treatment of this condition is therefore considered in the chapter 23 on emergencies, volume 3.

P. Urticaria (hives)

Urticaria appears as a local reddening of the skin which itches intensely and presently develops firm, elevated wheals. The condition may be temporary and may fade away within minutes or hours, or it may become chronic and last for a long time.

The cause of urticaria (hives) in most cases is an allergy to drugs, to certain foods, to insect stings, or to protein substances, such as pollens, that are inhaled. However, in more than 20 percent of the cases of urticaria the skin reaction is brought on by some emotional crisis rather than by an obvious allergy-producing contact. In a few cases it is triggered by such physical factors as exposure to cold, to heat, to sunlight, to pressure, or even to water.

The swollen spots appearing in urticaria resemble those that come from contact with nettles. The area around each one of the spots is usually reddened, but the spot itself appears almost white. A typical spot is from one quarter inch to one inch (0.6 to 2.5 cm.) in diameter.

Of the many drugs to which a person may become sensitive, penicillin and aspirin are the most common offenders. Inhaled substances that may cause the reaction of urticaria include pollens, molds, the dust from feathers, house dust, and animal dander. The insect stings most commonly productive of urticaria are those of bees, wasps, and hornets. In the case of a person sensitive to the substance which the insect injects into his skin, there may be a rather generalized appearance of urticaria over large areas of the skin.

It was formerly thought that a large number of cases of urticaria are the result of sensitivity to certain foods. It is now recognized that food sensitivity causes only a small percentage of such cases. Even so, when a genuine food sensitivity is present, the only relief is to determine the offending food and then omit it from the diet. The foods which may cause trouble are eggs, fish, shellfish, chocolate, certain nuts, tomatoes, cereals, berries, citrus fruits, pork, beef, and sometimes certain food additives.

Unresolved emotional problems, operating through the autonomic nervous system, render the tiny blood vessels within the skin more responsive to various insults. Many cases of persistent urticaria are benefitted by appropriate alterations in a person's way of life which relieve one's emotional crises.

There is a form of urticaria called angioedema (angioneurotic edema) which involves tissues deep in the skin. This form may affect the lips, the eyelids, the ears, or even areas of the arms or legs. In an occasional case, swelling develops in the membranes of the pharynx or larynx and interferes with the passage of air to and from the lungs. This situation requires emergency treatment. Otherwise, the treatment of angioedema is the same as for the common form of urticaria.

Care and Treatment

Identify, if possible, the substance or circumstance which causes the urticaria. Then avoid the offending substance or remove the troublesome circumstance.

For the immediate relief of the itching, the application of a thin paste of baking soda and water to the involved skin may give comfort. The application to the skin of a one-tenth of 1 percent solution of menthol in alcohol may have a similar soothing ef-

fect. A prescription which may be used in this same way is this:

Thymol	1
Glycerin	8
Alcohol (95%)	110
Water	100

Antihistamine drugs taken by mouth are often helpful in relieving a person's sensitivity to pollens and other protein substances contained in the inspired air. Because many brands of antihistamines abound, it may take some experimenting, even under the direction of a physician, to find the one that works best in the individual case. For the relief of severe acute attacks of urticaria, the physician may inject a dilute solution of epinephrine or may prescribe ephedrine to be taken by mouth or may administer corticosteroid by mouth or by injection.

Q. Nail Disorders

Nearly all abnormalities of the fingernails and toenails result from one or another of the following: congenital defects, accidental damage to the nail bed, bacterial infections, fungus infections, or some disease that affects the entire body or the skin in the region of the nails. Those abnormalities caused by systemic diseases usually correct themselves when these diseases are successfully treated. Brittleness of the nails may be caused by sluggish thyroid action, hypochromic anemia, or long use of fingernail polish.

NAIL DISEASES

The four involvements of the nails shown in the accompanying illustration are related to other skin diseases, or, in the case of koilonychia, to some systemic disease such as faulty iron metabolism. Onychomycosis is a manifestation of ringworm as considered in this chapter, page 374.

Care and Treatment

When the nails are thus involved, it may be necessary for the physician to

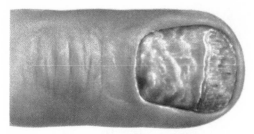

Onychomycosis. From fungi invasion.

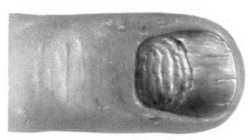

Psoriasis. Note typical depressions.

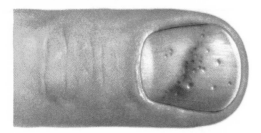

Eczema. Longitudinal splitting distinctive.

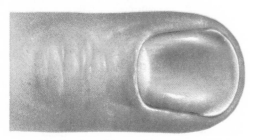

Koilonychia. Gives "spoon nail" effect.

remove a considerable portion of the affected nail and then use medications more potent than for the usual manifestations of fungus disease. When eczema (dermatitis) affects the nails, soothing lotions usually prove helpful. The more potent forms of treatment, such as the corticosteroid medications, are used only under a physician's supervision.

Sometimes simply anointing the nails nightly with olive or castor oil will help toughen them, especially if dressings are applied to keep the oil from being rubbed off during sleep. The following cream, which should be applied every night, is better than oil in some cases:

Lanolin	1
White wax	1
White petrolatum	2
Triethanolamine	3
Water q.s.ad.	30

INGROWING TOENAIL

In this condition the skin and flesh at one or both corners of the nail, usually the nail of the great toe, become tender and inflamed. The difficulty is usually caused by the wearing of shoes which force the toes into a crowded position.

Care and Treatment

In a mild case of ingrown toenail it is usually sufficient to use a probe to clean away the cuticle debris that has accumulated along the edges of the nail plate, making sure in the meantime, that no sliver or spur at the forward corner of the nail plate is gouging into the fleshy tissue. If such a sliver or spur is present, it should be removed by scissors. Attention should also be given to selecting the kind of footwear that allows sufficient room for the toes.

For the more severe case of ingrown toenail, in which the tissues have become inflamed or infected, it is desirable to work a small wisp of cotton under the edge of the nail plate, after loosening the tissues as described above, and moisten this wisp of cotton every few hours with a saturated solution of Epsom salts.

The use of an alternating hot and cold footbath each morning and evening, as described in chapter 25, volume 3, is helpful in relieving pain and inflammation. For cases in which the pain and infection become extreme, it may be necessary to have the physician remove a slender, lengthwise strip of the nail plate in the involved area.

PARONYCHIA

In paronychia the tissues which surround the fingernails, or occasionally, the toenails, become infected. The involved tissues are swollen and extremely tender and may exude pus. In the most persistent cases, the nail plate becomes thickened and discolored with transverse ridges. Often, several fingers are involved at the same time.

Paronychia usually develops in persons whose hands are immersed in water a great deal. In such, a slight injury to the finger allows bacteria or fungi to invade the tissues surrounding the nail. The susceptibility is greater in persons with diabetes or those whose nutrition is deficient.

Care and Treatment

Avoid as much as possible immersing the hands in water. After washing the hands, dry the fingers gently and thoroughly. When it becomes necessary to immerse the hands (as when washing dishes), wear cotton gloves next to the skin and cover these with rubber gloves. Before retiring at night, apply a medicated cream to the fingers, working it carefully into the tissues surrounding the fingernails. Suitable preparations for this condition include these: (1) Mycolog cream and (2) Castellani paint (carbol-fuchsin solution). For a persisting troublesome infection, the physician may prescribe an antibiotic medication.

HANGNAIL

Sometimes the cuticle which surrounds the nail at its base splits and creates a fissure which tears into the living tissue. The area becomes painful and may even be infected.

Care and Treatment

Gently trimming away the loosened tissue will usually allow the fissure to heal. For prevention, it is advisable to use a mild cream, massaging it into the nail margins so as to keep these tissues pliable.

R. Benign Tumors

BIRTHMARK (HEMANGIOMA, VASCULAR NEVUS)

Inasmuch as birthmarks appear in early life, this blemish of the skin is considered in chapter 17, volume 1.

MOLES (NEVI)

Practically everyone has at least a few moles located here and there in the skin. A mole develops even before birth as a cluster of melanocytes—the cells capable of producing the pigment melanin. Many moles do not become apparent until adulthood, even though their basic cells were present from before birth. In some moles, practically no melanin is produced, and therefore the mole remains the color of the surrounding skin. In others, the pigment melanin accounts for varying degrees

Some moles may become cancerous.

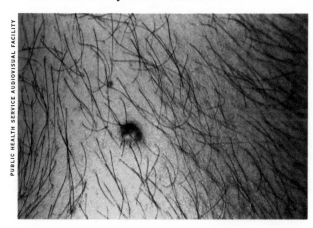

PUBLIC HEALTH SERVICE AUDIOVISUAL FACILITY

of darkness, even up to a purple-black color.

The possibility that a mole may, in an occasional case, transform into a malignant tumor is considered under the heading of Melanoma, in the next section of this chapter, page 402.

Care and Treatment

Except for the occasional possibility of a developing melanoma, as suggested in the previous paragraph, moles are harmless and require no treatment. Some persons desire that a mole appearing in a conspicuous place be removed. This can be done in a doctor's office by a simple procedure. Moles subject to irritation from clothing, such as at the belt line or under a bra strap should preferably be removed by the doctor even though, as yet, they may not show any tendency to be troublesome.

SEBORRHEIC KERATOSIS

Seborrheic keratosis is a condition in which many, small, slightly-raised lesions develop on the skin of a middle-aged or elderly person. The lesions are simple tumors, but they are not dangerous. They are not malignant and they have no tendency to become so. They are the most common type of skin tumor occurring in elderly persons.

The lesions of seborrheic keratosis are usually numerous. They occur on the face, including the forehead, on the neck, on the chest, and on the back. They vary in size, even in the same person, from a few millimeters in diameter to as much as several centimeters across. Most commonly they are only slightly darker than the surrounding skin, but some may be dark brown, even black. They are round (or oval) and are sharply demarcated from the surrounding skin. They are covered with a loosely attached, greasy crust. When the crust is removed, the base appears raw and pulpy and bleeds slightly. The surface of the lesion is smooth and shiny and may be crisscrossed by clefts. The lesion is soft and can be rolled between the fingers.

The lesions of seborrheic keratosis produce no symptoms except itching which, in some cases, is intense.

Care and Treatment

It is important for the person with skin lesions such as described above to see his doctor for a positive diagnosis. The lesions of a more serious skin condition may be mistaken for those of seborrheic keratosis. Once the diagnosis of seborrheic keratosis is confirmed, the only reason for the lesions to be removed is to relieve the itching, if present, or for cosmetic reasons. The lesions can be removed by a simple surgical procedure which leaves little or no scar.

SEBACEOUS CYST (WEN)

A sebaceous cyst is a harmless growth which results from the plugging of the outlet of a sebaceous gland—the oil gland associated with a hair follicle. Even with its outlet plugged, the gland continues to secrete the kind of oily material which it normally produces. Thus there develops a sac filled with an

Sebaceous cyst, called a wen, commonly appears on the neck or face.

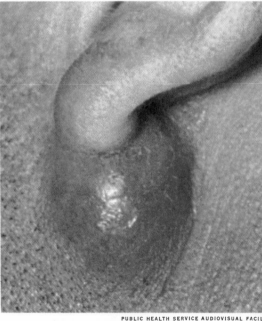

oily or fatty material. Sebaceous cysts usually appear on the scalp, the neck, or the face, but sometimes on other parts of the body. Growth of the cyst may continue for months or years. Growth eventually ceases, in some cases while the tumor is still small. Sebaceous cysts may range in number from one to several, and in size from a pea to an orange. They may be whitish, pinkish, or purplish in color. They may be either soft, doughy, elastic, or firm to the touch.

Sebaceous cysts seldom develop before middle age. They are rarely tender or painful, but may eventually become chronically inflamed and may even develop pus. When located on the scalp—where they are most often found—the skin over the cyst is usually bald.

Care and Treatment

Surgical removal of a sebaceous cyst is advisable, not only for the sake of appearance, but also to avoid its becoming inflamed. The operation is simple and is permanently successful when the entire sac is removed.

FATTY TUMOR (LIPOMA)

A fatty tumor is a benign, painless tumor, composed of fat cells, which develops in or just beneath the skin. It is soft, slowly growing, and freely movable. Occasionally, fatty tumors become large enough to interfere with the blood supply to the adjacent tissues.

Care and Treatment

The only satisfactory treatment for a fatty tumor is to have it removed by a simple surgical procedure.

KELOID

A keloid is a overgrowth of scar tissue or of tissue similar to that in scars, which continues to grow and form nodules or irregular tumor masses. A keloid usually follows an injury such as a burn or a laceration of the skin, which heals by scar formation. A keloid, fortunately, is not malignant and does not endanger life, but it may grow suffi-

ciently to involve adjoining healthy skin.

The tendency for keloid formation seems to run in families and is more common in blacks than in people with fair skin. A keloid may cause mild prickling and burning sensations and may become tender and painful.

Care and Treatment

When a keloid develops, a dermatologist (a physician who specializes in diseases of the skin) should be consulted. Treatment of a keloid is difficult because of its tendency to recur after removal. The injection of a particular kind of corticosteroid medication into the base of the lesion or into the surgical wound after the keloid has been removed by surgery probably gives the best prospect of avoiding a recurrence.

S. Malignant Changes

When we speak of malignant changes in the skin we refer to those circumstances in which a form of cancer develops. Cancer of the skin occurs more frequently than cancer in any other part of the body. Fortunately, a higher rate

Pipe smoker's cancer of the lip is a common form of skin cancer.

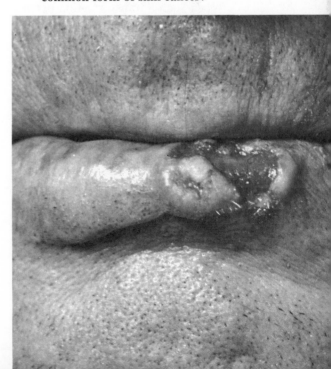

of success attends treatment of skin cancer than of any other kind of cancer—but it must be treated in order to avoid an unfavorable outcome.

The usual cancers of the skin develop in body areas exposed to sunlight over a long period of time. The development of actinic keratoses in such areas sets the stage for the later development of cancer. Not all actinic keratoses become cancerous, but because of the possibility of such a change, it is wise to have all such lesions (actinic keratoses) treated before opportunity for cancer develops.

Repeated or continuous irritation of a skin area predisposes to the development of cancer. Pipe smokers' cancer of the lip is a common form, caused by irritation by hot pipestems. Irritation by soot, paraffin, tar, or lubricating oils of petroleum origin is especially likely to cause cancer of the skin.

MELANOMA

The melanoma is a highly malignant form of cancer which often originates in the skin. Often it develops by way of changes within a pigmented mole. We emphasize it here because many persons have moles and because there are certain warning signs which a person may observe when a mole undergoes such an unfortunate transformation.

When such a transformation occurs, the melanocytes, the characteristic cells found in moles, take on characteristics of malignant tumor cells. They then tend to break away from the original mole and spread to invade other tissues. The melanoma is such a danger-

ous form of cancer that it behooves a person to take notice of any change occurring in a mole which might indicate that a malignant transformation is beginning. These are the changes to watch for:

1. A sudden increase in the surface area of a mole.

2. A change in the elevation of a mole; a change in texture—the mole's becoming nodular or thickened.

3. A change in the color of a mole as it becomes unevenly slate blue or rose colored. A mole which has always been black or very dark is not necessarily undergoing a transformation.

4. A change in a mole's characteristics, such as becoming scaly or manifesting a tendency to bleed.

5. The development of itching, burning, or tingling in a mole or in its vicinity.

Precautions to Take

Whenever there is a sore on the skin that refuses to heal over a period of more than three or four weeks or whenever there is a change in a mole as just described, a physician should be consulted promptly. He should make such examinations as enable him to determine whether cancer is developing. Most forms of cancer of the skin can be completely cured if the appropriate treatment is arranged early in the course of the cancerous change. Most of the tragedies that occur in connection with skin cancer are in cases in which there has been delay in seeking professional help.

SECTION VIII

Urinary and Sex Organs

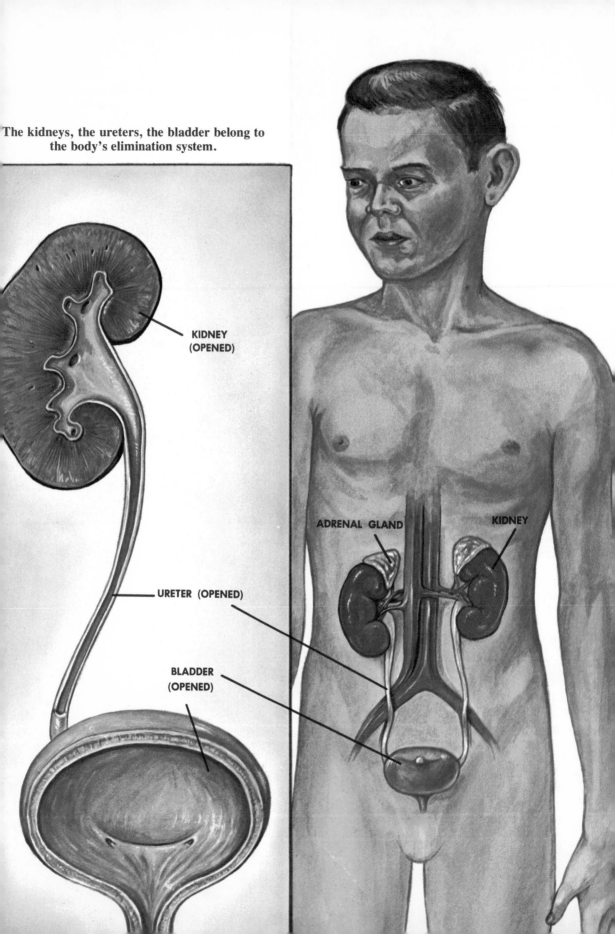

The kidneys, the ureters, the bladder belong to the body's elimination system.

KIDNEY (OPENED)

URETER (OPENED)

BLADDER (OPENED)

ADRENAL GLAND

KIDNEY

The Urinary Organs

The urinary organs produce urine and transmit it to the outside. They constitute the urinary system, which consists of the two kidneys; the ureters, which convey the urine from the kidneys to the urinary bladder; the bladder; and the urethra, which carries the urine from the bladder to the outside.

There are two kidneys, right and left, each shaped like a large bean and weighing between four and six ounces (115-170 gr.). They are located in the upper back part of the abdominal cavity, one on each side of the vertebral column, outside of (behind) the peritoneal sac which lines this body cavity. The upper end of each kidney reaches about the level of the twelfth rib, and an adrenal gland caps this upper part.

The concave part of the kidney faces toward the midline of the body. It is from this surface that the urine produced in the kidney is discharged. A close-fitting tissue funnel (the kidney pelvis) fits over this concave portion of the organ and carries the urine into the ureter, which is a small tube that extends to the urinary bladder. The bladder thus receives two ureters, one from each of the kidneys.

The bladder is a hollow organ with a thin, muscular wall which expands as the bladder fills, and contracts as it empties. It is located in the abdominal cavity just behind the pubic bone. Here it is protected from injury and is able to expand upward as it fills with urine. The outlet for the bladder is through the urethra, a single tube that opens to the outside. In the male the urethra passes through the prostate gland, which lies just beneath the bladder, and then extends through the length of the penis, at the end of which it opens to the outside. In the female, the urethra is a short, straight tube which opens into the vestibule, which is the cleft between the labia.

Functions of the Kidneys

The body requires many different substances in order to function normally. Food and drink and air supply these. Some essential substances occur in such abundance that the excesses must be thrown away along with the body's waste products.

It might seem that in eliminating substances from the body some essential materials may be lost. But a healthy body has a marvelous ability to keep what it needs. The kidneys are the organs that largely determine what shall stay and what shall go. Take the body's need for water as an example. A little more than half of the body's weight is due to the water it contains—water in the body fluids, water within the body's cells, and water in the spaces between the cells.

The body constantly loses water by several means. Exhaled air carries water vapor with it, accounting for the loss of almost a pint of water a day. Between one and two pints are lost each day from the skin, even during moderate weather. An average of three pints

Each kidney contains about one million nephrons similar to the one diagrammed below.

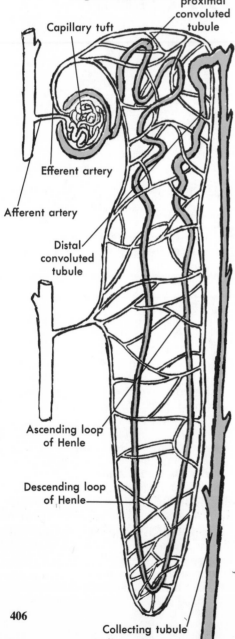

- Capillary tuft
- proximal convoluted tubule
- Efferent artery
- Afferent artery
- Distal convoluted tubule
- Ascending loop of Henle
- Descending loop of Henle
- Collecting tubule

goes out in the urine. The waste material expelled from the rectum contains a small amount of water. There is a considerable variation in the amount of water eliminated from the body, the exact amount depending on current conditions.

The body has three sources of water: (1) the water which a person drinks, (2) the water contained in food eaten, and (3) the water produced within the tissues as the result of processes of oxidation.

The exact amount of water which the body contains at any given time depends on the balance between the intake and the outgo. Loss of water occurs easily and may develop suddenly due to excessive perspiration, vomiting, diarrhea, or hemorrhage. When the supply runs low, thirst prompts the person to take a drink. When the loss of water from the body amounts to 10 percent of the body's weight, the situation becomes serious, and we speak of dehydration. When the amount of water in the body exceeds the need, the kidneys eliminate the excess.

The kidneys receive a generous supply of blood. We may say, from a practical standpoint, that all of the body's blood passes through the kidneys at one time or another during every ten minutes. While passing through the kidneys, the blood moves slowly through capillary structures constructed to permit some of the fluid portion of the blood to filter into the so-called kidney tubules. This fluid which enters the tubules contains no blood cells and no protein. It is called filtrate. During a 24-hour period the total filtrate amounts, on the average, to about 180 quarts (170 liters)—many times the volume of the body's blood. Obviously, then, most of this filtrate is returned to the blood before it leaves the kidneys.

How much of the water contained in the kidney filtrate is returned to the circulating blood depends upon the body's water balance. If the tissues and blood contain plenty of water, the kidneys allow the surplus of water to pass through the ureters into the bladder. If water is in short supply throughout the body, most of the water in the filtrate is returned to the circulating blood.

The exact amount of water which the kidneys allow to escape is controlled by the pituitary gland. When the blood becomes too concentrated, the pituitary gland secretes a chemical substance known as vasopressin. The blood carries this to the kidneys, where it brings about the return of as much water as possible to the blood.

This mechanism of control is similar to what takes place inside a chemical manufacturing plant. As we contemplate it, we can almost visualize a group of legendary dwarfs residing within the kidneys, waiting for signals from the pituitary gland. At the signal, they either close or open the figurative valves which regulate the amount of water that enters the urine.

But the kidneys have much else to do in addition to controlling the body's water balance. They not only permit the elimination of useless materials, but prevent the loss of valuable substances. To understand this function we must notice that each kidney contains about one million identical structures, called nephrons. A nephron consists of two parts—a renal corpuscle and a tubule. Each renal corpuscle consists of a tuft of blood capillaries surrounded by a delicate capsule, shaped like a funnel, which collects the fluid as it seeps out of the blood capillaries and pours it into the tubule. Tiny openings in the walls of these capillaries allow water and other substances to pass through. The openings are so small that the giant protein molecules contained in the blood plasma and the blood cells cannot squeeze through. There are many substances dissolved in the blood plasma which consist of small molecules. These include glucose (sugar), carbonates, sodium, chlorides, potassium, phosphate, calcium, sulphate, and urea. The urea is a waste product and is destined to be eliminated from the body as a constituent of the urine. But the other substances contained in

the kidney filtrate are valuable to the body and must be retained up to a certain amount.

Take for example the body's need for glucose. Glucose constitutes the body's fuel. By uniting with oxygen in the various cells of the body it provides the energy with which they carry on their activities. In a healthy person, under normal circumstances, all of the glucose contained in the kidney tubules is returned to the circulating blood for use throughout the body. Under some circumstances, however, the amount of glucose in the circulating blood becomes too great. In such cases, the kidneys reclaim only part of the glucose, allowing the excess to pass into the urine.

When a person has eaten too much candy or when for any reason a large allotment of sugar overwhelms the liver, the concentration of glucose in the blood reaches dangerous proportions. This is one of the circumstances under which the kidneys allow the excess of glucose to pass into the urine. A similar situation occurs in diabetes, in which the tissues fail to use glucose in the normal manner. Then glucose spills over into the urine. Thus the detection of glucose (sugar) in the urine (by a simple laboratory test) is an important aid in diagnosing diabetes or in the supervision of such a case under treatment.

The kidneys determine how much of the substances contained in the kidney filtrate shall be retained and how much eliminated. It is as though they put the molecules through a chute, saying to this molecule, "Go straight ahead," and to another, "Take the next exit."

It is ridiculous to assume that the infinitely large number of molecules in the kidney filtrate run single file past a solitary checkpoint. But remember there are a million nephrons in each kidney. The kidneys handle the task very much as ticket checkers at a large public performance check people as they enter. There are many ticket checkers and only a small number of people enter by any one gate. So, each nephron handles only one millionth of the filtrate of that kidney.

Protein, a substance for which the body has urgent need, does not become a part of the kidney filtrate. The openings in the walls of the capillaries in the renal corpuscles are so small that they do not permit the large molecules of protein to pass through. So protein does not occur, normally, in the kidney filtrate and hence not in the urine.

In certain forms of illness, however, protein does occur in the urine. When present, it indicates that the capillaries in the renal corpuscles are damaged, thus allowing the protein to seep through and become lost to the body. This sort of damage occurs in many cases of poisoning, in severe burns, in cases of very high blood pressure, in illnesses with sustained high fever, as a complication of some of the infectious diseases, in traumatic injuries to the kidneys, and in degenerative conditions of the kidney.

Another substance, if we may call it that, eliminated by the urine is hydrogen ions. The balance between acidity and alkalinity in the body's fluids is governed largely by the relative number of hydrogen ions present. It is the kidneys that maintain the proper acid-base balance in the body by eliminating the appropriate amount of hydrogen ions by way of the urine.

Certain of the cells lining the kidney tubules have the ability to eliminate ammonia, which also has its influence on the body's acid-base balance.

These vital functions of the kidney proceed automatically. How fortunate that we do not have to give conscious attention to the amount of water we should eliminate from the body on a given day! Neither do we have to count the sodium ions or the phosphate radicals or the calcium atoms to be sure that a sufficient number remain in the body. Normal eating and drinking supplies the body with a sufficient amount of materials which it needs, and the kidneys—credit to them—take care of the details of maintaining the right amount of these substances.

Kidney Replacement

It is fortunate that the body was designed with two kidneys rather than one. When injury or disease affects only one kidney, the remaining one has sufficient capacity to care for the body's needs. A person can maintain good health after one kidney has been removed, provided the remaining kidney is normal.

In some acute conditions of illness, as in some cases of poisoning, the kidneys become temporarily unable to carry on their usual functions. Without medical help, the individual would die from the accumulation of waste products and toxic substances. In such cases an artificial kidney may save life. By running the patient's blood through a complicated apparatus designed especially for this purpose and then returning the blood to the patient after the undesirable substances have been removed, his natural kidneys are given a chance to heal. This procedure is called hemodialysis.

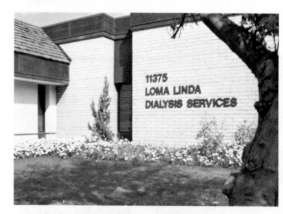

Ambulatory patients spend a few hours at a dialysis center for each hemodialysis treatment.

A somewhat simpler method of reducing the work load of diseased kidneys is the use of peritoneal dialysis, in which a "rinsing fluid" is injected into the periotoneal cavity and allowed to remain there 30 to 60 minutes while it dissolves some of the toxic substances that have accumulated in the blood.

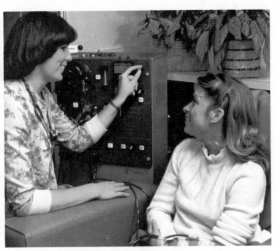

A child receiving a hemodialysis
treatment.

One of the marvels of modern surgery is the development of a method for transplanting a kidney from one person to another. The surgical procedure has been perfected so that the transplanted kidney begins to function once the operation is over. Certain problems remain in combating the body's tendency to reject a tissue or an organ from another person. In hundreds of cases, however, transplanted kidneys now function normally and thus prolong the lives of the patients who have received them. Thus far, kidney transplantation has been more successful than the transplantation of some other organs.

Emptying the Bladder

The kidneys produce urine continuously. The flow of urine enters the bladder through the ureters and is stored there. As the volume builds up, the bladder wall becomes stretched, and this stretching initiates nervous impulses which signal the need for urinating.

A person has willful control over the sphincter muscle that prevents urine from escaping through the urethra. If he deliberately abstains from urinating even when he receives the urge to do so, the detrusor muscle in the bladder wall will relax and permit the bladder to accommodate a little more urine before there develops another urge to urinate. When a person deliberately continues to abstain from urinating, the repeated urges to urinate become more frequent and more compelling.

When the individual chooses to urinate and allows the sphincter muscle to relax, urine flows through the urethra while the detrusor muscle in the bladder wall contracts. This action maintains pressure within the bladder sufficient to empty the bladder completely.

This combination of activity by which the sphincter relaxes and the detrusor muscle contracts is called the micturition reflex. Once the bladder is empty, the sphincter muscle contracts and the detrusor muscle relaxes, thus permitting urine to accumulate again within the bladder.

An adult receiving a hemodialysis
treatment.

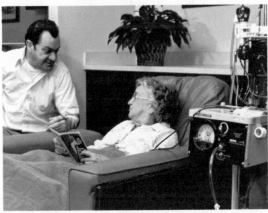

Diseases of the Urinary Organs

The organs of the urinary system and those of the reproductive system of either male or female are interrelated both anatomically and functionally. For example, the male urethra serves the urinary system and the reproductive system, because it is the passageway both for urine and for seminal fluid. Furthermore, some of the diseases that affect the urinary system are acquired by way of sexual activity. This is true of some of the ailments of the urethra, both male and female, and of certain ailments of the female bladder.

Because of this interrelationship of the two systems there is some overlapping of material contained in the present chapter with that in chapters 29, 30, 31, this volume, on the reproductive systems. In this chapter we consider the diseases of the kidneys, the ureters, the urinary bladder, and the female urethra. Diseases of the male urethra are included in chapter 29 with diseases of the male sex organs.

A. Diseases of the Kidney

The kidneys are vital organs in the sense that a person's life depends on their proper functioning. The various types of kidney disease produce a variety of symptoms, some of which do not even call attention to the kidneys as the source of difficulty.

Blood in the urine, frequency of urination, or the production of large volumes of urine, with accompanying thirst, signal that something is wrong with the organs which produce and eliminate urine. But even these do not prove the difficulty to be in the kidneys proper. Furthermore, diseases of the kidneys may produce such vague symptoms as unexplained fever, poor appetite, weakness, nausea, and anemia. High blood pressure or swelling of the tissues (edema) may be associated with kidney disease, but there can be other causes for these symptoms.

Therefore, in dealing with diseases of the kidney we must depend a great deal on laboratory tests of the urine and of the blood to help in determining whether the kidneys are performing their functions normally. For example, when urine tests indicate that albumin (a protein) is present in the urine, we have evidence that the kidneys are allowing the protein of the blood plasma to escape into the urine. This means that the kidneys are not performing normally.

X-ray examination of a kidney, especially when a dye is introduced, either through the ureter or by injection into the blood, indicates whether the shape, size, and structure of the kidney is normal.

In the remainder of this section, the more common kidney diseases are described, their symptoms listed, and treatment procedures suggested.

KIDNEY FAILURE AND UREMIA

The function of the kidneys is to remove the waste products from the blood. Normally, they provide a wide margin of safety. They contain much more functioning tissue than necessary to keep the concentration of waste products in the blood within safe limits. One kidney alone, if perfectly healthy, can care for the body's needs and still have functional capacity to spare.

Under certain conditions of disease or as the result of harmful chemicals or poisons circulating in the blood, the working capacity of the kidneys is reduced. If this reduction is gradual, the elimination of wastes will proceed normally for a time. Eventually a point is reached, however, beyond which the kidneys become unable to keep the concentration of the waste products in the blood at the desirable low levels. At first this inability occurs only under conditions of unusual demand, and at such times the concentration of the waste products in the blood increases above normal.

When the accumulation of waste products becomes so great that toxic symptoms occur, the condition is called uremia. The term *uremia* really means urine in the blood. What actually occurs is that the waste products which should normally be filtered out by the kidneys have increased to dangerously high levels in the blood because the kidneys are not functioning adequately. When damage to the kidneys is sudden and severe, the kidneys may cease to produce urine (oliguria). Acute kidney failure with uremia and/ or oliguria is a life-threatening condition.

Many conditions can cause kidney failure. Some of these act promptly, causing acute kidney failure, and others act cumulatively over a long time. It is important to detect these conditions, for in kidney damage, as in many other conditions, prevention is better than cure. Several chemical poisons are particularly prone to produce acute kidney failure. These include mercury, phenol (carbolic acid), and diethylene glycol (antifreeze). Recent observations indicate that a combination of aspirin and phenacetin, when used as a pain-killing medicine over a period of several years, is responsible for about 5 percent of the cases of kidney failure. Other forms of kidney disease, continuing over a period of time, can produce kidney failure. Persisting obstruction to the flow of urine, as may occur in the ureters or in the urethra, may cause sufficient back-pressure to damage the kidneys and eventually bring about kidney failure. Infectious diseases that involve the kidneys can do the same.

The symptoms that occur in cases of kidney failure are generalized symptoms, affecting the body as a whole. This overall involvement occurs because the accumulation of waste products in the blood affects the body very much as any poison affects it. And so we have involvements of the digestive organs, with nausea and vomiting; involvements of the cardiovascular system, with high blood pressure and anemia; involvements of the skin, with itching; involvements of the endocrine system, with an intolerance for glucose; and involvements of the nervous system, with headache, neuritis, convulsions, mental confusion, and, possibly, unconsciousness. Not all of these symptoms occur in a single case.

Care and Treatment

The doctor's first effort in handling a case of kidney failure is to determine the basic cause of the damage to the kidneys. Once this is determined, he will try to remove the cause. In some cases the kidneys will respond favorably when the cause of difficulty is removed.

In some cases, as in certain acute

poisonings, healing can occur in the kidneys if they are relieved for a time of their usual work load. This can be accomplished successfully in many cases by the temporary use of hemodialysis (the artificial kidney). In other cases, damage to the kidneys has been so extensive that return to normal kidney function is impossible. In such cases, life may be prolonged by placing the patient on a continuing program of hemodialysis, by which his blood is "rinsed" three or four times a week by the hemodialysis procedure.

Now that kidney transplantation has become feasible in many cases, the implanting of a normal kidney from some person who has died of another disease, may permit the patient who has had kidney failure to return to a normal way of life.

NEPHRITIS

The term *nephritis* covers a group of conditions in which both kidneys are involved in inflammatory or degenerative disease and in which some protein and some blood cells occur in the urine.

The normal kidney functions as a filtering device. Within the functioning units of the kidney (the nephrons) there are actually pores of microscopic size. As the blood passes by these pores, a certain amount of water and many of the smaller molecules contained in the blood pass through to become what is called urinary filtrate. The pores are normally so small that the larger molecules (principally those of protein) and the blood cells cannot pass through.

In nephritis the kidney's filtering mechanism does not work properly, and some of the large protein molecules (principally those of albumin) and some of the blood cells pass through the filter and eventually appear in the urine. The presence of the protein albumin in the urine is called albuminuria or proteinuria.

In many cases of nephritis there is edema (swelling of some of the body's tissues), elevated blood pressure, an accumulation of some of the nitroge-

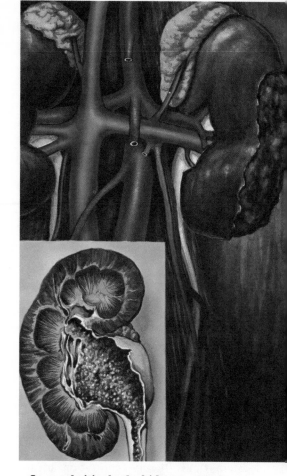

In nephritis both kidneys are involved. Lower left shows congestion inside the kidney.

nous waste products in the blood, and the presence of albumin in the urine (indicating that the kidneys are not functioning efficiently).

a. *Acute Nephritis (Acute Glomerulonephritis).* Acute infectious diseases such as scarlet fever, malaria, measles, and particularly sore throat caused by the streptococcus germ, may cause an acute inflammation of the kidneys. Phenol (carbolic acid), potassium chlorate, and turpentine are among the chemicals that can cause it. It may be a complication of pregnancy (in so-called toxemia of pregnancy). It occurs most frequently in children and is rare after middle age.

Contrary to common belief, a lame or painful back does not indicate kidney inflammation. One of the symptoms of acute inflammation of the kidneys is edema, although only the face and eyes may be puffy. Children with this disease may have convulsions. Headaches, nausea, and vomiting are other common symptoms. A severe headache may be the first warning of oncoming nephritis in a pregnant woman. There may be fever and great weakness. Changes in the urine are characteristic and significant. It becomes scanty, highly colored, turbid, and sometimes bloody. Albumin and pus are present in the urine, but these may be detected and measured only by a laboratory procedure.

Many people with acute nephritis can be completely cured. But if the condition is neglected, it may change into a chronic form, lasting over a period of several years before causing renal failure. In some cases, death comes within a few days.

Care and Treatment

The patient should have bedrest and be kept warm. Care by a physician is important. The diet should be planned by the physician to comply with the patient's particular condition. Salt and protein may need to be restricted. A warm bath may be given every day, but profuse perspiration should be avoided. No drugs should be used other than what the physician orders. As the acute stage of the disease subsides, more protein may be gradually added to the diet. Foods that can be added to good advantage are milk, cereals, and potatoes.

b. *Chronic Nephritis.* Chronic nephritis sometimes follows acute nephritis that does not progress to recovery. But usually chronic nephritis develops gradually from a low-grade infection of long standing or from protracted irritation by chemical substances. The damage done to the kidneys by toxemia of

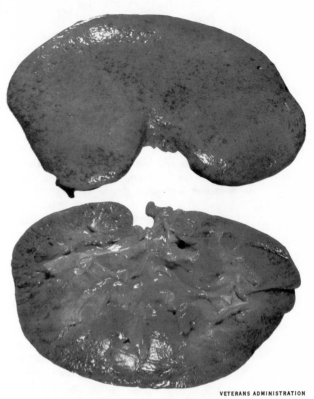

The human kidney as affected by nephritis, both external surface and interior being shown, this phase being between acute and chronic.

pregnancy may be permanent and may result in chronic nephritis.

A person with chronic nephritis may not realize that he has a serious kidney disease until it has progressed for several years. Incidental discovery of high blood pressure may be the first warning sign.

The kidney degeneration may have been progressing a long time before the characteristic headaches, loss of weight, weakness, shortness of breath, edema, and failing eyesight appear. The urinary symptoms are not so characteristic as in acute nephritis. The quantity of urine passed may be above normal, causing frequent urination, especially at night.

Chronic nephritis may run a course of from two to twenty years, and its victim may die of some other disease before the kidney damage becomes severe enough to cause death. The final event may be kidney failure with uremia, or it may be a stroke, coronary artery disease, or heart failure. The final stage of chronic nephritis may last a year or more.

Care and Treatment

Treatment aims at prolonging life and increasing comfort. It cannot cure the disease, because the kidney tissue has been damaged beyond repair.

It is advisable to have a physician in charge of the case. The progress of the disease and the dangers accompanying it cannot be judged satisfactorily without repeated careful examinations and special laboratory tests.

The patient should be protected from exposure to cold. A 30-minute tub bath at about 97° F. (36° C.) every evening just before retiring is beneficial. Drinking water freely is important unless there is edema (swelling of the tissues under the skin). The diet should consist chiefly of fruits and vegetables. Fruit juices and green leafy vegetables are especially good. Cases differ widely in their protein requirement, and it is wise to leave decision on this to the physician.

Many cases are greatly benefited by the judicious use of hemodialysis (artificial kidney). The surgical procedure of kidney transplantation has become quite successful. In this procedure, a healthy kidney from a live donor or from a person who has died from some other problem is surgically transplanted to the person whose kidneys are no longer functioning properly.

NEPHROSCLEROSIS (ARTERIOLAR NEPHROSCLEROSIS)

A combination of high blood pressure and hardening of the small arteries of the kidneys is likely to produce the characteristic symptoms both of systemic high blood pressure and chronic nephritis. The treatment should combine the essential features of the treatment for both conditions.

NEPHROSIS (NEPHROTIC SYNDROME)

This illness is characterized by pronounced edema (swelling of the tissues), protein (especially albumin) in the urine, and reduction of protein in the blood serum. Children (especially between the ages of 1 and 6) are affected more frequently than adults, and boys have this disease more commonly than girls.

The exact cause is not known, but it is sometimes associated with other diseases. It may be assumed that these or the prolonged effects of some poison has caused damage to the kidneys, which predisposes to nephrosis. Nephrosis may occur as one stage in the course of nephritis.

In untreated cases the illness persists for many months, sometimes with periods of partial remission. In some such cases eventual spontaneous cure occurs, but in many some other disease of the kidney develops, or a severe infection of the tissues sets in. Tissues swollen with edema are particularly susceptible to infection.

Care and Treatment

A physician should supervise the treatment and long-range care of the patient with nephrosis. Bed rest is generally necessary to restrict the patient's activities. The use of corticosteroid medications brings about almost magic improvement in the majority of childhood cases and permits a fair proportion of adult cases to heal. The use of antibiotic drugs serves very well to control the infections that otherwise cause many deaths. Of themselves, the antibiotic drugs do not change the course of the kidney involvement.

PYELONEPHRITIS

The pelvis of the kidney is the enlarged upper end of the ureter, which is the tube that conveys urine from the kidney to the bladder. Bacteria may come upward through the ureter from an infected bladder, or an infection in some other part of the body is sometimes the original source of the bacteria that produce pyelonephritis in which the kidney substance and the kidney pelvis are in an inflammatory process.

A tendency to frequent voiding of urine may be the only symptom with mild infections. At other times the inflammation is so great that the patient experiences a constant painful desire to void. There may be severe chills, high fever, headaches, nausea, vomiting, and extreme prostration for days at a time. The distress may be apparently confined to the bladder. Many people have had bladder treatments for a long time before realizing that the real trouble was in the kidneys. When pyelonephritis becomes chronic, destruction or degeneration of the kidney tissue may progress until it becomes so extensive that surgical removal of the kidney is the only feasible way to cure the disease. For this reason it is important to determine as early as possible whether one or both kidneys are involved and how far the infection has progressed. Obviously if both kidneys are infected, the removal of either one provides no benefit. Suitable treatment should be started early enough to make surgical removal of a kidney unnecessary.

Pyelonephritis seldom proves fatal unless neglected, but a cure often requires expert and persistent treatment. In some cases, it is helpful for the specialist to carry through the procedure of dilating the ureters so the urine can drain away from the kidneys more readily.

Care and Treatment

The treatment of pyelonephritis should be under the direct supervision of a physician. The treatment consists essentially of selecting and administering an effective antibiotic medication. Periodic examinations should be made to determine the effectiveness of the treatment.

FLOATING KIDNEY (NEPHROPTOSIS)

All kidneys are somewhat moveable. Sometimes one is sufficiently moveable

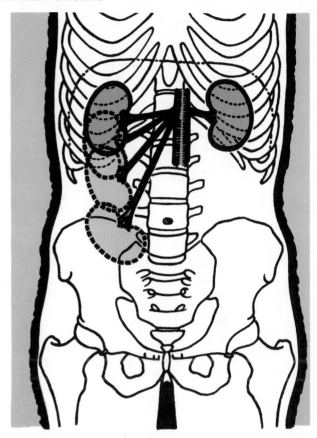

Prolapse of the kidney. Note different positions (dotted lines) a kidney can adopt in nephroptosis.

to make the organ easily felt through the abdominal wall. In most such cases no symptoms are caused. Occasionally a disturbance of the blood circulation to the kidney causes some congestion and pain. In other occasional cases the ureter may become kinked or otherwise partly or completely obstructed. In these complicated cases of prolapse the pain is usually a dull ache or a dragging sensation, but sometimes it is acute and colicky, especially in the case of an obstructed ureter.

Care and Treatment

Cases of mild floating kidney require no treatment other than reassurance of the patient. In the moderately severe cases which require

415

treatment it is advisable for the patient to increase the body weight so that the kidney can be surrounded by a pad of fat. The wearing of a kidney belt may also help to hold the kidney in its normal position. When such a belt is put in place, the patient should lie with feet elevated in order to keep the kidney in place while the belt is being fitted. In extreme cases, it is necessary to resort to surgery by which the kidney is anchored in its normal position.

KIDNEY STONES
(NEPHROLITHIASIS)

Kidney stones are masses of solid material that develop and enlarge within the pelvis of the kidney. They vary greatly in size, but their size tends to increase the longer they remain in the kidney pelvis. They also vary a great deal in chemical composition. The most common stones are composed of calcium oxalate. Others are composed of uric acid or of cystine. Kidney stones occur more commonly in certain geographic areas. Also, they are more frequent in certain family lines than in others.

Kidney stones are formed by a precipitation of some of the chemical substances normally dissolved in the urine. The exact cause of this precipitation is uncertain, but there are doubtless several causes which operate differently in various cases. Sometimes infection favors the development of kidney stones. Obstruction to the passage of urine may cause a stagnation which favors the development of stones. In some cases there seems to be a metabolic disorder, a physiological fact assumed to be the reason that uric acid stones are common in cases of gout. Dietary deficiencies are blamed for the formation of some kidney stones.

Very small stones that form in the pelvis of the kidney may pass down the ureters to the bladder, where they may lodge or from where they may be eliminated by passing through the urethra. Sometimes a small stone becomes lodged on its way through the ureter,

416

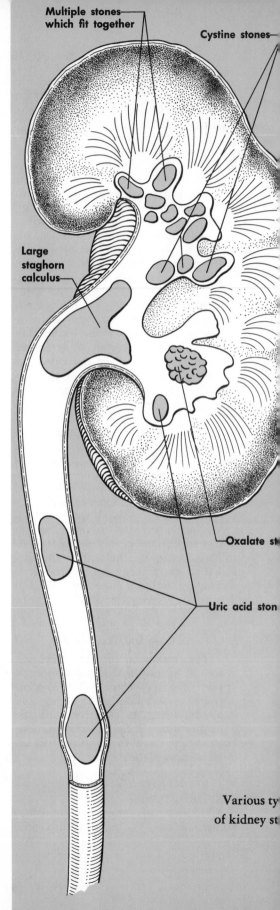

Multiple stones which fit together

Cystine stones

Large staghorn calculus

Oxalate st

Uric acid ston

Various ty of kidney st

causing extreme pain as the delicate muscle in the wall of the ureter contracts around the stone.

The presence of stones in the kidney pelvis favors the development of infection there, and this complication may cause symptoms. Some stones remain in the kidney pelvis for long periods of time without causing symptoms. Usually, however, the person with kidney stones suffers pain, which may vary from a dull ache in the lower part of the back to sharp, severe pain described as colic. This severe type of pain is usually intermittent, but the attacks may last for hours. Typically this severe pain is referred to the lower abdomen and groin. In many cases the stone injures the delicate lining of the kidney pelvis and blood appears in the urine.

The diagnosis of kidney stones can often be confirmed by X-ray examination.

Care and Treatment

The most important feature in the treatment of kidney stones is the passing of large volumes of water through the kidney. In other words, the patient should drink enough water so that he excretes at least four quarts (four liters) of urine within 24 hours. This may not dissolve existing stones, but it does serve in most cases to keep stones from becoming larger and, possibly, to prevent the formation of new stones. Physicians who specialize in urology use various medications in the hope of dissolving stones already present in the kidney pelvis. These attempts, however, are not uniformly successful. The final recourse in the treatment of kidney stones is to remove them by surgery.

POLYCYSTIC DISEASE

In some individuals, probably always happening before birth, segments of the kidney tubules fail to develop normally. These become blocked, forming closed sacs within which fluid accumulates. Such sacs are scattered throughout the kidney substance and are so numerous that they cannot be counted.

As time goes on, they gradually increase in size, causing a steady enlargement of the kidney and progressive damage by pressure on the remaining secreting tissue. In some cases kidney failure and death occur in early infancy. In others, the enlargement is so gradual that symptoms leading to the discovery of the condition may not show up before adulthood.

When the enlargement is sufficiently great, the kidney can be felt as an abnormal mass in the upper abdomen. Blood in the urine is common. Symptoms and treatment are like those for chronic nephritis. The condition is to some extent hereditary, nearly always involves both kidneys, and is incurable except by the surgical transplantation of a normal kidney to replace one of the polycystic ones.

TUMORS OF THE KIDNEY

Most tumors of the kidney are malignant. They may occur at any age. Even infants or young children may develop a rapidly growing, highly malignant cancer of the kidney.

Bloody urine is usually the first and most persistent symptom. The appearance of blood in the urine is an urgent indication that a physician should be consulted. If a kidney cancer is detected early, and if it is found that only one kidney is involved, surgical removal of the cancerous kidney may save life. For a more detailed discussion of cancer of the kidney, see chapter 11, volume 3.

B. Diseases of the Ureter

There are two ureters, one on the right and one on the left. These small-caliber tubes lead from the pelvis of each kidney directly downward to enter the urinary bladder by separate openings. In the adult, the ureter is about twelve inches (30 cm.) long, with a small lumen which, at the junction with the kidney pelvis, is about two millimeters in diameter. The wall of the ureter is composed essentially of smooth muscle which contracts in a peristaltic fashion. Rings of contraction move toward the bladder to propel about one milliliter of urine with each peristaltic wave.

URETERAL STRICTURE

In occasional cases a narrowing of the lumen of a ureter interferes with the passage of urine. Such a narrowing or stricture may follow a local infection of the ureter, may follow damage to the lining of the ureter caused by the presence or passing of a kidney stone, or may occur as the result of pressure from surrounding structures as may be caused by a tumor.

The symptom of ureteral stricture is pain in the lower back, which is referred to the region of the groin. Depending on the severity of the condition, this pain may vary from that of a dull ache to extreme, almost intolerable pain.

Care and Treatment

Treatment of a ureteral stricture requires the services of a urologist (a physician specializing in diseases of the urinary organs). In selected cases, the ureter may be stretched (ureteral dilation) by the passing of a small catheter from the bladder upward into the ureter. This requires a series of treatments at about fourteen-day intervals, with the size of the catheter being increased slightly at each treatment. The inserting of such a catheter requires the use of the cystoscope, an instrument which is passed through the urethra into the bladder.

The alternative in treating difficult cases of ureteral stricture, when stretching of the ureter is not feasible, is the surgical removal of the kidney and ureter on the affected side. Of course, it must be determined first that the opposite kidney and ureter are normal and functioning adequately.

URETERAL CALCULI

Ureteral calculi originate as kidney stones, the smaller ones of which may enter the ureter and move downward toward the bladder. The size and shape of such stones varies from case to case, the greatest damage to the ureter being caused by those stones which are rough or spiny. Ureteral calculi occur about twice as often in men as in women.

The caliber of the ureter is not uniform throughout its length. There are certain narrow places, and stones passing through the ureter tend to lodge at one or the other of these sites of narrowing. It is the continued peristaltic activity of the ureter that causes this lodgment of a stone to be painful. The pain may be very severe but is usually intermittent. In cases in which the stone fits snugly in the lumen of the ureter, the back pressure of urine, when sustained, may cause damage to the corresponding kidney.

Care and Treatment

The size and position of the ureteral calculus can usually be determined by X-ray examination. For the smaller stones, it is often possible by the use of medicines to relieve pain and relax the muscle of the ureter so that the stone will pass into the bladder. For large stones which lodge in the upper portion of the ureter, it may be necessary to perform a surgical procedure in which the ureter is opened and the stone removed. For larger stones lodging in the lower part of the ureter, it is possible in some cases to remove the stone by instruments manipulated through a cystoscope inserted into the bladder.

C. Diseases of the Bladder

URINARY INCONTINENCE (INABILITY TO HOLD THE URINE)

In urinary incontinence, a most troublesome symptom, the patient loses normal control of the passage of urine. This loss occurs commonly when either the bladder or the urethra is involved with local infections (cystitis or urethritis). There is a sudden urgency to empty the bladder, and if the desire is not gratified, urine may escape in spite

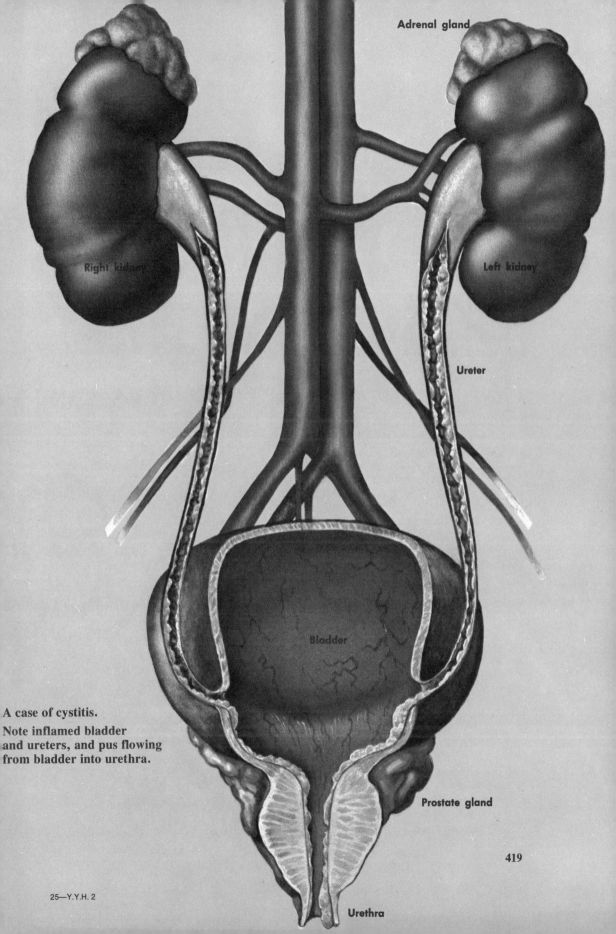

Adrenal gland

Right kidney

Left kidney

Ureter

Bladder

A case of cystitis.

Note inflamed bladder
and ureters, and pus flowing
from bladder into urethra.

Prostate gland

419

25—Y.Y.H. 2

Urethra

of efforts to retain it. The symptom occurs commonly in older men whose prostate gland has become enlarged. It occurs in women in whom tissue injuries sustained at the time of a difficult delivery of a child were not adequately restored. In such cases, coughing, sneezing, laughing, or sudden lifting may cause the urine to dribble.

Loss of urinary control also occurs in cases in which the spinal cord or the nerves to the bladder have been damaged by disease or injury, compressed by a tumor, or severed.

URINARY RETENTION

A partial obstruction to the outflow of urine may develop from a stricture of the urethra, an enlargement of the prostate gland, a developing tumor within the bladder, or the presence of a bladder stone. Whenever this happens the muscle in the wall of the bladder becomes stronger, at first, and forces the urine past the obstruction in a relatively normal manner. As the obstruction becomes more complete, a condition develops in which not all of the urine is emptied from the bladder at the time of voiding. That which remains in the bladder, called residual urine, reduces the bladder's effective capacity and makes it necessary for the person to void at more frequent intervals. Also, the presence of residual urine favors infection of the bladder lining, causing inflammation (cystitis). Continued back pressure from an obstructed bladder causes damage to the kidneys.

As such a condition of obstruction progresses, there comes a time—often a sudden event—when the person can no longer empty his bladder at all. The bladder continues to fill, producing distention and considerable discomfort. This type of complete urinary retention constitutes an emergency.

Care and Treatment

In a case of complete urinary retention in which no urine is passed, the physician will first arrange to drain the urine which is under pressure within the bladder and, second, discover and treat the basic cause of the condition. It is usually possible to provide temporary relief by passing a catheter into the bladder to drain away the impounded urine. When a physician is not immediately available, some relief can be provided by having the patient sit in a bathtub of hot water. Of course the patient should not drink more fluid during the time of waiting for the physcian to take over.

CYSTITIS (INFLAMMATION OF THE BLADDER)

Cystitis may occur as a complication of infection of the kidney (pyelonephritis).

In women, inflammation of the bladder often develops a day or two after sexual intercourse. The bacteria have traveled up the urethra to the bladder. In men, it may follow an inflammation of the prostate. Any partial obstruction

Various types of bladder stones

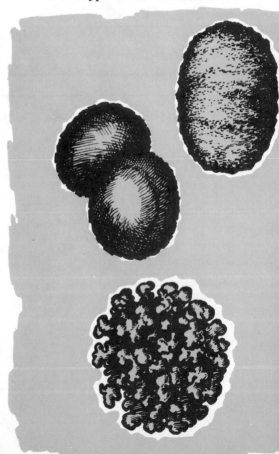

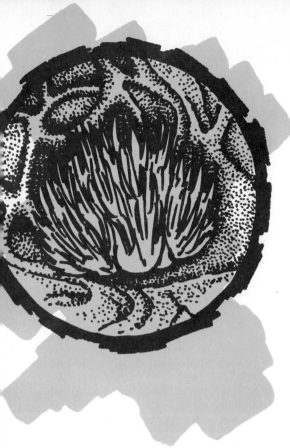

Tumor of the bladder as observed through a cystoscope.

to the outflow of urine, so that a residual amount of urine remains in the bladder, favors the development of infection within the bladder.

The symptoms of cystitis include burning on urination, a desire to void frequently, and an urgency to empty the bladder at once. General symptoms such as fever are usually caused by inflammations of other organs (as the kidneys or prostate) rather than by inflammation of the bladder itself.

Care and Treatment

The usual case of cystitis responds readily to appropriate antibiotic treatment. If the aggravating cause is an obstruction to the outflow of urine, as an enlarged prostate or a stricture of the urethra, such condition must be corrected. If cystitis subsides and recurs repeatedly, there is some underlying cause which should be discovered and corrected. It is impor-

tant for the person with cystitis to drink abundant fluid—up to ten glasses of water or fruit juice a day.

BLADDER STONES (VESICAL CALCULI)

Bladder stones occur more commonly in males than in females in a ratio of about twenty to one. They usually occur in the older age groups. Most bladder stones are formed right in the bladder, but a small proportion are stones that have originated in a kidney and descended through the ureter. Most of those that come from the kidney are small enough to pass through the bladder and on through the urethra to the outside.

Obstruction to the flow of urine and infection of the urinary organs are the important causes of stones forming within the bladder. The symptoms include difficulty in urinating, an urgency to urinate, and spasms of the bladder associated with pain which may be referred to the end of the penis. In some cases, the stone interferes intermittently with the flow of urine so that the urinary stream starts and stops.

Care and Treatment

Treatment in a case of bladder stone consists of removing the stone or stones by surgery and, second, of treating the condition responsible for the formation of stones in the first place.

TUMORS OF THE BLADDER

Tumors of the bladder are nearly three times as frequent in men as in women. Some tumors are benign and do not tend to recur after they have been adequately removed. Others are malignant and life-threatening. Various factors contribute to the development of bladder tumors. Long, continued irritation of the bladder, by whatever means, increases the probability of tumor formation. The occurrence of bladder tumors is more common among workers in certain coal-tar products. Also, smokers are more subject to tumors of the bladder than nonsmokers,

421

presumably because the chemical substances which contaminate the bloodstream in smokers are eventually eliminated through the urinary organs, and thus have opportunity to irritate the lining of the bladder.

The presence of blood in the urine is the most significant symptom of bladder tumor. There are other causes of blood in the urine, but the seriousness of a bladder tumor, when it occurs, justifies an examination by cystoscope (an instrument passed through the urethra for examination of the bladder).

Care and Treatment

It is urgent that an examination of the interior of the bladder (by cystoscope) be made in every case in which blood appears in the urine. If this symptom is caused by a developing tumor within the bladder, early treatment is indicated. The exact type of treatment will be determined by the particular kind of tumor that is present. In the case of malignant tumors, the patient's life is at stake, and it may be necessary to remove a considerable portion or all of the bladder along with the tumor and to follow the surgical procedure by some form of radiation. Even though it appears that the tumor has been completely removed, cystoscopic examination should be made every three months after the surgical treatment as a means of detecting possible recurrence of the tumor. In many cases it is possible to prolong the patient's life, even a matter of years, by making frequent cystoscopic examinations and planning the treatment program accordingly.

BLADDER FISTULAS

A fistula is an abnormal opening or channel between two organs of the body or between an organ and the skin surface. In the case of bladder fistulas, the abnormal opening is usually between the bladder and the colon (of the large intestine). Such an abnormal opening may develop as the result of an inflamed outpocketing (diverticulitis) of the colon, in which there develops an abscess that breaks through the wall of the bladder. In other cases, such a fistula may be caused by cancer of the bladder as it penetrates the surrounding tissues. A fistula may be caused by a mutilating injury.

The symptoms are usually those of cystitis (inflammation of the bladder), which include a sensation of burning on urination and a frequency and urgency for passing urine. The telltale symptom is the passing of gas through the urethra at the end of urination (pneumaturia). Such gas originates in the colon and passes through the fistula into the bladder.

Care and Treatment

Very occasionally bladder fistulas heal spontaneously. In the usual case the treatment is by surgical repair, which involves the removal of the affected portion of the colon as well as closure of the fistulous opening.

CYSTOCELE

Cystoceles occur in women. A cystocele is a protrusion of the base of the bladder into the vagina. It is usually the result of injury at the time of childbirth which weakens the normal support which retains the bladder in position. Cystocele is often accompanied by a protrusion of the rectum as well (rectocele). In mild cases of cystocele, there may be no symptoms. When symptoms occur, they are the result of the retention of urine in the bladder, and the symptoms consist of the usual evidences of cystitis: frequency of urination, burning on urination, and urgency to void.

Care and Treatment

For the less severe cases of cystocele, the muscular support of the bladder may be strengthened by consistently daily exercise of the sphincter muscles that control the passage of urine and of feces. For this, the patient deliberately contracts and relaxes these muscles over a period of several minutes, performing the exercises at least twice a day. Other than this, and particularly when symptoms of cystitis have developed, the treatment for cystocele is the surgical repair of the perineal structures so as to strengthen the support of the bladder.

D. Diseases of the Urethra

As mentioned in the previous chapter, the structure and relations of the urethra differ somewhat in the male as compared with the female. Correspondingly, the diseases and their treatment when the urethra is involved are different in the two sexes. The diseases of the male urethra are considered in connection with the diseases of the male sex organs in chapter 29, this volume. In the present chapter we are concerned with the involvements of the female urethra.

URETHRITIS IN THE FEMALE

Urethritis is an infection of the urethra. It may be a complication of cystitis (inflammation of the bladder) or of an infection of the vagina. The urethra often becomes involved in cases of gonococcal infection, which is discussed in chapter 29, this volume, and in chapter 31, this volume.

The symptoms often include those of cystitis (inflammation of the bladder), but in addition there is discomfort, burning, and mild pain, especially when urine is passed and immediately after.

Infections of the urethra typically cause changes in the delicate membrane lining this passageway that may even lead to some scar formation and a shrinkage of the urethral tube. The small glands in the wall of the urethra may become infected, and this aggravates and prolongs the symptoms.

Care and Treatment

The nature of the infection must be determined, and when this is accomplished, the proper antibiotics must be used to combat the infection. Usually it is necessary also to stretch the urethra where it has been narrowed by the formation of scars, and this requires the passing of instruments of gradually increasing size. In many cases it is necessary to cauterize the lining of the urethra by the use of a dilute silver nitrate solution to destroy the infected glands in the lining of the urethra.

URETHROCELE

In urethrocele there is a displacement of the female urethra, which occurs as part of the condition of cystocele as described in the previous section. This displacement of the urethra, along with that of the bladder, usually occurs as a result of damage to the perineum at the time of a difficult childbirth. This damage weakens the support to the bladder and related structures so that they project downward into the vestibule (the space between the labia). This displacement often interferes with the complete emptying of the bladder, which sets the stage for infection to develop.

Care and Treatment

The treatment of urethrocele requires a surgical procedure by which the bladder and urethra are returned to their normal position and the supporting tissues of the perineum are reinforced by reconstructive surgery.

the prospect of pregnancy during the next month.

The Vagina. The vagina is a soft tissue tube, nearly four inches (9 cm.) long, which extends downward and forward from the cervix of the uterus to its external opening at the vulva. It is into the vagina that the seminal fluid is deposited at the time of sexual intercourse. The walls of the vagina are sufficiently pliable so that at the time of childbirth the tube becomes stretched to form a portion of the birth canal.

In the virgin, the opening into the vagina is often partially closed by a crescent-shaped fold of firm tissue called the hymen (maidenhead). It used to be thought that the absence of a hymen was proof that the individual had previously engaged in intercourse. In some young women, however, the hymen is naturally absent and in others it has been stretched to the point of disappearance by the use of vaginal tampons for personal hygiene at times of menstruation. Some physicians instruct the young woman, at the time of her premarital examination, on the means of dilating the hymen so that it will not cause discomfort during the honeymoon period. Even without such preparation for marriage, the hymen stretches progressively at repeated attempts at intercourse or breaks apart if the attempts are too vigorous. The slight bleeding which this may bring about is not serious, and healing occurs readily.

The Vulva. The vulva consists of the external genital area and includes the major and minor labia, the clitoris, and vestibule, and certain glands located in the walls of the vestibule.

The labia are folds of tissue which extend inward on the right and left sides of the vulva, the minor labia being located just inside the area embraced by the major labia.

The clitoris is a small sensory organ located at the forward part of the vulva where the minor labia join each other in the midline. It contains many sensitive nerve receptors, as does the glans of the penis in the male. Contact with the clitoris, as at the time of sexual intercourse, activates reflex mechanisms which prepare a woman to participate in the sex act.

The vestibule is the cleft-like space between the minor labia and behind the clitoris. Within this space there are the openings of the urethra, about one inch (2.5 cm.) back of the clitoris, and the opening of the vagina just back of the urethral opening.

The glands located in the walls of the vestibule produce a viscid secretion which serves as a lubricant to protect the sensitive tissues of the vulva from irritation and to facilitate intercourse.

The Breasts. The breasts are usually described in connection with the reproductive organs because their production of milk is related to childbearing and because certain of the nervous impulses initiated in the nipples activate the sexual reflexes.

They consist of complicated glandular structures supported by connective tissue and covered by skin. The ducts which drain the gland units find their way to the nipple where they open to the outside through fifteen or twenty small openings. The proportions of gland tissue and supporting tissue within the breast vary from one individual to another. It is not possible to estimate the milk-producing capacity of a breast on the basis of its total size, some being small yet capable of producing a greater volume of milk than larger ones.

The pigmented area of modified skin which surrounds the nipple contains small glands which secrete an oily material which lubricates and protects the nipple while the babe is nursing.

The breasts are especially subject to disease, particularly cancer. Most tragically, the kind of cancer that involves the breasts is often highly malignant and spreads quickly to other parts of the body. It is very important, then, for a woman to consult her doctor when any lump appears in the breast, for only as breast cancer is treated in its very early stages is the outcome relatively satisfactory.

Inability to Have Children

Facts about conception, presented in the earlier parts of this chapter, make it clear that anything which interferes with the meeting of the male and female sex cells within the oviduct of the wife renders conception impossible.

Damages resulting from such diseases as mumps or gonorrhea may interfere either with the production of male sex cells or with their passage through portions of the reproductive system. Minor imbalances of function among the endocrine glands may make a husband less fertile than normal.

With respect to the wife, any interference with the production of sex cells or with their passage through the oviducts may make it impossible for her to become a mother. In some cases, even though union between the male and female sex cells occurs in the oviduct, conditions within the uterus may be unfavorable to the continued development of the embryo. In a woman as well as in a man, dysfunctions of the endocrine organs may interfere with the reproductive functions.

There are some cases in which miscarriage terminates a pregnancy before the babe has developed far enough to survive. In certain women there is a tendency to miscarriage with each pregnancy. These cases require special care by the physician throughout the period of pregnancy.

The "Change of Life"

Our descriptions of the functions of the reproductive organs in the earlier parts of this chapter have been based upon what normally takes place during the prime of life. There comes a time, however, in the experience of both men and women, when sexual desire, sexual abilities, and the possibility of parenthood decline or even fade away. This waning of sexual desire varies greatly from individual to individual. There is usually a diminution during the forties and fifties as compared with the twenties. But often, the husband and wife retain their desire and capacity for sexual intimacies even past sixty.

With respect to the prospect of parenthood, a woman usually loses the capacity to become a mother earlier than a man loses his capacity to become a father. In women there comes a time, usually during the late forties, when the female sex cells are no longer liberated from the ovaries. Obviously, then, she is no longer able to become pregnant. At about this same time the monthly menstrual cycle ceases. We speak of this as the "change of life" or menopause.

Although a man may continue to produce male sex cells past the age of sixty and seventy years, the number and vitality of the cells he produces is usually decreased.

Diseases of the Male Sex Organs

A. Involvements of the Penis

IMPOTENCE

Impotence is the inability of a man to perform the sex act satisfactorily. It may consist of weak erection, inability to gain an erection, loss of the normal sensation at the time of ejaculation, or loss of sexual desire. In the normal course of life's events, a man's sexual ability and even his sexual desire gradually diminish as he becomes older. This decline in sexual ability may be noticed in some cases as early as during the forties. But in exceptional cases, a man may retain his sexual ability even into his eighties and nineties.

Most men take the natural decline in sexual ability as a matter of course. If the ability declines faster than the desire, however, a man feels thwarted and will usually seek his doctor's advice.

Certain conditions of health, both physical and mental, may interfere with a man's ability to perform the sex act. Infections of certain of the sex organs may thus interfere. Surgery on the prostate gland may cause a decline in sexual ability. Even arteriosclerosis, if it reduces the blood supply to the sex organs, may cause a decline in sexual ability. Certain endocrine distur-

bances, especially those which reduce the production of the male sex hormone, may have this effect. Certain diseases of the nervous system, such as those affecting the spinal cord, can reduce a man's sexual ability. The persistent use of drugs and the condition of chronic alcoholism are responsible for their share of impotence.

Far more than half of the instances of impotence are caused by psychological factors. Persisting fatigue, feelings of insecurity or of inferiority, or fear of the consequences of intercourse can interfere with a man's potency. Lack of cooperation by the sexual partner or a recurring sense of guilt because of a previous sexual indiscretion may reduce a man's sexual capacity.

Care and Treatment

When impotence develops suddenly or unrelated to any psychological factor, a physician should be consulted to determine whether some disease of the sex organs or of the nervous system may now require attention. Inasmuch as the majority of the cases of impotence are caused by psychological factors, the treatment in these cases requires a review of the person's life-style, preferably in cooperation with a counselor.

PHIMOSIS AND PARAPHIMOSIS

These are conditions in which the foreskin of the penis (prepuce) in a male who has not been circumcised becomes so tight as to interfere with keeping the glans clean (in phimosis) or with the circulation of blood to the glans (paraphimosis). In phimosis, the foreskin is in a forward position, covering the glans; in paraphimosis, the foreskin is in a retracted position just behind the glans and causes a constricting band in that position.

In the forward type (phimosis) the resulting difficulty is that the space between the glans and the foreskin becomes contaminated, and this may lead to actual infection. In paraphimosis, an emergency condition develops in which the glans is deprived of adequate blood, with the possibility that ulceration or even destruction of tissue may result. In paraphimosis, the pain is severe and the involved tissues are very tender.

Care and Treatment

In both of these conditions, the ultimate treatment is to have the foreskin removed by the surgical procedure of circumcision. The palliative treatment for phimosis is to retract the foreskin backward from the glans and clean the involved tissues gently with soap. Then, after the area has been gently dried, the foreskin should be pulled forward over the glans. The emergency treatment for paraphimosis involves exerting firm but gentle pressure against the glans so as to reduce the amount of blood which it contains, following which the foreskin may be pulled forward. Failure of this emergency treatment for paraphimosis requires that the physician make an incision through the foreskin, followed, as soon as circumstances permit, by the complete operation of circumcision.

GENITAL HERPES SIMPLEX

There are two types of the herpes simplex virus. Type 1 is the causative agent in the cold sores that commonly appear around the lips. Type 2 of the herpes simplex virus is responsible for lesions that occur in the delicate skin and membranes of the genital areas of both male and female. This virus infection is spread by person-to-person contact and is therefore usually acquired by sexual intercourse. The virus, once it enters a person's tissues, remains latent for the remainder of life and causes mild recurrences of the lesions on the skin and membranes from time to time throughout life. When the virus is first acquired, the lesions appear within about six days following exposure. The lesions usually disappear spontaneously within three to six weeks. In the subsequent attacks, the symptoms are less severe and do not last as long.

Genital herpes simplex is manifested in the male by the appearance of clusters of small vesicles on the glans of the penis, on the foreskin if present, and, occasionally, along the shaft of the penis. As these vesicles rupture, they leave small, shallow ulcers. In the recurrent attacks, the lesions occur at the same sites as those of the primary illness and tend to heal more quickly—within seven to ten days.

Care and Treatment

Genital herpes simplex is a sexually transmitted disease. Its care and treatment is therefore considered in chapter 31, volume 2.

SYPHILIS AND OTHER VENEREAL INFECTIONS

Syphilis and some other sexually transmitted infections cause a solitary lesion, often on the glans of the penis, which becomes ulcerated. For a further consideration of syphilis and other sexually transmitted infections, see chapter 31, volume 2.

CANCER

Cancer of the penis usually makes its first appearance on the glans or the foreskin. It begins as a thickening of the delicate skin, which may then appear wartlike. When allowed to progress, ulceration soon develops.

Any such lesion developing on the

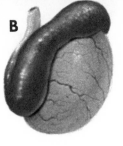

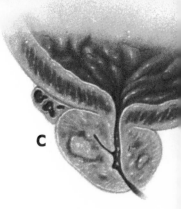

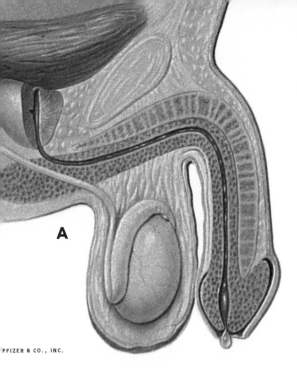

A. The male sex organs, showing inflammation of the urethra such as occurs in nonspecific urethritis. B. The inflammation may extend into the epididymis and (C) also to the prostate.

penis deserves prompt attention by a physician. The earlier the treatment, the less the possibility of spread to other parts of the body and the less will be the loss of functionality.

B. Involvements of the Urethra

GONOCOCCAL URETHRITIS

In gonococcal urethritis the lining of the urethra becomes inflamed because of an infection by the gonococcus—the germ of gonorrhea, usually acquired by sexual contact. The symptoms appear within two to six days after contact with a person already infected with gonorrhea. The severity of the symptoms varies from person to person. In the milder cases there is itching at the terminal portion of the glans followed by the production of a thick, yellow discharge from the urethra. Usually there is pain in the urethra and a burning sensation when urine is passed. When treatment is delayed, the infection extends upward to the bladder with symptoms of painful and frequent urination and bladder spasm.

Care and Treatment

The treatment of gonorrheal urethritis consists of the use of antibiotic medications given in large doses. See chapter 31, volume 2, page 470.

NONGONOCOCCAL URETHRITIS (NONSPECIFIC URETHRITIS)

An inflammation of the urethra in which a discharge escapes at the end of the penis raises the question of the possibility of a gonorrheal infection. However, in more than half of such cases the inflammation is caused by something other than gonorrhea. About half the cases of nongonococcal urethritis are caused by one of the chlamydial organisms, as mentioned in chapter 31, volume 2. The ingestion of certain poisons such as turpentine and wood alcohol may cause the urethra to become inflamed. Even alcoholic beverages sometimes have this effect. When the urethra becomes irritated from trauma or from irritating medicines that have been instilled into the urethra, ordinary bacteria may enter the delicate membrane and set up an infection there. An infection of the prostate gland or of the bladder may extend into the urethra, causing inflammation.

The symptoms of nongonococcal urethritis may be so mild as to consist only of a slight watery discharge from the urethra, or they may be so severe as to consist of a bloody, purulent discharge accompanied by a burning sensation and frequency of urination.

Care and Treatment

The treatment program is directed toward finding and removing the cause of the inflammation. For cases caused by chlamydia, the recommended treatment is tetracycline administered by mouth in specified doses over a period of about three weeks. The patient's sexual partner should receive the same treatment at the same time. Other than this, local treatment by the physician consists of instilling into the urethra a mild antiseptic or soothing solution and, in persistent cases, of instilling a very dilute solution (1:1000) of silver nitrate to aid in eradicating areas of persistent infection.

URETHRAL STRICTURE

Urethral stricture consists of a narrowing of the urethra such as may result from the healing of an injury or from a neglected case of urethritis. The most common cause of urethral stricture is a gonorrheal infection which has not been adequately treated.

The symptoms are those of obstruction to the flow of urine. In a typical case, the urinary stream gradually becomes reduced in size. As the stricture becomes more severe, urination becomes more frequent and is associated with pain in the penis. In some cases the stricture is associated with a per-

sisting infection so that there may be a purulent discharge from the urethra, and the urine, when passed, is cloudy.

Care and Treatment

The treatment of urethral stricture requires the services of a physician, as he gradually stretches the urethral passage by a series of treatments in which instruments of proper size and shape are inserted into the urethra.

C. Diseases of the Prostate

PROSTATITIS (INFECTION OF THE PROSTATE)

The anatomical location of the prostate gland makes it vulnerable to infections from the urethra. The prostate surrounds the urethra at its exit from the bladder, and many ducts carrying prostatic secretion open into the urethra.

Infections involving the prostate (prostatitis) are usually secondary to an infection of the urethra (urethritis). In a minority of cases, however, the infection has been brought to the prostate by way of the blood from an infection in some other part of the body.

In cases of acute prostatitis, there is pain at the base or even at the tip of the penis; uncontrolled dripping of cloudy fluid from the urethra (originating in the prostate); and, usually, fever. There may be slowness of the urinary stream. In some cases the urine contains small

The prostate surrounds the urethra just beneath the bladder.

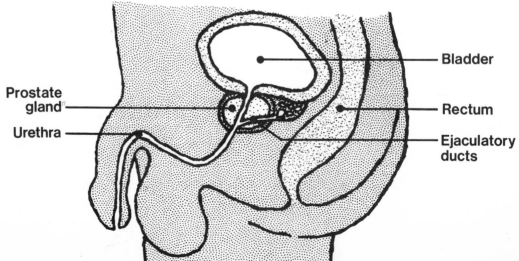

Prostate gland

Urethra

Bladder

Rectum

Ejaculatory ducts

amounts of blood and pus. In some cases of chronic prostatitis no actual infection can be proved. These may be the result of congestion of blood and stagnation of prostatic secretion.

Care and Treatment

The treatment of acute prostatitis consists of the use of appropriate antibiotic medications to correct the infection. Hot sitz baths taken for twenty minutes at a time three or four times a day will help to relieve the symptoms. In such a bath, the patient sits in a tub of water as hot as he can tolerate with ice bags applied to the forehead and over the heart. For cases of chronic prostatitis, hot sitz baths even without the use of antibiotic medications constitute the treatment of choice.

PROSTATIC ENLARGEMENT (BENIGN PROSTATIC HYPERTROPHY)

Prostatic enlargement occurs commonly in elderly men. Even at age forty about 10 percent of men have some enlargement of the prostate. By age 60, this is true of most men.

As the prostate increases in size it tends to reduce the caliber of the urethra as it passes through the prostate. This stricture interferes with the flow of urine, producing the typical symptoms of difficulty in starting the urinary stream, reduced force of the urinary stream, and dribbling of urine after voiding. There is usually increased frequency of urination, especially at night.

There are two hazards associated with enlargement of the prostate: (1) the possibility that the bladder is not emptied completely at the time of voiding (this sets the stage for infection within the bladder) and (2) the possibility that there may be a sudden complete blockage to the flow of urine.

Care and Treatment

Inasmuch as the symptoms of prostatic enlargement develop gradually, a man with this problem should depend upon the advice of his physician on whether the time has come for the prostate to be removed by surgery. The usual surgical procedure (transurethral resection) requires the skill of a urologist—a physician trained in handling diseases of the urinary organs.) The tissue of the prostate is removed through a specially designed instrument inserted through the urethra. This type of surgery usually does not cause impotence.

CANCER OF THE PROSTATE

Cancer of the prostate is one of the common forms of cancer occurring in older men. Fortunately, it is usually a slow-growing type. However, there is also a fast-growing type.

The prostate can be examined satisfactorily by the physician passing his gloved finger through the anal canal and determining the size, shape, and consistency of the prostate as it is felt through the forward wall of the rectum.

Inasmuch as cancer of the prostate in its early stages produces no particular symptoms, it is important for men above 50 years of age to have periodic examinations in which the examining physician determines the state of the prostate. When the prostate is enlarged, this examination should be made at least once a year.

Care and Treatment

When cancer of the prostate develops, it is important for the patient to be placed under the care of a urologist. He must exercise his judgment in deciding whether to remove the prostate by surgery, treat it by radiation, or monitor the progress of the cancer for the next few months. The fast-growing type of cancer of the prostate must have immediate treatment.

D. Involvement of the Seminal Vesicles

SEMINAL VESICULITIS

The seminal vesicles, right and left, are located adjacent to the prostate at

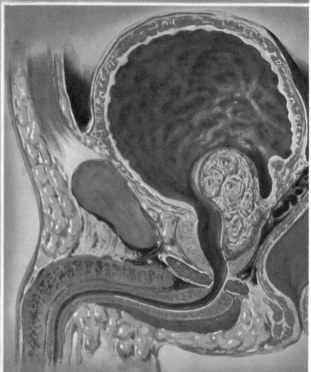

LATERAL LOBES
WITH MEDIAN
COMMISSURE

MEDIAN LOBE

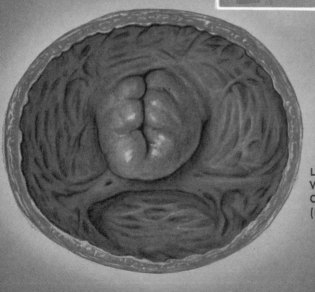

LATERAL LOBES
WITH MEDIAN
COMMISSURE
(Intravesical View)

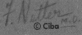

the under surface of the bladder. Their ducts drain through the prostate and into the ejaculatory ducts which carry the seminal fluid into the urethra. Inflammation of the seminal vesicles occurs commonly in association with prostatitis. The causes are the same as those that give rise to prostatitis. The symptoms are the same as in prostatitis, with the usual addition of pain which seems to originate in the groins or in the testes.

Care and Treatment

The treatment for seminal vesiculitis is the same as for prostatitis, including the use of antibiotic medications and hot sitz baths three or four times a day. Infection in the seminal vesicles is difficult to control, and even when the inflammation subsides, future recurrences are common.

E. Involvement of the Epididymis

EPIDIDYMITIS

Inflammation of the epididymis most commonly results from infection which makes its way from the prostate gland, moving through the ductus deferens to the epididymis. Neglected gonorrhea is a frequent cause of epididymitis, though not the only possible cause. Infection and inflammation of the epididymis give rise to swelling, pain, and tenderness within the scrotum. Usually there is fever. The symptoms are made worse by physical activity.

Care and Treatment

The usual case of epididymitis requires no specific treatment beyond what is useful for controlling the infection in the prostate from which the infection in the epididymis was derived. The care of the patient consists of quiet bed rest for at least a week. The pain within the scrotum is relieved somewhat by providing a pillow to support the scrotum so that the testis and the related epididymis do not hang loosely within the scrotum. Antibiotic medications may be useful.

F. Involvements of the Testis

ORCHITIS

Orchitis is the name given to inflammation of the testis. The testis may become involved along with the epididymis in a case of epididymitis. More commonly, however, involvement of the testis is secondary to a systemic infection such as scarlet fever or, especially, mumps.

Orchitis produces severe local pain in the scrotum, with an enlargement of the involved testis. The scrotum is red and swollen. The patient feels ill and typically has a fever. Orchitis may involve one or both testes.

A serious aspect of orchitis is the permanent damage, following severe cases, to those cells of the testis that produce the male sex cells (spermatozoa). When both testes are involved, the patient may be rendered sterile (incapable of becoming a father) because the male sex cells are no longer produced.

Care and Treatment

The patient with orchitis usually feels so ill that he prefers to remain in bed during the few days of the acute phase of the inflammation. Ice packs applied to the scrotum help to relieve the pain. Even while the patient is in bed, it is helpful to support the scrotum by placing a small pillow between the thighs. When the patient is able to walk, it is helpful to support the scrotum by a soft bandage so that the testes do not hang loosely within the scrotum. Attention should be given to treating the systemic disease, such as mumps, when the orchitis is secondary to such an illness.

In an occasional severe case of orchitis, an abscess develops within the affected testis. When this occurs, surgical drainage of the abscess becomes necessary.

INFERTILITY (STERILITY)

Infertility in the male is the inability to bring about conception in the wife. In order for conception to occur and pregnancy to follow, both the husband and the wife must be able to perform their respective roles in producing sex cells. In years past it was often assumed that the wife was primarily at fault when conception did not occur. Current data indicates that in cases where conception does not occur, the man is responsible in about 30 percent of cases, the woman in approximately 40 percent, and both partners in the remaining 30 percent. Here we are dealing with a condition in which the husband is not capable of causing his normal, healthy wife to become pregnant.

Many possible factors cause infertility in a man. A few cases are due to some developmental defect of the male sex organs. These may be impossible to correct. Other cases are due to deficiencies of the endocrine organs and such may or may not be correctable. Damage by disease of the male sex organs, such as prostatitis, may be treatable. In such conditions as those caused by venereal disease or by severe orchitis, the damage may be permanent. Still other cases of infertility are functional in that they can be corrected by removing such factors as intense fatigue, smoking, use of alcohol, excess sexual indulgence, and the psychological conditions contributing to impotence.

Care and Treatment

The first effort must be to determine the particular cause of infertility in a given case. When it is some correctable organic condition, treatment must be planned accordingly. For those cases in which the individual's life-style has interfered with his ability to produce normal sex cells, the remedy consists of improving one's pattern of living. Reform may require the avoidance of alcohol, tobacco, and even caffeine. It requires that the man be temperate in his sexual activities so as to avoid the kind of fatigue that might interfere with the normal function of his sex organs. He should obtain adequate sleep and engage in

regular physical exercise. He should make sure of an adequate diet. And if he is overweight, he should bring his weight within reasonable limits.

TUMORS OF THE TESTES

Tumors of the testes, when they occur, are very subtle in their early development and may be highly malignant as they spread early to other parts of the body. Their highest incidence is in males under 40 years of age. Even the so-called less malignant type of testicular tumor carries an average mortality rate of about 50 percent.

The first evidence of the development of such a tumor is a gradual painless enlargement of the testis. In tumors permitted to continue, the size of the testis increases and the patient notes a feeling of weight in the scrotum. Pain in the affected testis eventually develops. The tumor, as it grows, can be felt through the scrotum and is hard and firm to the touch.

Care and Treatment

The only hope for a favorable outcome is by early detection and prompt surgical removal of the entire testis. When a man has any question prompted by an enlargement of a testis, he should consult his physician promptly.

G. Involvements of the Scrotum and Contents

INGUINAL HERNIA

Hernias are discussed in chapter 17, volume 2. One of the common sites for the development of a hernia is in the inguinal region, that area of the lower part of the abdominal wall just above the scrotum through which the blood vessels and the vas deferens pass on their way to and from the abdominal cavity. In some persons, this area is a weak spot in the abdominal wall that permits the protrusion of a loop of bowel. As such a hernia protrudes, it finds its way into the scrotum causing a significant enlargement there. The protruding mass is soft to the touch, and there may be an associated sensation of pain. The sex organs are not directly affected by such a development, but the hernia should be cared for, preferably by surgical repair of the weak place in the abdominal wall.

HYDROCELE

A hydrocele is an accumulation of clear, light-yellow fluid in the membranous sac around the testis and epididymis and within the scrotum. This condition may develop at any age. It is caused by some mild irritation of the lining of the sac. It may occur in both sides, but more often in only one side. Hydrocele sacs vary greatly in size. Some are so small as to be hardly noticeable. There is a tendency for a hydrocele to increase in size. It causes little or no pain. It does not seem to injure the general health. Verification of a hydrocele as contrasted to a solid tumor is made by placing a bright light behind the enlarged scrotum. In the case of hydrocele, the light is seen to pass quite readily through the clear fluid.

Care and Treatment

A small hydrocele requires no treatment. For those that become large enough to be inconvenient, the physician may remove the fluid from time to time by inserting a needle. The preferable treatment, however, requires surgical correction.

VARICOCELE

A varicocele is a dilitation or varicosity of the veins that carry blood from the testis and epididymis to the large veins of the abdomen. It is a common condition, most men having a mild varicocele on the left side, especially during the years immediately following puberty. The right side is less frequently affected. The dilated veins feel somewhat like a bunch of earthworms at the side of the testis and above it. Varicocele may sometimes cause a slight sensation of weight and a mild, dragging pain; but it does not shorten life or cause a serious threat to health.

Care and Treatment

When a varicocele is not large, no treatment is required. In moderately severe cases, it is helpful to wear a support which suspends the scrotum so that the weight of the varicocele will not be troublesome. In the more severe cases, the condition can be corrected by the surgical removal of a portion of the dilated veins.

Diseases of the Female Sex Organs

A. Breast Diseases

The human breast is subject to many normal changes in size, structure, and function. First there is the marked change that occurs during adolescence when the breast of childhood develops into the breast of young womanhood. This so-called virgin breast is not yet capable of producing milk, but its fundamental structure is established and ready for further development should pregnancy occur. The virgin breast is responsive to the cyclic changes in the endocrine balances throughout the body and typically responds prior to each menstruation by a slight enlargement, which in some persons produces mild discomfort.

When pregnancy occurs, the glandular tissue within the breast undergoes rapid development, and the breast enlarges. Even before the child is born there may be a slight production of secretion which escapes from the nipple. Once the child is born, the glandular tissue within the breast becomes active in the production of milk.

If the baby nurses at the breast, the glandular tissue remains active for a number of months or until nursing at the breast is discontinued. The breast then regresses in size and in functional capacity, only to be activated again should another pregnancy occur. This readiness to produce milk persists until the late forties when, at the time of the menopause, the glandular components within the breast gradually disappear. The fatty tissue within the breast preserves the normal contour, with a slight reduction in size, throughout the remainder of life.

Most of the abnormal conditions that affect the female breast are classed as benign in contrast to cancer of the breast, which is classed as malignant. In some cases it is difficult to determine by a simple external examination whether a condition of the breast is benign or malignant.

Signs to Consider

1. *Discharge From the Nipple.* It is normal for a small amount of milk to be produced in the breasts of a pregnant woman just prior to the delivery of her child. This should cause no concern. In cases in which the breast becomes infected (mastitis) there may be a discharge of pussy fluid from the nipple. In such a case there will be pain and swelling and other evidences of infection within the breast. A bloody discharge from the nipple surely indicates an unhealthy condition within the

breast. A bloody discharge sometimes accompanies benign conditions, but it also occurs in certain cases of cancer of the breast.

2. *Pain in the Breast.* Many women experience mild discomfort in the breasts prior to each menstrual period. Significant pain in the breast is noticed, of course, when an infection develops (mastitis) and in some cases of mammary dysplasia. Early cancer of the breast is usually not accompanied by pain. Perhaps this is unfortunate, for the absence of pain may be falsely reassuring to the woman with an early cancer of the breast.

3. *Changes in Appearance.* In many healthy women one breast is slightly higher than the other and this should cause no concern. But when a change occurs in the shape or appearance of a breast it should be examined by a physician to determine whether disease is developing. Retraction or deviation of one nipple as compared with the other should raise a woman's suspicion. Also, the dimpling of skin over any part of the breast is probably caused by the development of an abnormal condition within the breast.

4. *Detection of a lump.* A woman should make a self-examination of her breasts at least every month. The method of performing this is explained in chapter 11, volume 3, where there is a detailed discussion of cancer of the breast. Many times a lump in the breast is caused by a benign form of disease. However, a lump in the breast is often the first evidence of cancer. Therefore, the finding of a lump in the breast should be taken very seriously, and professional advice should be obtained at once.

ACUTE MASTITIS (INFLAMMATION OF THE BREAST)

Acute mastitis is an infection usually caused by invasion of the staphylococcus germ through a fissure in the delicate skin that covers the nipple. The in-

fection typically occurs a few days or a few weeks after childbirth in a case where the mother is nursing her infant. The infection tends to find its way into some particular area of the breast. The skin over this area becomes red, tender, and firm to the touch.

In the early stage of this infection, the progress of the infection can be halted by the appropriate use of antibiotic medication. When the infection is allowed to progress, the patient develops fever, and a strong possibility exists that an abscess will develop within the breast. Once an abscess forms, a surgical incision must be made so that the abscess can be drained.

When the infection is controlled reasonably early by antibiotic medication, it is acceptable for the infant to continue drawing milk from this breast.

MAMMARY DYSPLASIA (CHRONIC CYSTIC MASTITIS)

This is a condition in which cystic (hollow, fluid-filled) nodules develop within the breast. The condition develops in about 20 percent of women in the 30-to-50 age bracket. It usually involves both breasts, and the cystic nodules of varying sizes are easily felt by the examining fingers.

There may be no symptoms other than the discovery of the nodules, but in many cases pain or tenderness call attention to the presence of these nodules. There may be a slight discharge from the nipple. In some cases, the cysts tend to enlarge just before the time of menstruation. The exact cause of mammary dysplasia is not known, but the fact that the cysts tend to disappear at the time of the menopause without later recurrence, suggests that their development is caused by an imbalance of the endocrine system.

Mammary dysplasia, of itself, is harmless except for the inconvenience and discomfort. But the seriousness of this condition is that it may be easily confused with beginning cancer of the breast. It is tragic, of course, when a beginning cancer is mistakenly considered to be mammary dysplasia and

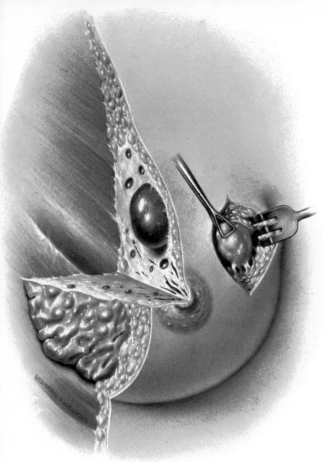

CHAS. PFIZER & CO., INC.

Lower left, chronic cystic mastitis; center, cystic disease with single large cyst; right, benign tumor.

valuable time is lost for treating the cancer. The findings on examination of the breast in mammary dysplasia resemble those in cancer so closely that it is imperative when lumps develop within the breast to make sure which condition is present. This certainty is accomplished by the minor surgical procedure of removing one or more of the lumps for microscopic examination.

Care and Treatment

Once it is made certain that the condition in the breast is that of mammary dysplasia, the larger lumps can be reduced by the physician inserting a small needle and withdrawing the fluid which the cysts contain. Also, appropriate endocrine preparations may reduce the cyst formation. Oral contraceptives, containing hormones as they do, may be of help. Even so, the patient with mammary dysplasia should be examined at frequent intervals (every six months) as a means of detecting any development of cancer. The woman with mammary dysplasia carries twice the prospect of developing cancer of the breast as does the woman without mammary dysplasia. The pain and the tenderness associated with the presence of cysts in this disease can be partially relieved by the wearing of a brassiere which gives good support and protects, somewhat from mechanical injury.

FIBROADENOMA

A fibroadenoma is a true tumor of the breast, a disease slightly less common than cancer of the breast. It tends to occur in relatively young women—in the 15- to 35-year age group. It is not classed as malignant, because it does not tend to spread. It typically occurs as a single, round, rubbery, painless mass which may be up to two inches (5 cm.) in diameter. A fibroadenoma may increase in size during a pregnancy.

Care and Treatment

The treatment for a fibroadenoma is surgical removal of the tumor. This is accomplished rather simply because this type of tumor is enclosed within a capsule of fibrous tissue.

CANCER OF THE BREAST

Cancer of the breast is considered in chapter 11, volume 3. It is a serious disease because of the tendency to spread to other parts of the body. Cancer of the breast is highly malignant. It occurs quite commonly, involving, on the average, one out of every thirteen Caucasian women. Many studies have been made to determine what factors predominate in making a woman susceptible to this disease. In summary, cancer of the breast occurs most commonly under the following conditions.

1. Caucasian race.
2. Age above 50.

3. History of cancer in other family members such as mother or sister.

4. Previous cancer of the lining of the uterus or of the other breast.

5. Previous development of mammary dysplasia.

6. Early adolescence—first menstruation prior to age 12.

7. Never married.

8. Never pregnant.

9. First child born after age 30.

From the above list it is clear that most women carry a certain risk of developing breast cancer. Those with the greatest number of risk factors obviously are in greatest danger of developing this disease. A woman who has several risk factors should be consistent in making self-examination of her breasts once each month and should report to her doctor any changes that might signal the development of a beginning cancer.

B. Disorders of the Ovaries

FUNCTIONAL DISORDERS

The ovaries have two functions to perform: the production of female sex cells (ova) and the production of sex hormones. Hormones regulate the secondary sex characteristics and, to some degree, the cyclic functioning of the sex organs. When the hormones produced by the ovaries are either in short supply or in superabundance, the symptoms consist of alterations in the secondary sex characteristics (the female characteristics) or in changes in the usual monthly menstrual cycle. The exact changes thus produced will be different in the various age groups: in childhood before the onset of puberty, during the active sex life of the woman, or after the menopause.

1. *Hypofunction of the Ovaries.* There is a genetic disorder called gonadal dysgenesis (Turner's syndrome) in which the ovaries do not develop adequately. In this condition the transformation from girlhood to womanhood is defective. The breasts fail to de-velop. Hair in the pubic and axillary areas is sparse. Usually, there is an absence of the usual monthly cycle so that menstruation does not occur. The logical treatment for this condition is the administration of estrogen hormones as a replacement for what the ovaries are not producing. This form of treatment will stimulate the development of the secondary sex characteristics but will not bring about the production of normal female sex cells (ova).

In the early or middle fifties, the ovaries normally cease their production of female sex cells and, at the same time, reduce their production of female sex hormones. Thus it is a reduction in the function of the ovaries that brings about the menopause ("change of life"), discussed later in this chapter.

The ovaries are interrelated functionally with other endocrine organs. Therefore, the function of the ovaries may decline in response to disorders of such other endocrine organs as the pituitary, the adrenal, or the hypothalamus. It is doubtless this interrelationship of the endocrine organs that accounts for the cases of temporary lack of menstruation in young women under emotional stress.

2. *Hyperfunction of the Ovaries.* Certain tumors may develop within the ovaries that cause them to produce an excess of female sex hormones. When such a tumor develops during girlhood, the girl takes on the characteristics of womanhood at an unusually early age. The breasts develop and menstruation begins perhaps as early as six or eight years of age. When the feminizing tumors develop during the sexually active years of life, the symptoms consist essentially of irregular uterine bleeding. When the ovaries become hyperactive after the menopause, the symptom consists of false menstruation (bleeding from the uterus at the time of life when there should be no such bleeding).

The usual treatment for hyperfunction of the ovaries is the surgical removal of the involved ovary or of both ovaries when both are involved. Such an operation is called an oophorectomy.

INFLAMMATORY DISEASE OF THE OVARIES

Inflammatory disorders affecting the ovaries (oophoritis) typically occur as a part of a general infection of the pelvic organs designated as pelvic inflammatory disease. The problem may be caused by one or more of several kinds of germs. Many of the serious cases are associated with a neglected gonorrheal infection. The severity of the infection and the eventual outcome vary from case to case. Of course, cases recognized and treated early fare best. In neglected cases the possibility exists of future infertility (inability to bear children) and even death.

Usually inflammation of the ovaries is combined with inflammation of the oviduct (salpingo-oophoritis). The symptoms in acute cases include lower abdominal pain, abdominal tenderness, back pain extending down one or both legs, pussy discharge from the vagina, fever, chills, and rapid heartbeat.

Care and Treatment

The treatment must be adapted to the conditions of the individual case and includes the use of appropriate antibiotic medications and, perhaps, extensive pelvic surgery.

There is further discussion of pelvic inflammatory disease in the latter part of this chapter.

FOLLICLE CYSTS OF THE OVARIES

In the normal course of ovarian function during a woman's sex life, several follicles develop at the surface of each ovary during each month. Each of these contains a female sex cell in addition to a little fluid. Normally one of these follicles, sometimes in the right ovary and sometimes in the left, bursts and allows the female sex cell (ovum) to escape from the ovary and begin its passage through the oviduct toward the uterus. As soon as this one follicle ruptures, the endocrine influences shift, and the remaining follicles, which did not rupture, soon disappear.

In some cases the fluid in the follicles which have not ruptured disappears slowly, so there remain several blister-like structures (fluid-filled) at the surface of the ovaries. These constitute the follicle cysts of which we speak here. Usually these disappear spontaneously within about two months.

In some cases the presence of these cysts causes aching pelvic pain and is occasionally responsible for abnormal bleeding from the uterus. In such cases, appropriate treatment with ovarian hormones will usually reestablish normal ovarian function and hasten the disappearance of the persisting cysts. Ovarian cysts which persist longer than two months are probably associated with some other disorder of the ovaries.

POLYCYSTIC OVARIAN DISEASE (SCLEROCYSTIC OVARIAN DISEASE)

Polycystic ovarian disease is an uncommon ailment in which multiple cysts develop in both ovaries. It occurs typically between ages 15 and 30, and may be responsible for the failure of the ovaries to produce female sex cells. The typical symptom consists of periods of time in which menstruation does not occur.

Care and Treatment

Hormone therapy may help to reestablish the normal menstrual cycle. In some cases, the surgical removal of portions of each ovary is helpful.

OVARIAN TUMORS

The majority of tumors that develop in the ovaries contain fluid-filled cavities (cysts). Tumors of the ovaries are divided into two classes: benign and malignant. The benign tumors do not tend to spread to other parts of the body and are not life-threatening. However, certain of these benign tumors, if not removed by surgery, grow to enormous size. One type of benign ovarian tumor is the teratoma or dermoid cyst.

It is peculiar in that various body structures, such as bones, teeth, or hair, are found in the cysts.

There are several types of malignant tumors of the ovary, all of which are dangerous because of their tendency to spread to other parts of the body. Most of the malignant tumors of the ovary develop within the ovarian substance, but about 20 percent develop as the result of tumor cells which have migrated to the ovary from some other part of the body.

One of the problems in dealing with ovarian tumors, particularly with malignant ones, is that they may not produce symptoms in the early stages of their development. When symptoms do develop, they consist of abdominal swelling and, as they grow larger, of difficult breathing, indigestion, frequency of urination, and the development of varicose veins in the legs. Some ovarian tumors interfere with the normal endocrine balances and thus produce symptoms relating to the menstrual cycle.

Care and Treatment

Ovarian tumors which are benign are treated successfully by surgical removal. Malignant ovarian tumors, however, carry a high mortality rate, largely because they do not produce symptoms in their early stages and therefore do not receive early treatment. Surgical removal followed by chemotherapy (medications which destroy cancer cells) is the usual method of treatment.

C. Diseases of the Oviducts (Fallopian Tubes)

INFLAMMATORY DISEASE OF THE OVIDUCTS (SALPINGITIS)

Inflammation of the oviducts occurs in connection with three kinds of infection: (1) that of gonorrhea (the most frequent cause), (2) that produced by streptococcic and staphylococcic organisms, and (3) that of tuberculosis (the least frequent cause). An inflammatory involvement of the oviducts is called salpingitis.

The germs of gonorrhea gain access to the female sex organs by way of sexual intercourse with a partner already infected with this disease. The germs first cause an infection of the tissues of the vulva, the vagina, and the cervix of the uterus. The infection then follows the lining of the uterus and enters the oviducts, where it causes greater tissue damage than in the interior of the uterus. This infection may move on through the length of the oviducts and involve the lining of the pelvic cavity and the ovaries in what is described as pelvic inflammatory disease. (See the discussion of pelvic inflammatory disease in the latter part of this chapter.) Gonorrheal involvement of the oviduct may occur promptly after the initial gonorrheal infection, or it may occur some time later. Whenever it occurs, the lining of the oviduct is virtually destroyed and an abscess may possibly develop. The usual, unfortunate complication is that the lumen of the oviduct becomes narrowed or even obliterated, interfering with the passage of the female sex cells (ova) to the uterus. Thus, sterility (inability to become pregnant) usually follows.

Infection by streptococcic or staphylococcic organisms may begin as a puerperal infection (occurring following childbirth) in which the germs enter the tissues of the cervix of the uterus following an injury to these tissues. Such an infection may occur following an abortion. The germs find their way into the tissues that surround the uterus and are then carried by veins and lymphatic vessels to the oviducts. The lining of the oviducts is not always destroyed in this type of infection, and thus in some cases it is still possible for the patient to become pregnant after the infection subsides.

Involvement of the oviducts by tuberculosis occurs infrequently, but when it does occur it is secondary to a tuberculous infection in some other part of the body, the germs having been carried by the blood.

The symptoms of salpingitis vary somewhat with the type of infection. In acute gonorrheal salpingitis the patient experiences severe pain in the lower abdomen, with distension of the abdomen. There is nausea, vomiting, fever, and rapid pulse. In the septic infections (those produced by streptococcus or staphylococcus organisms) the patient is weak and has pelvic pain and perhaps chills and fever. There may be a pussy discharge from the vagina.

Care and Treatment

The treatment of salpingitis should be prompt and adequate, in the hope of preventing a further extension of the infection. The patient should be under the supervision of a physician who will first make the necessary examinations and tests to determine what type of germ is causing the infection. He will then prescribe the appropriate antibiotic medications. In the meantime, the patient should rest in bed, preferably with the head of the bed raised 18 to 20 inches higher than the foot (Fowler position). Precautions should be taken to prevent the patient from becoming dehydrated. This is especially important if the patient is losing fluid by vomiting. It may even be necessary to administer fluid by vein in order to prevent dehydration.

Resistance to the infection can be promoted by the use of hot sitz baths in which the patient sits in hot water with the temperature being gradually increased to the patient's tolerance. The sitz bath should last about 20 minutes and be repeated two or three times a day.

In some cases of salpingitis, once the acute infection is under control, the physician will advise the surgical removal of the tissues involved. Removal is especially necessary when an abscess has developed. The surgical removal of an oviduct is called salpingectomy.

TUBAL ECTOPIC PREGNANCY

In an occasional case of early pregnancy the ovum now united with a male sex cell (spermatozoan) fails to make its way as it normally should through the entire length of the oviduct (fallopian tube) and into the interior of the uterus. In such an event, the unborn child will begin its development wherever the united sex cells happen to lodge. This eventuality constitutes a so-called ectopic (misplaced) pregnancy. By far the most common site for an ectopic pregnancy is within one of the oviducts, where it constitutes a tubal pregnancy. The usual cause of a tubal pregnancy is that the oviduct has been previously inflamed and the lumen has become so narrow that the ovum does not have room to pass through.

The hazard of tubal pregnancy is that the tissues of the oviduct are not designed to stretch as much as those of the uterus. Thus, after about three months of development, the fetus has grown to such size that it causes the oviduct to rupture, producing a life-threatening hemorrhage for which emergency surgical treatment is the only satisfactory remedy. In the meantime, the unborn child perishes. It is very desirable to detect a tubal pregnancy during the three-month period before spontaneous rupture occurs. The evidences are simple and few:

1. Indications of early pregnancy including (a) a missed menstrual period, (b) "morning sickness" (in about half of early pregnancies), (c) tenderness and enlargement of the breasts, and (d) a positive pregnancy test as may be arranged by the physician.

2. Scanty "spotting" through the vagina of dark-colored blood.

3. Cramping pain in one side of the lower abdomen beginning soon after the first menstrual period is missed.

In cases of tubal pregnancy not detected and treated before rupture occurs, there develop startling symptoms of an emergency situation. It is important that these be recognized for what they mean. Immediate surgery is necessary to control the profuse bleeding occurring at the site of rupture. The

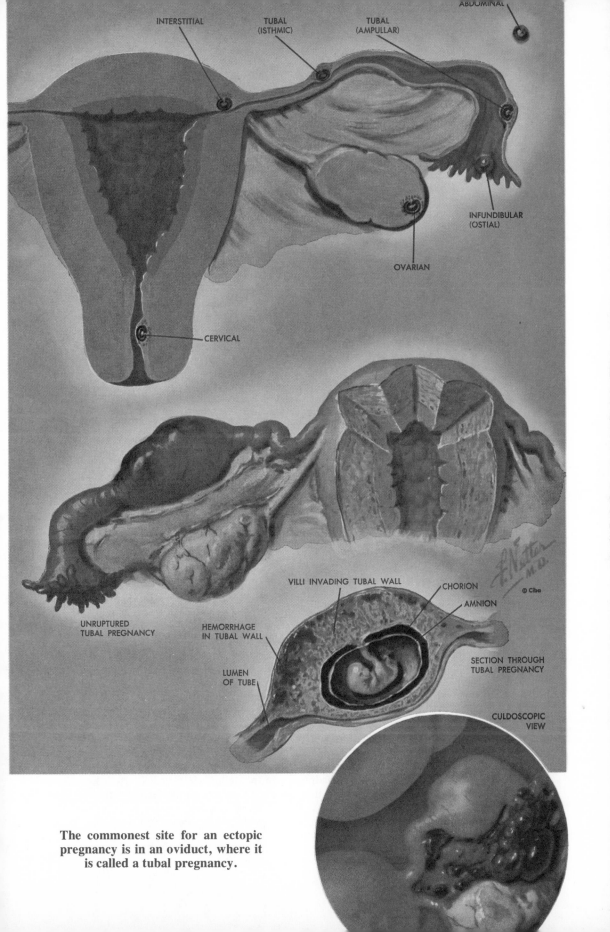

INTERSTITIAL

TUBAL (ISTHMIC)

TUBAL (AMPULLAR)

ABDOMINAL

INFUNDIBULAR (OSTIAL)

OVARIAN

CERVICAL

UNRUPTURED TUBAL PREGNANCY

VILLI INVADING TUBAL WALL

CHORION

AMNION

HEMORRHAGE IN TUBAL WALL

SECTION THROUGH TUBAL PREGNANCY

LUMEN OF TUBE

CULDOSCOPIC VIEW

The commonest site for an ectopic pregnancy is in an oviduct, where it is called a tubal pregnancy.

evidences of rupture of a tubal pregnancy are these:

1. Previous indications, as mentioned above, that a tubal pregnancy exists.

2. Marked, sudden, lower abdominal pain.

3. Evidences of sudden hemorrhage even though in this situation the blood is still contained within the abdominal cavity. These evidences of severe hemorrhage may include fainting, shock, extreme weakness, thirst, profuse sweating, air hunger, and a failure to pass urine.

Care and Treatment

Tubal ectopic pregnancy requires surgical intervention. It is never possible to preserve the fetus. In the fortunate cases in which the diagnosis has been made before the oviduct ruptures, the surgeon may find it feasible to remove the fetus and its membranes from the oviduct and then repair the oviduct.

In the emergency situation in which the oviduct has already ruptured, the surgeon's concern is to control the profuse bleeding from the torn tissues at the site of rupture and restore the volume of blood that has been lost from the patient's vascular system. The blood that has escaped from the torn tissues is now "at large" within the abdominal cavity. This pool of blood must be removed. In some cases it is possible to salvage this blood and return it to the patient by so-called autotransfusion. Otherwise, the patient will need to receive donor blood by transfusion.

D. Uterine Diseases

MENSTRUAL DISORDERS AND UTERINE BLEEDING

First we need to mention the normal sequence of events in the menstrual month so there will be a basis for comparison when we consider the disorders that may occur. Menstruation is a normal circumstance in which part of the delicate lining of the uterus becomes loosened from its attachment and, together with a certain amount of blood and tissue fluid, passes through the cervix of the uterus, then through the vagina, and escapes to the outside. For the average woman, menstruation occurs about every 28 days, but in some perfectly normal persons the interval may be as short as 20 days or as long as 48 days. The process of menstruation lasts for a period of three to seven days—shorter in some women and longer in others. The process is accompanied by a certain amount of discomfort because the muscle in the wall of the uterus contracts as the shedding of the lining takes place.

In the life history of a woman, menstruation occurs first at about 12 years of age and continues at "monthly" intervals until about age 50, when it ceases at the time of menopause. Menstruation normally ceases during periods of pregnancy. Women in good health may occasionally fail to menstruate at the expected time. Such a missed period suggests the possibility of a beginning pregnancy, but it may also occur when a woman is excessively tired or when she has been under excessive emotional stress.

The days of the menstrual month are numbered from the first day of the occurrence of menstruation. For our present purpose, we will use the average 28-day menstrual cycle as an illustration. Beginning with day 1, menstruation occurs and lasts for a few days—in some women only three days and for others as much as seven days. About day 14, one of the ovaries liberates a female sex cell (an ovum). In the meantime, the lining of the uterus is being restored, following the few days of menstruation, so that it will be ready to receive and nourish the combined sex cells should conception take place. If conception and consequent pregnancy do not occur there is a sudden decline in the production of the ovarian hormones which have stimulated the restoration of the lining of the uterus. This decline occurs on about the twenty-eighth day, allowing the next menstruation to begin on day 1 of the following cycle.

Now that we have reviewed the normal events that take place in the uterus each month, we are prepared to draw the line between the normal and the abnormal in uterine function. Bleeding from the uterus must be considered abnormal if it occurs during childhood prior to the time that a girl reaches her time of puberty (when menstruation normally begins). Bleeding from the uterus is abnormal if it occurs in later life after menstruation has ceased at the time of the menopause. Also, the pattern of menstruation must be considered abnormal if the amount of blood lost at menstruation is either less or greater than the usual amount. Extreme degrees of discomfort (extreme cramps) must also be considered as abnormal.

Amenorrhea. Amenorrhea is a condition in which menstruation does not occur. In primary amenorrhea a girl who has reached the age of puberty (when the sex organs become active) does not menstruate month by month. The cause may be some failure of normal development of the sex organs that interferes with the discharge of the menstrual flow from the uterus through the vagina. It may be the result of an endocrine disorder in which the ovaries, the pituitary gland, or the thyroid gland are not functioning normally. It may be caused by unfavorable conditions of health, such as crash dieting, obesity, or some debilitating illness. It may be caused by emotional stress or by the use of certain drugs.

Secondary amenorrhea is a symptom in which a woman who has previously menstruated normally now fails to menstruate over a period of three or four months. The difficulty may be caused by faulty function of the endocrine organs or by some systemic disease that interferes with the normal processes of metabolism or nutrition. It may be caused by adhesions or disease that interfere with the normal passage of the menstrual flow.

Amenorrhea is a symptom, not a disease. Therefore the remedy consists of identifying and treating the basic cause. In many cases the family physician can make necessary examinations. In some cases he may refer the patient to a physician who specializes in gynecology or endocrinology. Once the underlying cause is determined, attention should focus on the treatment of this condition.

Dysmenorrhea. Dysmenorrhea consists of severe suffering as compared with the moderate discomfort that normally accompanies the process of menstruation. In dysmenorrhea there occur intermittent, sharp, cramping pains which begin in the lower abdomen and are reflected to the lower back and the thighs. The symptoms may be so severe as to be accompanied by nausea, vomiting, and diarrhea. The symptoms usually reach their peak within 24 hours after the beginning of the menstrual flow. Dysmenorrhea is said to be the most common of all of the complaints relating to the female sex organs. It is classified as primary or secondary. Primary dysmenorrhea includes the majority of cases. In these there is no actual disease or abnormality of the sex organs. In secondary dysmenorrhea the pain at the time of menstruation is caused by disease such as inflammation of the sex organs, tumors of the ovary or uterus, or obstruction to the flow of menstrual fluid caused by scar tissue or tumor formation.

Care and Treatment

There are several means by which the symptoms of primary dysmenorrhea may be relieved. The simplest and the least hazardous is the application of heat by the placing of fomentations or a heating pad over the lower abdomen and lower part of the back. Such applications of heat should be used for 20 to 30 minutes, three or four times a day until the symptoms are relieved. For details of the use of heat in such cases, see chapter 25, volume 3.

Many women use aspirin as a pain-relieving medication at the time of menstruation. Best results are obtained by beginning the use of aspirin (One or two five-grain tablets every four hours) a few hours before the menstrual flow begins and continuing it until the symptoms are relieved. When aspirin is used for this purpose, the family doctor should be so informed so that he can be on the watch for unfavorable effects of this type of treatment. Stronger pain-relieving medications are not advisable because of the danger of establishing drug dependence, the prelude to drug addiction.

Many women with dysmenorrhea obtain relief by the use of birth control pills. For the relief of dysmenorrhea, the birth control pills are used in the same pattern of dosage as is used for the prevention of pregnancy.

A recent development in the treatment of dysmenorrhea depends on the observation that the chemical substance prostaglandin, produced by the tissues which line the uterus, has the effect of causing painful menstruation when present in excessive amounts. Certain medications are available which inhibit the production of prostaglandin. These are expected to relieve the pain of dysmenorrhea in a majority of cases. They sometimes produce unfavorable side effects, so their use should be under the direction of a physician.

Cases of secondary dysmenorrhea are best treated, of course, by discovering and correcting the disease of the female sex organs responsible for causing menstruation to be painful. This requires examination, diagnosis, and treatment by a physician.

Abnormal Bleeding From the Uterus. Excessive bleeding from the uterus most often occurs in connection with the menstrual period, in which case it is called *menorrhagia*. Bleeding at other times is called *metrorrhagia*. The most frequent causes of abnormal uterine hemorrhage are the following: tumors of the uterus, cancer of the uterus, overgrowth of the tissue which lines the uterus, ovarian cysts, retention of a portion of the placenta following childbirth, and disturbances of the endocrine glands.

LACERATION OF THE CERVIX OF THE UTERUS

Childbirth is often attended by some injury to the cervix (the outlet of the uterus). Small lacerations (breaks of tissue) usually heal without trouble. Extensive lacerations, however, may cause much discomfort and ill health. Chronic inflammation of the membrane lining the uterus, and a disagreeable discharge from the vagina are common complications of neglected lacerations of the cervix. Old, unrepaired, eroded lacerations predispose to cancer.

Care and Treatment

About six weeks after childbirth, every mother should return to her physician for a pelvic examination, at which time, if needed, treatment may be given to the cervix to prevent development of possible chronic trouble.

PUERPERAL INFECTION ("CHILD-BED FEVER")

The puerperium (postpartum period) is that period of a few days following the delivery of a child during which the female sex organs are returning to their usual, nonpregnant condition. Because of the disruption of tissue at the time of childbirth, germs may enter the tissues temporarily unprotected. The serious possibility of puerperal infection exists in connection with a regular childbirth and even after a miscarriage or an abortion.

Because of the advances made in medical science and the careful procedures followed by those who now attend mothers at the time of childbirth, the incidence of puerperal infection has been greatly reduced. But it is still practically impossible to keep the vulva and vaginal tissues entirely free from germs. Symptoms, when puerperal infection develops, appear about the third day after childbirth and consist of fever, rapid heartbeat, tenderness in the lower abdomen, and a foul-smelling discharge from the vagina. When not treated promptly and adequately, puerperal infection may lead to such serious complications as abscess formation, thrombophlebitis, and septic shock.

Care and Treatment

The patient should receive hospital care under the supervision of a physician. The treatment consists essentially of the use of such antibiotic medications as will control the particular infection. The patient must be given abundant fluids, even by the intravenous route. A padded icebag applied to the patient's lower abdomen 20 minutes out of each hour, during the period of treatment, helps to prevent the spread of the infection.

DISPLACEMENTS OF THE UTERUS

The uterus is normally held in position by four pairs of ligaments, by muscles and fascia, and by the fat contained in the tissues of the pelvis. Even so, the uterus may be displaced backward, sideways, or downward. A tumor of the uterus may drag or push it into some abnormal position. A tumor

Displacement of the uterus.

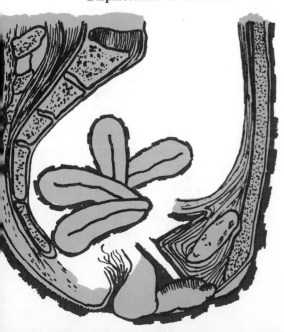

located in one of the surrounding structures may displace the uterus by pressure.

A settling downward of the uterus is called prolapse. Prolapse of the uterus may be so extreme that the cervix protrudes from the vulva. Loss of weight, weakening of the ligaments, and unrepaired lacerations that occurred at childbirth are the chief causes of such downward sagging. Backward tipping of the uterus is called retroversion. Displacements of the uterus may cause pelvic pain, backache, abnormal menstrual bleeding, and inability to become pregnant.

Care and Treatment

When the uterus becomes displaced, it may be possible for the physician to perform a so-called bimanual manipulation to bring the organ into a more favorable position. In the more serious cases the physician may recommend a surgical procedure in which the ligaments which hold the uterus are reinforced so as to retain the organ in normal position.

TROPHOBLASTIC DISEASE

A curious condition occasionally develops in connection with a pregnancy in which cells belonging to the placenta grow excessively and at the expense of the fetus. In the United States this condition occurs once in about 2000 pregnancies. Strangely it is more common in Asian countries, in which it occurs once in about 200 pregnancies. In about 80 percent of these cases, the abnormal growth of tissue remains within the cavity of the uterus and constitutes what is called an hydatidiform mole. It consists of a mass of grapelike vesicles. In about 15 percent of cases of trophoblastic disease the growth of tissue invades the muscular wall of the uterus and is then called a chorioadenoma destruens. In the remaining 5 percent of cases, the abnormal tissue not only invades the wall of the uterus, but cell clusters migrate to remote parts of the body where they establish highly malignant tumors. This highly malignant

455

abnormal discharge, (B) those causing ulcers, (C) those associated with lumps or bumps in the affected areas, (D) those transmitted by lice or mites, and (E) those, other than the above, in which there is inflammation of the vagina.

A. Diseases Characterized by Discharges

GONORRHEA

Gonorrhea is the most subtle of the serious diseases transmitted by sexual contact. Because of the very contagious nature of gonorrhea, the physician who treats a case is required by law to report it to the Public Health Department. However, many cases go unreported and, unfortunately, untreated. Estimates vary on the percentage of cases actually reported, one being as low as 15 percent and another, 32 percent. Even so, the number of reported cases runs between one million and two million new cases per year in the United States. No wonder gonorrhea is a major concern of health-promoting agencies!

The symptoms of gonorrhea vary greatly from case to case and from time to time in a case not adequately treated. In a woman, the first symptoms typically appear three to ten days after intercourse with an infected man and consist of pain on urination, pain in the vagina, and a profuse discharge from the vagina, yellow-green in color and fetid in odor. In a man, the initial symptoms typically appear in two to six days—a little sooner than in a woman. They consist of itching at the outlet of the urethra, burning on urination, and the appearance of a yellow, thick, pussy discharge from the urethra. When the infection is allowed to progress untreated, there may develop frequency and urgency of urination.

One of the subtle features of gonorrhea is that some persons with this infection have no symptoms even when the disease is active. Up to 50 percent of infected women harbor the infection without realizing they have it. Up to 10 percent of infected men are "silent carriers" without symptoms. Without symptoms, they neglect treatment. These people present a continuing hazard to others and are themselves candidates for the serious complications that occur in untreated cases. By carelessness in the bathroom and about the home they may transmit the germs to children in the family, causing such miserable infections as those that cause blindness. Infants and young girls are particularly susceptible to gonorrheal infections carried by contaminated hands, clothing, or towels.

One of the common complications of gonorrhea in women is salpingitis and the lamentable prospect of ectopic pregnancy or the permanent inability to become pregnant. Gonorrhea is one of the important causes of pelvic inflammatory disease, as described in the preceding chapter.

In men the gonorrheal infection easily spreads to the prostate or to the epididymis, causing prostatitis or epididymitis. Also, there is the prospect in untreated men of the later occurrence of stricture of the urethra.

In both men and women, but more commonly in women, the danger lurks that the germs that cause gonorrhea may be carried by the blood throughout the body, thus causing skin lesions, septic arthritis of various joints, and even involvements of the heart or liver.

Gonorrheal infections may occur in the pharynx or in the anorectal region. In these cases the transmission of the germs is usually by way of aberrant sexual relations. The membranes of the eye are especially susceptible to infection by the germs of gonorrhea. Formerly, some of the most tragic cases of blindness occurred when a newborn baby's eyes were thus infected at the time of birth. Now the law requires that the eyes of all babies must be treated appropriately at the time of birth.

The diagnosis of gonorrhea is usually made by the physician's examination of discharges from the urethra, vagina, or other affected tissues. It may be neces-

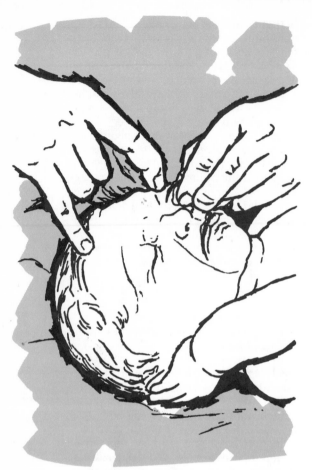

Treatment of the newborn against gonorrheal infection prevents possible blindness from such infection.

sary to have the specimen cultured in the laboratory to confirm the diagnosis. But the mere finding of the germs of gonorrhea in a given case does not rule out the possibility that some other sexually transmitted disease may also be present. Hence the physician usually requests other tests so as to detect any other condition that may deserve treatment.

Care and Treatment

The treatment of gonorrhea is by the prompt and intensive use of appropriate antibiotic medications. Persistence in the program of treatment is often necessary because various strains of the germ react in various ways to the medications. In recent years there have developed so-called resistant strains of these germs. For the successful treatment of infections with such strains, the physician will have to use other types of medications than those ordinarily found effective. Even when the symptoms have abated, it is advisable to repeat the laboratory tests to determine whether the germs may still be present.

NONGONOCOCCAL URETHRITIS

Nongonococcal urethritis is so named because (1) this disease, though it resembles gonorrhea, is not caused by the germ that causes gonorrhea; (2) it affects both men and women, but the symptoms are usually more conspicuous among affected men than among affected women; and (3) in men it is the urethra that is involved in the early stages of the disease. The number of cases of nongonococcal urethritis has increased enormously in recent years. It may be caused by any one of several kinds of germs, but in more than half of the cases the responsible germ is *Chlamydia trachomatis*.

For nongonococcal urethritis the incubation period (elapsed time from sexual contact until symptoms appear) is longer than in gonorrhea, being from one to three weeks, or even longer. The symptoms are similar but usually milder than those of gonorrhea. The possible complications in both male and female are about the same as with gonorrhea. In the male there may develop urethral stricture, epididimytis, and even arthritis. Relapses are common, but many supposed relapses are probably caused by reinfection. In the female, the infection commonly involves the vagina and cervix of the uterus. Salpingitis and pelvic inflammatory disease may develop as complications. When a pregnant woman harbors this infection, the baby may become infected as it passes through the birth canal, with possible infections of the membranes of the eyes and/or the pharynx.

Care and Treatment

Cases of nongonococcal urethritis do not respond to the use of penicillin, the mainstay for treating gonorrhea. Instead, most of these cases are treated by the use of tetracycline administered by mouth in specified doses over a period of about three weeks. For cases that do not tolerate tetracycline, erythromycin is an effective alternative. It is very important that the patient's sexual partner be treated also, even though the partner may not be having symptoms at the time.

B. Diseases Characterized by Ulcers

GENITAL HERPES SIMPLEX

Genital herpes simplex is a sexually transmitted disease caused by a virus quite similar to the virus responsible for chicken pox and for the common herpetic lesions around the mouth (cold sores). The virus which attacks the genital organs is designated as herpes simplex virus, Type 2. In the female, genital herpes simplex causes painful lesions on the delicate skin of the vulva and the membrane lining the vagina. In the male the lesions appear on the penis. This disease accounts for 10 to 15 percent of all sexually transmitted diseases.

The lesions develop in about a week (from 2 to 20 days) after sexual contact with a person who is in an active phase of the disease. The skin or membrane of the affected area first becomes reddened and then develops many tiny vesicles which soon break down to form small, painful ulcers. The ulcers tend to heal spontaneously in about 10 days.

The virus, once acquired, tends to remain latent in a person's tissues for life, causing milder recurrences of the lesions from time to time when the individual's general vitality is at low ebb. The lesions of the recurrent attacks shed the virus just as readily as do those of the original attack. Therefore the disease is contagious whenever the lesions occur.

In addition to its being contagious, there are two other serious considerations with respect to genital herpes simplex as it affects women. First is the grave possibility of its being transmitted to a newborn child. When lesions are present in the mother's cervix or vagina at the time of delivery, the prospects of the child becoming infected are variously estimated at between 10 and 50 percent. The newborn's defenses against infection are not yet fully developed, and the infant death rate from such infection approaches 50 percent. Because of this possibility physicians usually recommend delivery by cesarean operation for expectant mothers who have active genital herpes simplex.

The second serious complication for women is the increased prospect of cancer of the cervix of the uterus. Genital herpes simplex increases a woman's susceptibility to cancer of the cervix by about five times. It is therefore recommended that the woman who has this infection should arrange for an examination which includes a Pap test at least once a year, this as a means of detecting cancerous changes at an early stage.

Care and Treatment

Inasmuch as genital herpes simplex is caused by a virus, there is, as yet, no real cure. Treatment is still aimed at relieving symptoms. The treatment for the initial attack, when the virus is first acquired, differs from that of the recurrent attacks that follow from time to time throughout life.

For the initial attack acyclovir (Zovirax), a synthetic drug available in a 5 percent ointment, is now recommended. It was approved in 1982 for use in the United States. It has proved effective in hastening the healing of the ulcers that occur in the delicate tissues of the genital region during the initial attack. The ointment is applied to the lesions every three hours, six times a day, for seven days.

For a male who has not been circumcised, the foreskin should be retracted so that all areas of the delicate skin are treated. Acyclovir will not prevent later recurrences, and it is not recommended for treatment of the recurrent attacks.

For the recurrent attacks the involved areas should be bathed three or four times a day with a salt solution (1 teaspoonful of salt to the pint of water) or with a mild antiseptic solution (such as benzalkonium 1:4000). Following this treatment, the area should be dried and then dusted with aluminum acetate powder. Should the lesions become infected with ordinary bacteria, treatment with an antibiotic medication is indicated.

SYPHILIS (LUES VENEREA)

Syphilis has long been considered the most serious of the sexually transmitted diseases because of its persistence in the human body when the infection is untreated and because of its various destructive and incapacitating effects on the body's tissues and organs. Syphilis has been known as a sexually transmitted disease since the late 1400s when it was disseminated in Europe in epidemic proportions by the sailors and soldiers of that era.

The advent of penicillin, remarkably effective in the treatment of syphilis, has partially controlled the spread of this disease; but still nearly 100,000 new cases are reported each year in the United States, with an estimated backlog of more than 300,000 untreated cases. The responsible germ is the *Treponema pallidum,* a spiral-shaped organism that multiplies rapidly in human tissues.

The germs of syphilis can enter the body either through some break in the skin or by passing directly through an intact moist membrane such as lines the vagina or mouth. The lesions of syphilis, described later, occur in either the skin or in a moist membrane, and these lesions teem with the germs. The disease is most frequently acquired by sexual intercourse with a person in

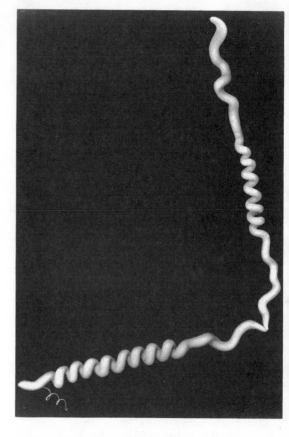

The corkscrew appearance of the syphilis germ (highly magnified).

whom a lesion or lesions are present. It can also be acquired by the accidental injection into the skin of contaminated material. During the last five months of pregnancy it is readily transmitted from an infected mother to her unborn child. The disease is rarely transmitted by a person who has harbored the infection longer than four years, for in this late stage usually no lesions remain in the skin or the moist membranes.

The time interval between the entrance of germs into a person's tissues and the appearance of the primary lesion (the first evidence that the person has acquired the infection) varies in different cases from as few as ten days to as many as sixty days, with an average of three to four weeks. Once the germs have entered, they not only multiply in the local tissues at the site of entrance, but they travel through the lymphatic vessels and blood channels throughout the body. But this early dissemination of the germs causes no symptoms. The first discernible evidence that an infection has occurred is the appearance of a single papule at the site of entrance, which then ulcerates to form the so-called chancre or primary lesion.

The chancre is a round ulcer with raised edges and a firm texture. It varies in size, being as small as one fourth inch (6 mm.) in diameter in some cases or as large as three fourths inch (19 mm.) in diameter in others. It is painless. Usually there is just one. In women the chancre typically occurs in the vagina or on the cervix of the uterus. In men it occurs usually on the skin of the penis. It may occur in the mouth in either sex. A chancre tends to heal spontaneously in one to six weeks, but this does not mean that the disease has abated. It only means that the disease is progressing from its primary stage (the stage of the chancre) to its secondary stage. The disease is extremely contagious during this primary stage, for the ulcerated area of the chancre contains many germs.

If the person infected with syphilis has not been adequately treated during the primary stage, the evidences of the secondary stage begin about six weeks after the chancre heals. These consist of multiple lesions on the skin and membranes, plus enlargement of the lymph nodes and one or more of various problems in the internal organs and nervous system.

The so-called mucocutaneous lesions (in membranes and skin) of the secondary stage constitute a generalized rash which lasts for two to six weeks. Pink macules appear in the skin and membranes, often even of the palms and soles. The scalp is often affected with a resulting spotty loss of hair—a "moth-eaten alopecia." Round, slightly raised, painless gray plaques appear on the lips, in the mouth, and on the delicate skin of the vulva or of the glans of the penis. Even though these skin lesions heal within a few weeks, they tend to recur one or more times in about one fourth of cases. These lesions contain the germs of syphilis, and thus the condition continues to be contagious. The various organs that may be affected during this secondary stage include the spleen, the liver, the meninges, and the eye.

Following the secondary stage, syphilis becomes quiescent for a variable time in the so-called latent stage. Early in this latent stage there may be a transient return of the mucocutaneous lesions which characterize the secondary stage. The disease may continue to be contagious during the first four years or so of this latent stage. For the most part the person is symptom-free during this time, even though the germs of syphilis are still present in his tissues.

In the untreated case this latent period may be as short as two years or it may last for the remainder of life. In the usual case it is followed in about twenty years by the late stage (tertiary stage) in which serious, destructive lesions develop in the nervous system and/or in the cardiovascular system.

In about one fourth of untreated cases the germs of syphilis invade the nervous system during the secondary stage of the disease (from three to eighteen months after the infection is acquired). The germs lie dormant here throughout the latent phase only to cause such tragic complications as general paresis and tabes dorsalis during the late stage of the disease. For a description of these complications, see the section on "Syphilis of the Nervous System," in chapter 4, volume 3.

Complications of late syphilis affecting the cardiovascular system cause a destructive process in the tissues of the first portion of the aorta, resulting in aortitis, thoracic aortic aneurysm, and aortic insufficiency of the heart.

Another dreadful manifestation of untreated syphilis is its involvement of the unborn child. The fetus is not susceptible to the syphilis which may be

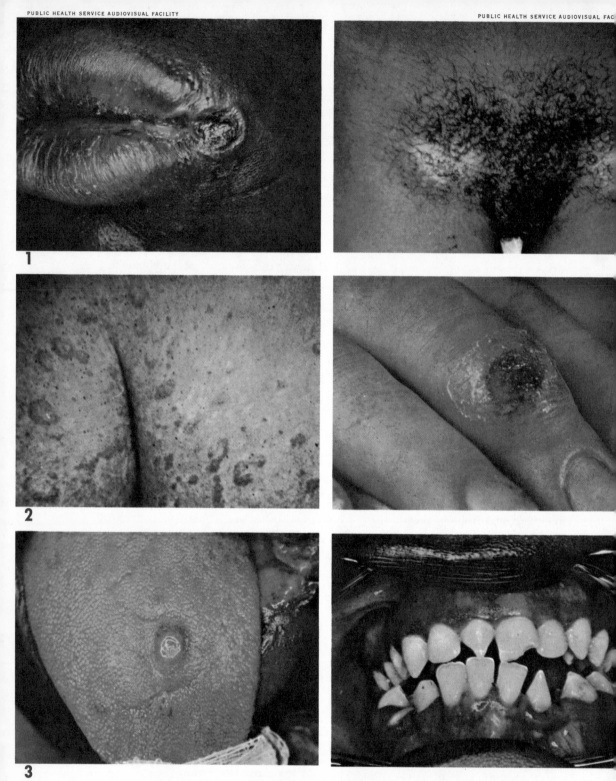

Manifestations of syphilis as they appear on various parts of the body: (1) chancre on the lip; (2) blotches on the skin; (3) chancre on the tongue; (4) swollen lymph nodes of the groin; (5) chancre on finger; and (6) notched, peg-shaped teeth (the latter a condition typical of syphilis acquired prior to birth).

present in its mother's body until after the fourth month of fetal development. Thus there is compelling reason for the expectant mother to submit to tests for syphilis very early in her pregnancy and to receive adequate treatment, when indicated, during the first four months of pregnancy. An unborn child carried by a syphilitic mother during the last five months of pregnancy has a 70 to 95 percent chance of acquiring congenital syphilis. The manifestations of congenital syphilis appear during the first two years of a baby's life and include skin lesions, blood-stained "snuffles," hydrocephalus, convulsions, mental retardation, bone changes, blindness, deafness, and malformed teeth.

Detection of syphilis. Medical scientists have developed sophisticated serologic tests by which a sample of blood or cerebrospinal fluid is processed in the laboratory to detect the presence of an active syphilitic infection. Such a test becomes positive for syphilis during the primary phase of the disease. It will indicate the presence of the disease even during its latent phase. In the early stage of the chancre the serologic test will not yet be positive. In this early stage the physician may make a microscopic examination of a fluid sample from the raw area of the chancre and actually observe the germs of syphilis when present.

Care and Treatment

The preceding descriptions make it clear that the consequences of syphilis become more serious the longer adequate treatment is delayed. At best syphilis is a tragic disease. But delay compounds the tragedy. Furthermore, the treatment becomes progressively less effective the longer it is delayed.

Appropriate forms of penicillin are effective in controlling and eliminating a syphilitic infection. But the treatment must be continued over a period of time in order to be com-

pletely effective. Periodic tests should be used during and after the treatment to check on the treatment's effectiveness.

Syphilis can be acquired from a person who has no symptoms at the time the infection is transmitted. It is important for the doctor to inquire what personal contacts his patient has had and to insist that such person or persons be properly treated. Only thus can the epidemic tendencies of syphilis be controlled.

CHANCROID

Chancroid is a less common sexually transmitted disease, of which there are about two thousand reported cases per year in the United States. It is caused by the germ *Hemophilus ducreyi*. The incubation period for this disease is about ten days, following which there develop painful ulcers on the genital organs. The ulcers are not firm (in contrast to the syphilitic chancre), they have undermined borders, and they are covered by a pussy exudate. The tissue surrounding the ulcers is swollen, and the lymph nodes in the groin become tender and may even develop abscesses.

The diagnosis of this disease requires a microscopic search of the material derived from an ulcer, or a laboratory culturing of this material to identify the germs.

Care and Treatment

Sulfonamide or tetracycline administered by mouth in appropriate doses over a period of two or three weeks are usually effective.

GRANULOMA INGUINALE

This is a relatively rare sexually transmitted disease caused by a germ called *Calymmatobacterium granulomatis* and characterized by a long incubation period and the development of a spreading ulcer in the genital or perianal area. Nodules tend to form around the ulcer as it extends. In severe cases there is much tissue destruction with eventual scarring. The diagnosis requires the removal of a specimen of tissue and a microscopic search for germ-laden cells.

Care and Treatment

Tetracycline in appropriate, divided doses over a period of two to four weeks is effective.

C. Diseases Characterized by Lumps and Bumps

LYMPHOGRANULOMA VENEREUM

This disease of worldwide distribution is most prevalent in the tropical areas and relatively rare in the United States. It is usually transmitted by sexual contact and is caused by a microorganism called *Chlamydia trachomatis*. The incubation period is about three weeks. The infection is first manifested by a small papule or painless ulcer on the external genital organs, which heals rapidly and may even go unnoticed. Following this the lymph nodes in the groin for male patients and around the anus in female patients become swollen and tender. The swollen nodes are designated as buboes. The overlying skin turns purplish and may break down to form persistent, painful, draining ulcers. The healing process in untreated cases is slow, and in female patients there may develop a troublesome stricture of the anus or rectum.

The diagnosis is confirmed by any one of several laboratory tests, the most popular of which is the Frei test, in which a small amount of test material is injected into the patient's skin.

Care and Treatment

The treatment is by the use of tetracycline administered by mouth in appropriate doses each day for a period of about three weeks.

CONDYLOMA ACUMINATUM (GENITAL WARTS)

The lesions of condyloma acuminatum are soft, pink clusters of wartlike overgrowths that develop in the moist areas of the genitalia. They are caused by a virus related to that which causes common skin warts. The virus is transmitted by sexual contact, and the lesions develop within about three months of the time of exposure to a person who has this infection. In the female the lesions may become so extensive as to interfere with the process of childbirth.

Care and Treatment

Successful treatment requires first attention to other conditions such as urethritis or vaginitis that may promote the condition of moisture in the genital area. The cautious, local application of a 25 percent solution of podophyllum resin in tincture of benzoin compound is usually effective. Otherwise the surgical removal of the overgrown lesions may be necessary.

D. Diseases Transmitted by Lice and Mites

PEDICULOSIS PUBIS

This ailment, caused by germs transmitted by lice, can be conveyed from one person to another by sexual contact. The ailment is described in chapter 25, volume 2.

SCABIES

Scabies or "the itch" is transmitted by mites and, in occasional cases, is carried from one person to another at the time of sexual contact. The disease is discussed in chapter 25, volume 2.

E. Other Types of Sexually Transmitted Vaginitis

Such infections of the vagina as trichomoniasis and candidiasis are readily acquired by sexual contact. These are discussed in chapter 30, volume 2.

PROMINENT ACHIEVEMENTS IN MEDICINE

(a pictorial supplement)

Medical practice keeps moving from the past and present to the future tense. In a world where knowledge doubles at least every seven years, it is not surprising that medicine too is in the midst of an information explosion.

Physicians and medical educators who gaze into the crystal ball see amazing new developments in the offing: mankind free from infectious disease, enjoyment of physical and mental life up to age ninety or a hundred, replacement of defective parts of the body with artificial devices, diagnosis by computer (even "penny-in-the-slot" medical checkups), surgery by laser beams, improvement of memory by drugs, and on and on.

But progress in medicine, whether past, present, or future, is and always will be associated with individual men and women—gifted people who rise to prominence and contribute of their talents to the betterment of their fellows. Illustrious and long is the roster of names of people who have thus contributed, and the list continues to grow.

Readers of current literature have admired the biographical profiles of great people in medicine as presented by Parke, Davis & Company in their *History of Medicine in Pictures*. Reproductions of paintings in full color, and historical articles covering the history of medicine from antiquity to the present day, appeared in the company's *Therapeutic notes*, and in other magazines, beginning with 1957.

Great names responsible for great breakthroughs include Hippocrates, Galen, Vesalius, Edward Jenner, William Harvey, Philippe Pinel, Louis Pasteur, John Hunter, Benjamin Rush, and many others. Here we present paintings of seven of these persons, with a condensation of the write-up about each one. Parke, Davis & Company undertook this project as a service in behalf of the profession of medicine, and also as a means of promoting understanding and appreciation for what medicine throughout the centuries has meant to better health and welfare.

The authors and publishers of *You and Your Health* acknowledge their indebtedness to Artist Robert A. Thom for the paintings, to George A. Bender and his associates for the text, and of course to Parke, Davis & Company for permission to reproduce this material.

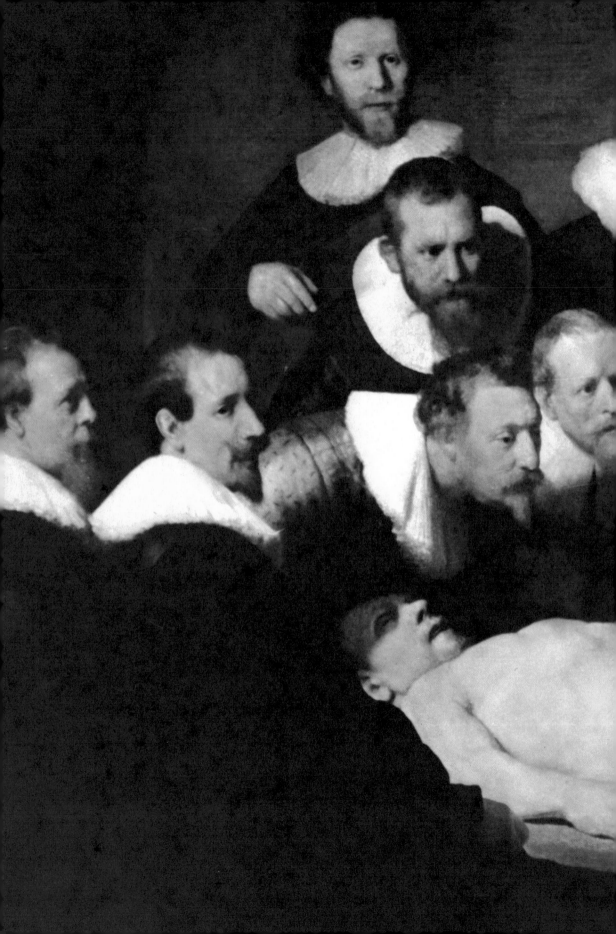

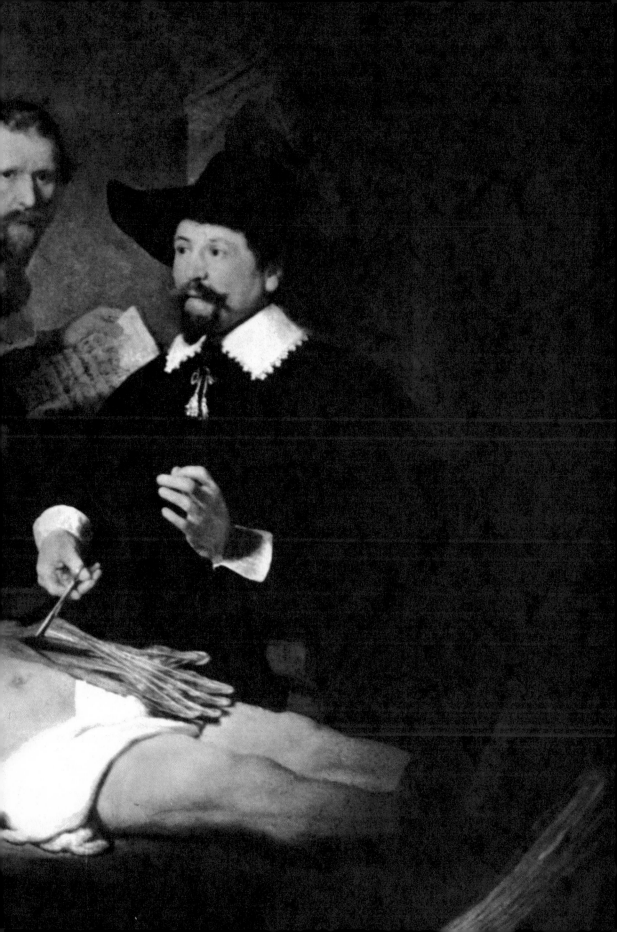

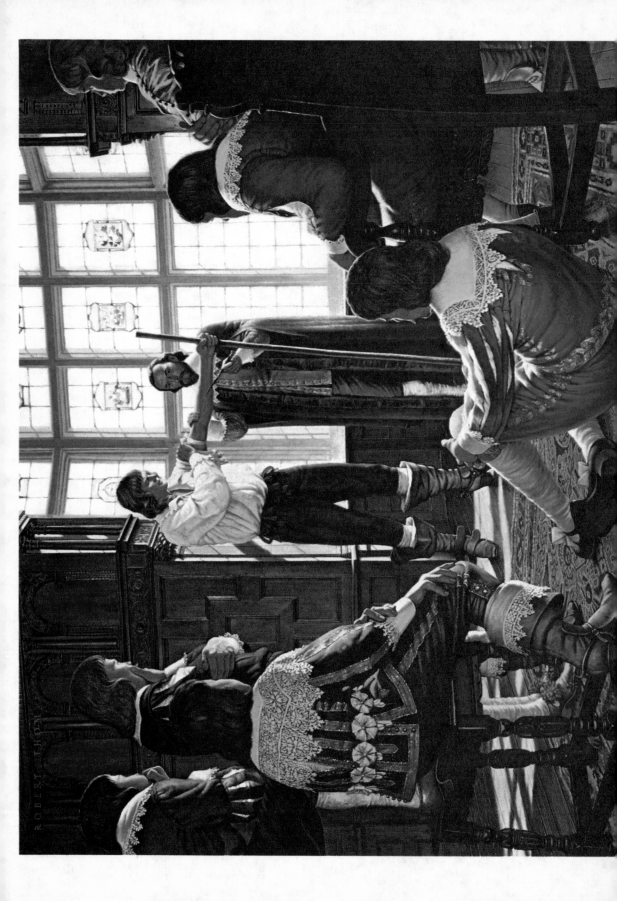

HARVEY AND THE CIRCULATION OF THE BLOOD

William Harvey (1578-1657) demonstrated proof of his revolutionary theory of the circulation of the blood during anatomical lectures before London's College of Physicians. His *De Motu Cordis* upset Galenic tradition and introduced new concepts of anatomy.

What has been called the greatest discovery ever made in physiology—the circulation of the blood—was quietly announced early in the seventeenth century as a part of a series of lectures in anatomy. The man who brought about this discovery was William Harvey, a short, slight, dark-complexioned Englishman, with flashing, spirited eyes and a wealth of nervous energy.

William Harvey was born at Folkestone, England, April 1, 1578, the eldest son of a large well-to-do family. He was given every educational advantage and was graduated with a bachelor of arts degree from Caius College at Cambridge University in 1597. Shortly thereafter Harvey enrolled in the University of Padua's famed medical school and studied under Fabricius of Aquapendente. In later years Harvey was to acknowledge his debt to the great teacher, crediting Fabricius's work on the valves in veins for having stimulated him to investigate the mystery of blood circulation.

Harvey received the degree of doctor of medicine from the University of Padua in 1602 and returned to England the same year. Quickly rising to prominence, he was appointed physician to St. Bartholomew's Hospital in 1609 and held this important position until 1643. He also was

early elected a Fellow by the College of Physicians, and continued close association with this distinguished group throughout his life.

Harvey began his lectures on anatomy in April, 1616, in the College of Physicians' new headquarters at Amen Corner, at the end of Paternoster Row. Of great significance among his first lecture notes is the first clue to Harvey's convictions concerning blood circulation and the heart.

It was not until twelve years later, in 1628, that Harvey saw fit to publish his great work—a book which revolutionized the thinking of medical men in anatomy and therapeutics. The title: *Exercitatio Anatomica de Motu Cordis et Sanguinis in Animalibus*—"An Anatomical Treatise on the Movement of the Heart and Blood in Animals."

In essence, Harvey's observations were: The heart is a muscular organ that contracts and relaxes; at each contraction of the auricles, blood is forced into corresponding ventricles, and thence into the great arteries as the ventricles contract; once in the arteries, blood cannot return directly to the heart because of the heart valves.

Harvey's experiments were at once simple and illuminating. One was made by having an assistant grasp a staff firmly in his hand. Harvey, then, by depressing visible veins with one or two fingers, could demonstrate the single direction of flow of venous blood.

Death came to William Harvey on June 3, 1657, in his eightieth year. Thus was closed one of the most fruitful careers in medicine of the seventeenth century, contributions of which were to benefit all mankind thereafter.

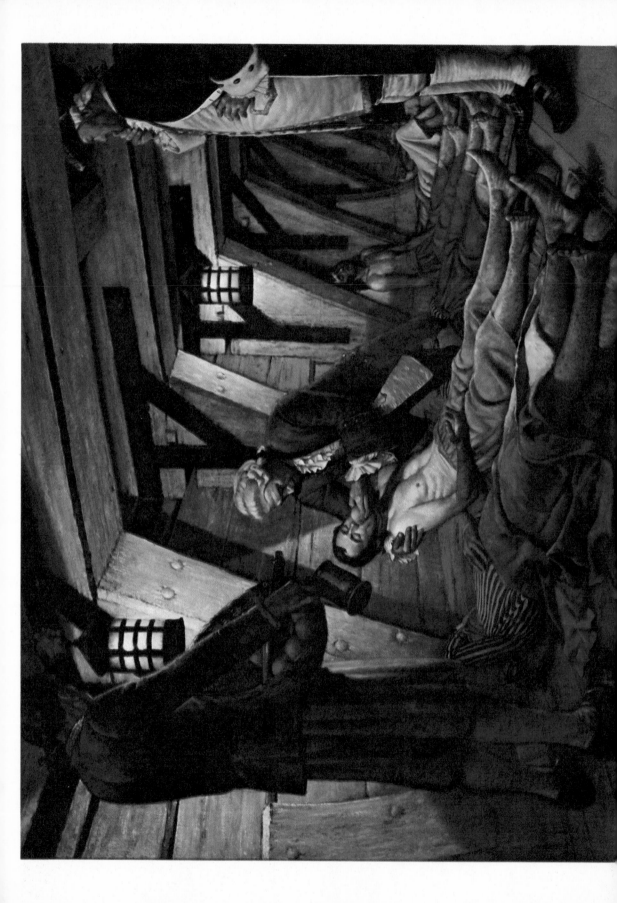

GOLDBERGER: DIETARY DEFICIENCY AND DISEASE

Dr. Joseph Goldberger (1874-1929), United States Public Health Surgeon, began studies of pellagra in 1914 near Jackson, Mississippi, in orphanages, asylums, and prisons. His research proved dietary deficiency the cause and directed other scientists toward discovery of vitamins.

When Dr. Joseph Goldberger, Surgeon, United States Public Health Service, and his assistant, Dr. C. H. Waring, began studies of pellagra at the Methodist and Baptist orphanages near Jackson, Mississippi, in 1914, they faced puzzling questions: Why were the adults, the older children, and the very young in these institutions free of the disease? Why, every year, did it strike children aged three to twelve? Dr. Goldberger ruled out infection and toxic foods as causes. With cooperation of Director J. R. Carter and House Mother "Miss Ida," the doctors added fresh meat, eggs, milk, oatmeal, peas, beans (foods commonly reserved for older people), and other vegetables to children's diets. Pellagra disappeared. By bold experiments Dr. Goldberger proved dietary deficiency the cause of pellagra and pointed the way toward discovery of health-sustaining vitamins.

Joseph Goldberger was born July 16, 1874, on a peasant farm near Giralt, Austria-Hungary (now a part of Czechoslovakia). When he was only seven years old, he came with his parents to America, the family settling in New York City. He chose medicine for his career; and after graduating from Bellevue Hospital Medical College, he entered the Public Health Service as an assistant surgeon and gained the reputation of being a "health detective."

Having scored successes in his study of measles, diphtheria, and other diseases, he was sent in 1914 by the surgeon general to the cotton country of the South to take over investigations of pellagra, a problem so widespread there that it was seriously affecting the economy.

Dr. Goldberger and his assistant set out to learn all they could about the disease. They went to cotton-mill towns; to the cotton fields; to the hills and valleys. They found hundreds of people afflicted with skin lesions, weakness, digestive upsets, diarrhea, and mental disturbances—typical signs of pellagra. But it was the suffering among the children in the two orphanages that challenged Dr. Goldberger most of all to discover the cause of the disease.

It was not long before the inquiring mind of the medical detective began to visualize patterns in the puzzle. Although the children's diet was adequate caloriewise, adults received considerably more meat and protein foods. The little children during their first two years received plenty of milk; but after that age, the children's diet was largely carbohydrate: corn bread, grits, cane syrup, and molasses.

To check his suspicions that the problem lay in a nutritional deficiency, Dr. Goldberger requested supplementary foods for the children in the age group most afflicted. Soon he noticed the signs of pellagra disappearing from the little faces. He launched similar studies at the Georgia State sanitarium and at the Mississippi State penitentiary. All tests proved pellagra could be prevented or cured by diet. His work prepared the way for other men to discover vitamin B and the part it plays in prevention of disease.

Selective Atlas of
Normal Anatomy

Anatomy of the Heart

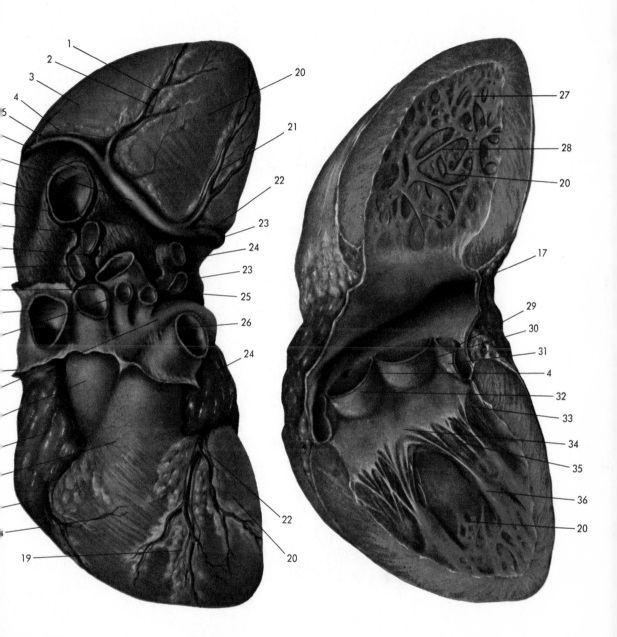

Middle cardiac vein
Posterior descending branch of right coronary artery
Right ventricle
Right coronary artery
Small cardiac vein
Inferior vena cava
Coronary sinus
Right auricle
Left atrium
Right pulmonary vein
Right branch of pulmonary artery
Innominate artery

13 Superior vena cava
14 Left common carotid artery
15 Pericardium
16 Aortic arch
17 Ascending aorta
18 Conus arteriosus
19 Anterior descending branch of left coronary artery
20 Left ventricle
21 Posterior vein of left ventricle
22 Great cardiac vein
23 Left pulmonary vein
24 Left auricle

25 Left subclavian artery
26 Left branch of pulmonary artery
27 Trabeculae carneae
28 Trabecula tendinea
29 Left coronary artery
30 Posterior semilunar valve
31 Left semilunar valve
32 Right semilunar valve
33 Posterior cusp of mitral (bicuspid) valve
34 Anterior cusp of mitral (bicuspid) valve
35 Chordae tendineae
36 Papillary muscle

Anatomy of the Stomach

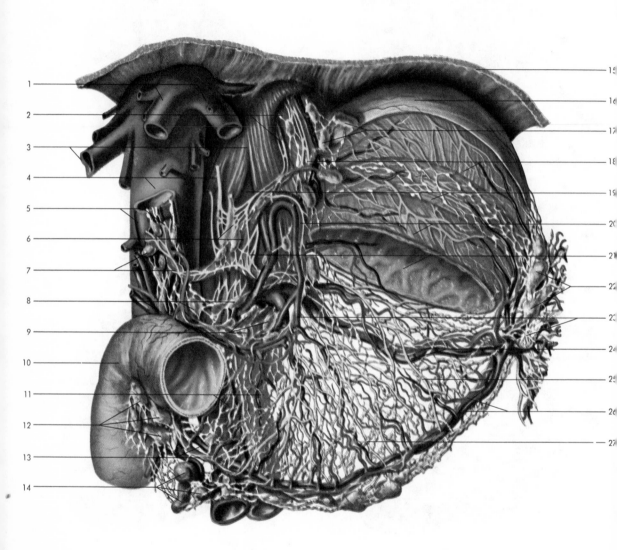

1 Middle and left hepatic veins
2 Right vagus nerve and esophagus
3 Right hepatic vein and crura of diaphragm
4 Inferior vena cava and greater splanchnic nerve
5 Portal vein and hepatic artery
6 Celiac plexus and celiac artery
7 Hepatic lymph node and hepatic rami of vagus nerve
8 Gastroduodenal artery and suprapyloric lymph nodes

9 Superior gastric lymph nodes
10 Duodenum
11 Superior mesenteric artery and vein
12 Subpyloric lymph nodes
13 Right gastroepiploic artery and vein
14 Inferior gastric lymph nodes
15 Diaphragm
16 Serosa
17 Paracardial lymph nodes
18 Left vagus nerve and longitudinal muscular layer

19 Abdominal aorta and circular muscular layer
20 Left gastric artery and oblique muscular layer
21 Celiac rami of vagus nerve and gastric mucosa
22 Splenic lymph nodes
23 Left gastric (coronary) vein and splenic rami of vagus nerve
24 Splenic artery and vein
25 Gastric rami of vagus nerve
26 Left gastroepiploic artery and vein
27 Gastric lymphatic plexus

The Sympathetic Nervous System

ABDOMINAL PORTION

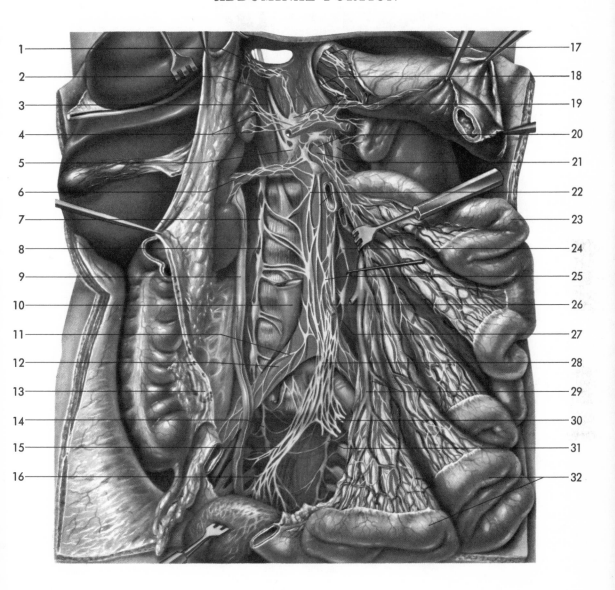

1 Phrenic ganglion and plexus
2 Greater splanchnic nerve
3 Lesser splanchnic nerve
4 Suprarenal plexus
5 Aorticorenal ganglion
6 Right renal artery and plexus
7 Right lumbar sympathetic ganglion
8 Right sympathetic trunk
9 Ureter
10 Vena cava
11 Iliac plexus

12 Right common iliac artery
13 Mesocolon (cut)
14 Right sacral sympathetic ganglion
15 Right pelvic plexus
16 Pudendal plexus
17 Left vagus nerve
18 Right vagus nerve
19 Celiac plexus and right celiac ganglion
20 Superior mesenteric ganglion and plexus
21 Left celiac ganglion; superior mesenteric artery

22 Abdominal aortic plexus
23 Jejunum
24 Left lumbar sympathetic ganglion
25 Inferior mesenteric ganglion
26 Inferior mesenteric plexus
27 Left sympathetic trunk
28 Hypogastric plexus
29 Branches of superior mesenteric artery and vein
30 Left pelvic plexus
31 Left sacral sympathetic ganglion
32 Ileum

The Sympathetic Nervous System

CEPHALIC, CERVICAL AND THORACIC PORTIONS

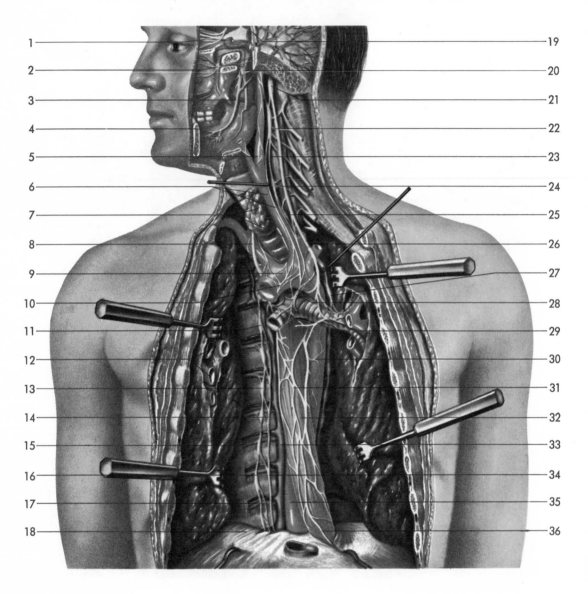

1 Ciliary ganglion
2 Sphenopalatine ganglion
3 Lingual nerve
4 Submandibular ganglion
5 Internal carotid artery
6 Common carotid artery; superior cardiac nerve
7 Thyroid gland; recurrent laryngeal nerve
8 Right vagus nerve
9 Aortic arch
10 Superficial cardiac plexus
11 Fifth thoracic sympathetic ganglion

12 Pulmonary artery and vein
13 Seventh thoracic sympathetic ganglion
14 Greater splanchnic nerve
15 Intercostal artery, vein and nerve
16 Tenth thoracic sympathetic ganglion
17 Lesser splanchnic nerve
18 Diaphragm
19 Trigeminal nerve
20 Otic ganglion
21 Nodose ganglion
22 Superior cervical sympathetic ganglion
23 Cervical sympathetic trunk
24 Middle cervical sympathetic ganglion

25 Inferior cervical sympathetic ganglion
26 Left vagus nerve
27 Fourth thoracic sympathetic ganglion
28 Cardiac ganglion
29 Anterior pulmonary plexus
30 Aortic plexus
31 Esophageal plexus
32 Esophagus
33 Azygos vein
34 Splanchnic ganglion
35 Aorta
36 Anterior gastric cord of vagus

The Coronary Arteries

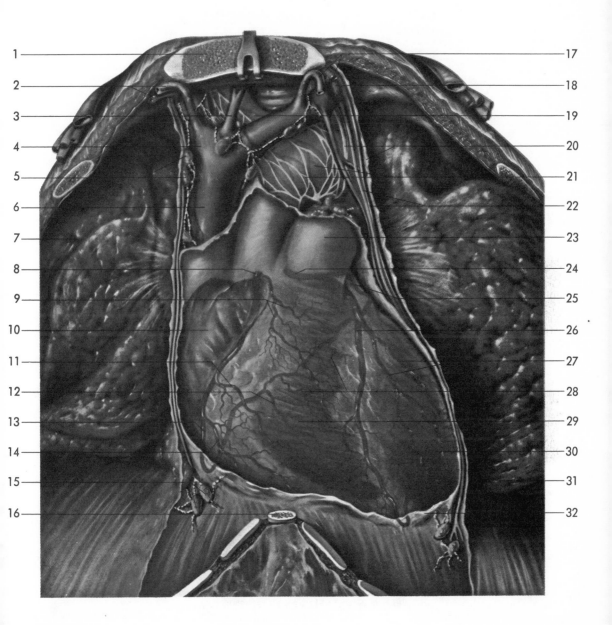

1 Manubrium
2 Right internal mammary artery and vein
3 Thyreoidea ima vein
4 Right brachiocephalic vein
5 Anterior superior mediastinal lymph nodes
6 Superior vena cava
7 Right lung
8 Right coronary artery
9 Preventricular arteries
10 Right atrium
11 Lateral branch of right coronary artery

12 Posterior descending branch of right circumflex artery
13 Right circumflex artery
14 Right marginal artery
15 Anterior inferior mediastinal lymph nodes
16 Xiphoid process
17 Left internal mammary artery and vein
18 Left brachiocephalic vein
19 Brachiocephalic trunk
20 Vagus nerve; mediastinal pleura (Cut)
21 Superficial cardiac plexus; arch of aorta

22 Pericardiacophrenic artery; phrenic nerve
23 Pulmonary artery
24 Left coronary artery
25 Left circumflex artery
26 Anterior descending branch of left coronary artery
27 Left marginal arteries
28 Left ventricular branches
29 Right ventricle
30 Left ventricle
31 Left lung
32 Pericardium (cut)

Anatomy of the Ear

FRONTAL SECTION SHOWING COMPONENT PARTS OF THE HUMAN EAR

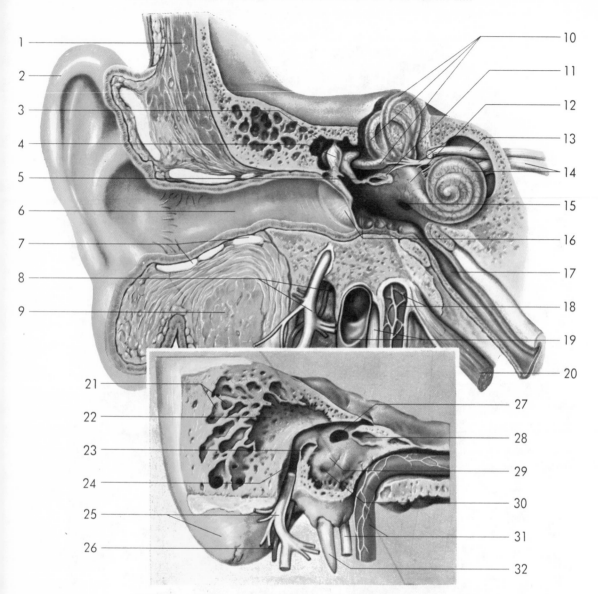

SECTION THROUGH RIGHT TEMPORAL BONE SHOWING RELATIONSHIP BETWEEN MASTOID CELLS AND TYMPANIC CAVITY

1 Temporal muscle
2 Helix
3 Epitympanic recess
4 Malleus
5 Incus
6 External acoustic meatus
7 Cartilaginous part of external acoustic meatus
8 Facial nerve and stylomastoid artery
9 Parotid gland
10 Semicircular canals
11 Stapes
12 Vestibule and vestibular nerve

13 Facial nerve
14 Cochlea and cochlear nerve
15 Cochlear (round) window
16 Tympanic membrane and tympanic cavity
17 Auditory (Eustachian) tube
18 Internal carotid artery and sympathetic nerve plexus
19 Glossopharyngeal nerve and internal jugular vein
20 Levator veli palatini muscle
21 Mastoid cells
22 Tympanic antrum

23 Cavity of the pyramidal eminence for the stapedius
24 Facial canal
25 Facial nerve and mastoid process
26 Stylomastoid artery
27 Vestibular (oval) window
28 Cochleariform process
29 Promontory
30 Cochlear fenestra
31 Internal carotid artery and glossopharyngeal nerve
32 Styloid process

Region of the Mouth

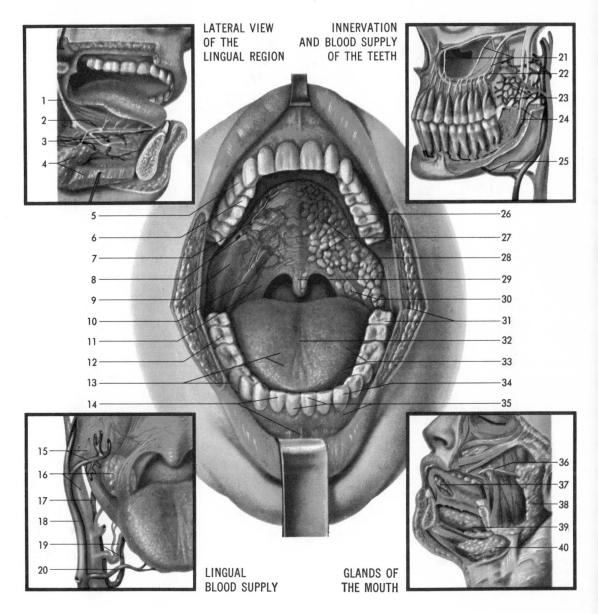

LATERAL VIEW OF THE LINGUAL REGION

INNERVATION AND BLOOD SUPPLY OF THE TEETH

LINGUAL BLOOD SUPPLY

GLANDS OF THE MOUTH

1 Lingual nerve
2 Submaxillary duct
3 Sublingual branches of lingual artery and vein
4 Submaxillary gland; mylohyoid muscle
5 First premolar
6 Second premolar
7 Greater palatine artery and nerve
8 Lesser palatine artery and nerve
9 Pterygomandibular raphe
10 Glossopalatine muscle
11 Pharyngopalatinus muscle
12 Second molar
13 Filiform papillae; second premolar
14 Lateral incisor; frenulum of lower lip

15 Internal maxillary artery and vein
16 External carotid artery; palatine tonsil
17 Internal jugular vein
18 Posterior facial vein
19 Lingual artery and vein
20 Ranine vein
21 Anterior, middle and posterior superior alveolar nerves
22 Posterior superior alveolar artery
23 Pterygoid venous plexus
24 Inferior alveolar nerve and artery
25 External maxillary artery; anterior facial vein
26 First molar
27 Palatine glands

28 Cut edge of mucous membrane
29 Uvula
30 Palatine tonsils
31 Third molar; buccinator muscle
32 Median sulcus of tongue
33 Fungiform papillae
34 Canine
35 Central incisors; gingiva
36 Parotid duct
37 Anterior lingual gland
38 Parotid gland
39 Sublingual gland
40 Submaxillary gland

Anatomy of the Lung

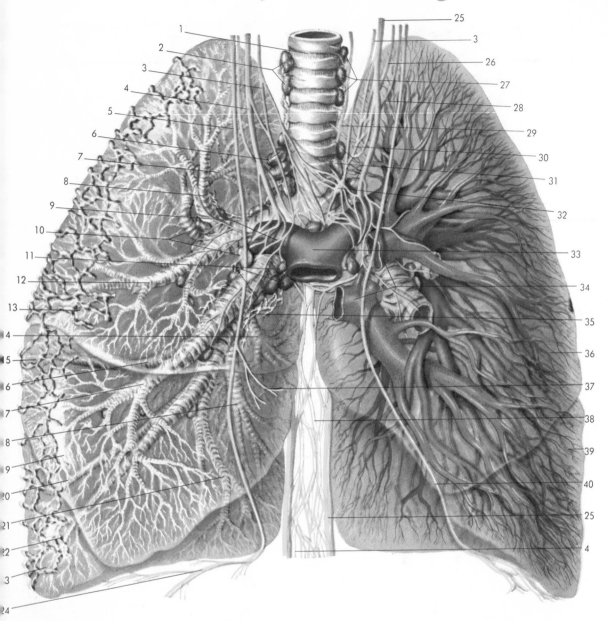

1 Trachea
2 Right tracheal lymph nodes
3 Superior cardiac nerve
4 Right vagus nerve
5 Right phrenic nerve
6 Right superior tracheobronchial lymph nodes
7 Posterior bronchial branch, upper lobe
8 Apical bronchial branch, upper lobe
9 Anterior pulmonary plexus
10 Interbronchial lymph nodes
11 Inferior tracheobronchial lymph nodes
12 Anterior bronchial branch, upper lobe
13 Upper lobe of right lung
14 Superior bronchial branch, lower lobe

15 Superficial lymphatic plexus
16 Lateral bronchial branch, middle lobe
17 Medial bronchial branch, middle lobe
18 Posterior basal bronchial branch, lower lobe
19 Middle lobe of right lung
20 Lateral basal bronchial branch, lower lobe
21 Medial basal bronchial branch, lower lobe
22 Anterior basal bronchial branch, lower lobe
23 Lower lobe of right lung
24 Phrenicoabdominal branch of phrenic nerve
25 Left vagus nerve
26 Middle cardiac nerve

27 Left tracheal lymph nodes
28 Inferior cardiac nerve
29 Recurrent laryngeal nerve
30 Superficial cardiac plexus
31 Left superior tracheobronchial lymph nodes
32 Inferior cardiac ganglion
33 Pulmonary artery
34 Left pulmonary veins
35 Deep lymphatic plexus
36 Upper lobe of left lung
37 Pericardial branch of phrenic nerve
38 Esophageal plexus
39 Lower lobe of left lung
40 Left phrenic nerve

The Intervertebral Disks

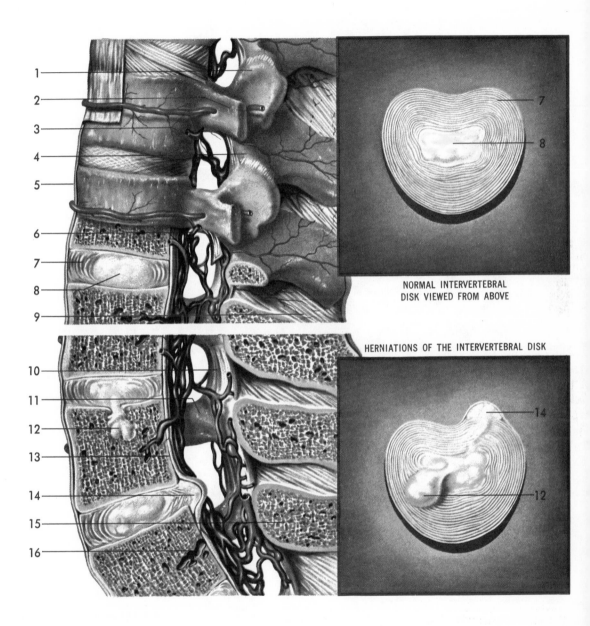

NORMAL INTERVERTEBRAL
DISK VIEWED FROM ABOVE

HERNIATIONS OF THE INTERVERTEBRAL DISK

1 Superior articular process
2 Transverse process
3 Lumbar artery and vein
4 Inferior articular process
5 Anterior longitudinal ligament
6 Internal vertebral venous plexus

7 Fibrous ring of intervertebral disk
8 Nucleus pulposus
9 Interspinous ligament
10 Ligamentum flavum
11 Lamina
12 Herniation of nucleus pulposus into
the spongiosa (Schmorl lesion)

13 Posterior longitudinal ligament
14 Herniation of nucleus pulposus beneath
the posterior longitudinal ligament
15 Spinous process
16 Basivertebral vein

Anatomy of the Brain

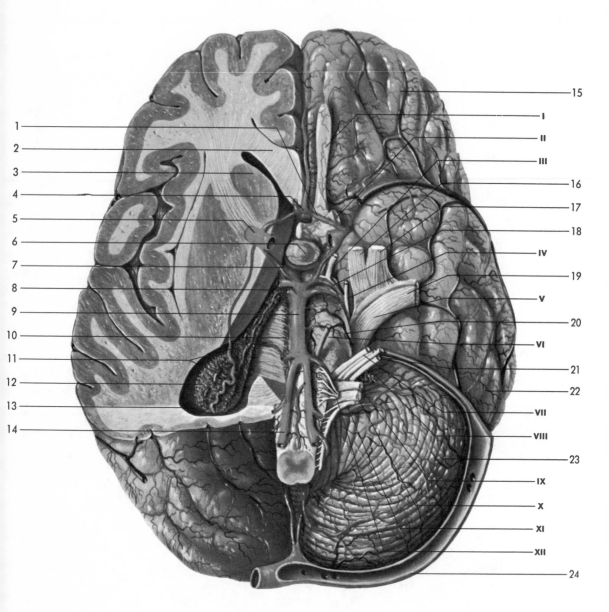

1 Anterior cerebral artery	13 Inferior cornu of lateral ventricle	**CRANIAL NERVES**
2 Trunk of corpus callosum	14 Vertebral artery	I. Olfactory nerve
3 Head of caudate nucleus	15 Frontal lobe	II. Optic nerve
4 Anterior communicating artery	16 Ophthalmic nerve	III. Oculomotor nerve
5 Middle cerebral artery	17 Maxillary nerve	IV. Trochlear nerve
6 Hypophysis	18 Posterior cerebral artery	V. Trigeminal nerve
7 Posterior communicating artery	19 Mandibular nerve	VI. Abducens nerve
8 Superior cerebellar artery	20 Pons	VII. Facial nerve
9 Basilar artery	21 Intermediate nerve	VIII. Acoustic nerve
10 Internal cerebral vein	22 Temporal lobe	IX. Glossopharyngeal nerve
11 Choroid artery and vein	23 Cerebellum	X. Vagus nerve
12 Choroid plexus of lateral ventricle	24 Left transverse sinus	XI. Accessory nerve
		XII. Hypoglossal nerve

Anatomy of the Ankle

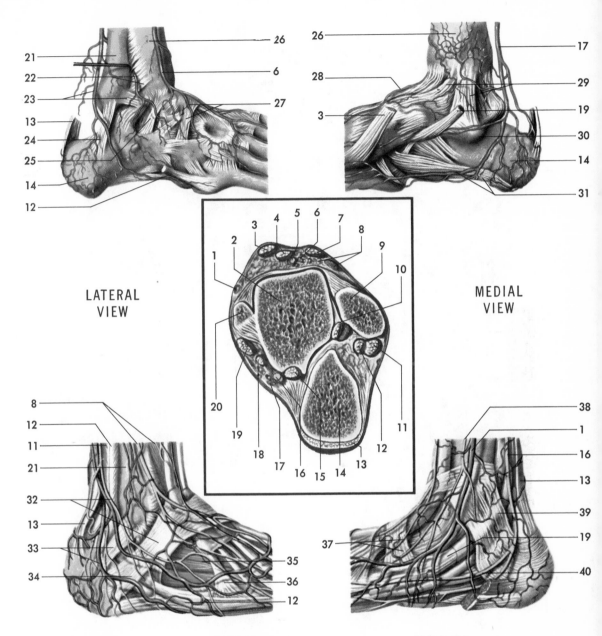

LATERAL VIEW

MEDIAL VIEW

1 Great saphenous vein
2 Talus
3 Tendon of tibialis anterior
4 Tendon of extensor hallucis longus
5 Deep peroneal nerve
6 Anterior tibial artery
7 Tendon of extensor digitorum longus
8 Peroneus tertius muscle and superficial peroneal nerve
9 Lateral malleolus
10 Posterior talofibular ligament
11 Tendon of peroneus longus
12 Tendon of peroneus brevis
13 Calcaneal tendon
14 Calcaneus
15 Tendon of flexor hallucis longus

16 Tibial nerve
17 Posterior tibial artery
18 Tendon of flexor digitorum longus
19 Tendon of tibialis posterior
20 Medial malleolus
21 Fibula
22 Perforating peroneal artery and anterior ligament of external malleolus
23 Peroneal artery and anterior talofibular ligament
24 Calcaneofibular ligament
25 External talocalcaneal ligament
26 Tibia
27 Lateral tarsal artery and dorsal cuboideo-navicular ligament
28 Dorsal pedis artery

29 Deltoid ligament
30 Sustentaculum tali
31 Long plantar ligament and lateral plantar artery
32 Sural nerve and cruciate ligament
33 Superior peroneal retinaculum and small saphenous vein
34 Inferior peroneal retinaculum
35 Extensor digitorum brevis muscle
36 Tendon of peroneus tertius
37 Medial dorsal cutaneous nerve and cruciate ligament
38 Saphenous nerve
39 Laciniate ligament
40 Medial plantar nerve

Pelvis and Hip Joint

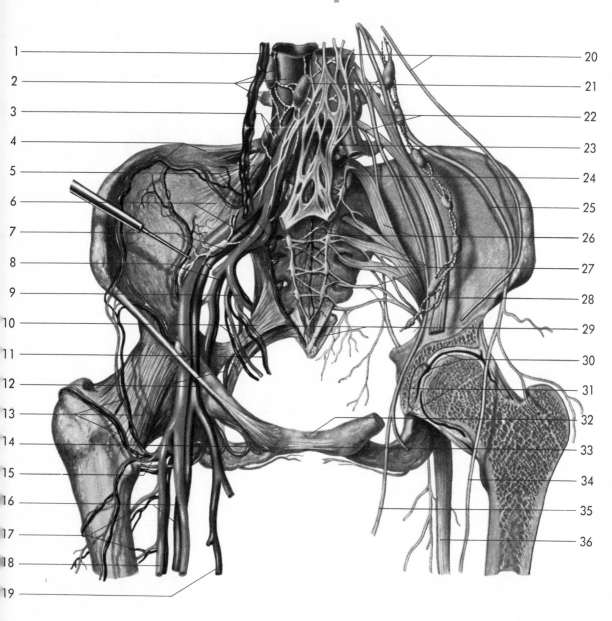

1 Ovarian artery and vein
2 Vena cava; lumbar lymph nodes
3 Right common iliac artery and vein
4 Iliolumbar ligament; branches of iliolumbar artery and vein
5 Lumbosacral ligament; superior gluteal artery and vein
6 Anterior sacroiliac ligament; internal iliac (hypogastric) artery
7 External iliac artery and vein
8 Obturator artery and vein
9 Inferior gluteal artery and vein
10 Sacrospinous ligament; uterine artery and vein
11 Sacrotuberous ligament; vaginal artery and vein

12 Inguinal ligament; internal pudendal artery
13 Iliofemoral ligament; branches of lateral femoral circumflex artery and vein
14 Lacunar ligament
15 Lateral femoral circumflex artery and vein
16 Femoral artery and vein
17 Perforating arteries and veins
18 Deep femoral artery and vein
19 Great saphenous vein
20 Aorta; ilioinguinal nerve
21 Lateral aortic lymph nodes
22 Lumbar nerves
23 Hypogastric sympathetic plexus
24 Sympathetic trunk

25 Lateral femoral cutaneous nerve
26 Middle sacral artery and vein; lumbosacral trunk
27 Sacral nerves
28 Femoral nerve
29 Lateral sacral artery and vein; anterior sacrococcygeal ligament
30 Lunate articular cartilage; joint cavity
31 Acetabular fat pad; ligamentum teres
32 Interpubic fibrocartilage
33 Superior pubic ligament
34 Anterior branch of lateral femoral cutaneous nerve
35 Obturator nerve
36 Great sciatic nerve

Anatomy of the Hand

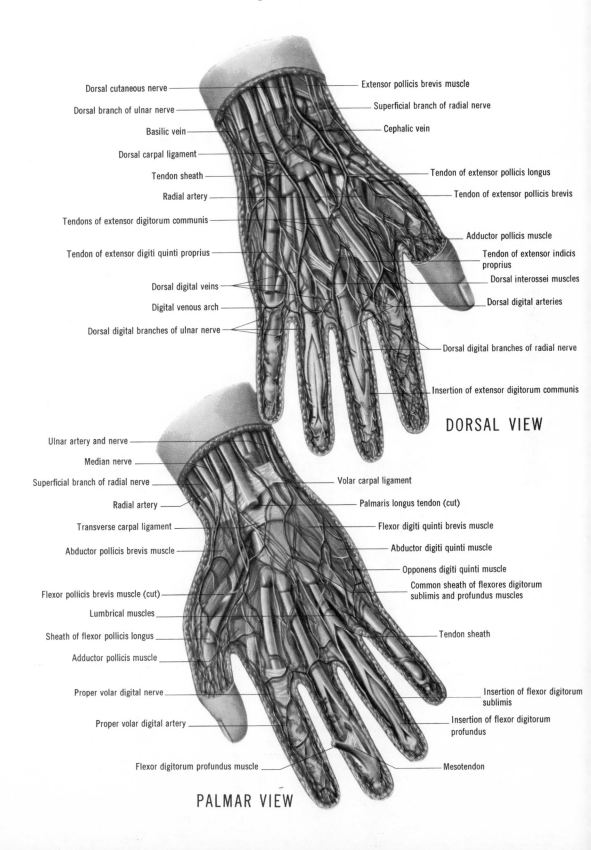

Dorsal cutaneous nerve

Dorsal branch of ulnar nerve

Basilic vein

Dorsal carpal ligament

Tendon sheath

Radial artery

Tendons of extensor digitorum communis

Tendon of extensor digiti quinti proprius

Dorsal digital veins

Digital venous arch

Dorsal digital branches of ulnar nerve

Extensor pollicis brevis muscle

Superficial branch of radial nerve

Cephalic vein

Tendon of extensor pollicis longus

Tendon of extensor pollicis brevis

Adductor pollicis muscle

Tendon of extensor indicis proprius

Dorsal interossei muscles

Dorsal digital arteries

Dorsal digital branches of radial nerve

Insertion of extensor digitorum communis

DORSAL VIEW

Ulnar artery and nerve

Median nerve

Superficial branch of radial nerve

Radial artery

Transverse carpal ligament

Abductor pollicis brevis muscle

Flexor pollicis brevis muscle (cut)

Lumbrical muscles

Sheath of flexor pollicis longus

Adductor pollicis muscle

Proper volar digital nerve

Proper volar digital artery

Flexor digitorum profundus muscle

Volar carpal ligament

Palmaris longus tendon (cut)

Flexor digiti quinti brevis muscle

Abductor digiti quinti muscle

Opponens digiti quinti muscle

Common sheath of flexores digitorum sublimis and profundus muscles

Tendon sheath

Insertion of flexor digitorum sublimis

Insertion of flexor digitorum profundus

Mesotendon

PALMAR VIEW

Anatomy of the Male Genitalia

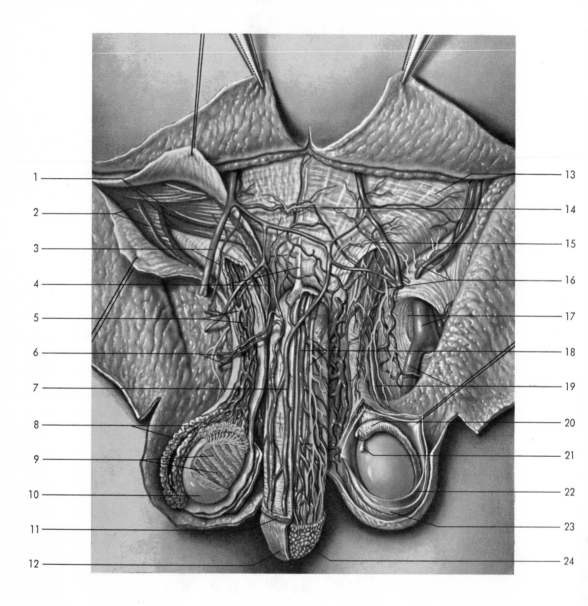

1 Transversus abdominis muscle and iliohypogastric nerve
2 Obliquus abdominis internus muscle and ilioinguinal nerve
3 Superficial epigastric artery and vein
4 Genital branch of genitofemoral nerve and suspensory ligament of penis
5 Internal spermatic artery and pampiniform plexus
6 External pudendal artery and vein
7 Superficial dorsal vein of penis
8 Vas deferens and deferential artery

9 Lobules of testis
10 Testis (covered by visceral tunica vaginalis)
11 Prepuce
12 Glans penis
13 Abdominal aponeurosis
14 Anterior cutaneous branch of subcostal nerve
15 Subcutaneous inguinal ring
16 Ilioinguinal nerve and superficial iliac circumflex artery and vein

17 Fossa ovalis and femoral artery and ve
18 Dorsal artery and nerve, and deep dorsal vein, of penis
19 Cremaster muscle and great saphenous vein
20 Head of epididymis
21 Appendix of testis
22 Parietal layer of tunica vaginalis
23 Infundibuliform fascia
24 Plexus cavernosus

Anatomy of
the Female Genitalia

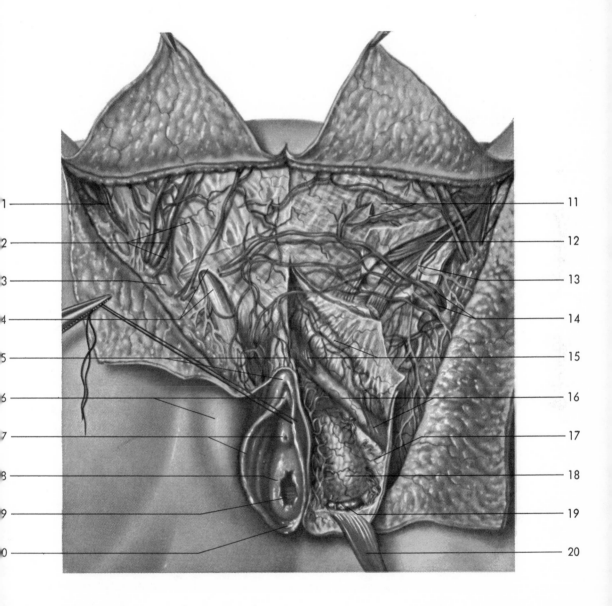

1 Superficial iliac circumflex artery and vein

2 Tela subcutanea and superficial epigastric artery and vein

3 Inguinal lymph node

4 Subcutaneous inguinal ring and round ligament of uterus

5 Prepuce and dorsal vein of clitoris

6 Clitoris and labium majus

7 External urethral orifice and labium minus

8 Hymen

9 Vaginal orifice

10 Navicular fossa

11 Abdominal aponeurosis and anterior cutaneous branch of subcostal nerve

12 Obliquus abdominis internus muscle

13 Ilioinguinal nerve

14 Superficial external pudendal artery and vein

15 Fascia lata and bulbocavernosus muscle

16 Ischiocavernosus muscle and crus of clitoris

17 Inferior fascia of the urogenital diaphragm

18 Vestibular bulb

19 Major vestibular (Bartholin's) gland

20 Bulbocavernosus muscle

Photo and Illustrations

Sandoz Pharmaceuticals, pages 12, 51; Lederle Laboratories, pages 14, 46, 92, 104; Lucille Innes, pages 15, 18, 19, 20, 39, 90, 99 (lower), 100, 106, 107, 130, 240, 370; James Converse, pages 16, 83, 118, 152, 157, 192, 194, 216, 224, 323, 349, 352, 356, 357, 358 (lower), 359, 360, 361, 365, 374, 376, 377, 378, 379, 383, 384, 388, 389, 391, 392, 394, 395, 408, 411, 416, 424, 425, 428 (lower), 429, 432, 436, 438, 439, 444, 445, 447, 448, 449, 453, 457, 458; Robert Eldridge, pages 24, 48, 114, 351, 358 (upper), 428 (upper); Kelly Solis-Novarro, page 24, 26, 57, 117, 154, 160, 231; United Press International, pages 25, 215, 295; Public Health Service Audiovisual Facility, pages 28, 29, 55, 59, 190, 191, 198, 207, 231, 247, 249, 251, 253, 254, 256, 259, 260, 261, 262, 265, 266, 271, 273, 275, 277, 279, 281, 284, 289, 291, 302, 304, 306, 314, 317, 323; Chas. Pfizer & Co., Inc., pages 34, 160, 306, 308, 309, 310, 311, 312; Margery Gardephe, pages 36, 37, 41, 94, 95, 103, 135, 147; F. Netter, M.D., © Ciba Pharmaceuticals, pages 69, 197, 300, 321; D. Tank, pages 85, 123, 135, 142, 204, 234, 326, 332, 337, 343, 422; Joan Walter, page 86; The Upjohn Company, pages 97, 159, 165, 169, 217; Ichiro Nakashima, pages 112, 121, 125, 139, 241, 243, 245, 375, 400, 404, 427; Howard Larkin, pages 146, 148, 234; Doho Chemical Company, page 161; Review & Herald Publishing Association, page 164; Elias A. Papazian, page 172; Three Lions, Inc., pages 172, 367; American Cancer Society, page 176; Gene Ahrens, page 198; Lester Quade, pages 226, 237; Eric Kreye, pages 234, 268; A. Devaney, Inc., page 242; Loma Linda School of Medicine, pages 247, 250; Joe Maniscalco, pages 257, 363, 413; Black Star, page 282; Clay Adams, pages 283, 285; Paul R. Nelson, Samuel Myslis, Robert H. Wright, page 296; Ron Polacsek, page 332.

General Index

(All numbers along with entries refer to pages in one of the three volumes. All cross references refer to other entries in this index)